Steppingstones to professional nursing

KATHRYN W. CAFFERTY
R.N., Ed.D.
Formerly Chairman, Department of Nursing,
Bakersfield College,
Bakersfield, California

LEONE K. SUGARMAN
R.N., B.S.Ed., M.S.
Formerly Instructor in Medical-Surgical
Nursing, Sinclair Community College,
Dayton, Ohio

Steppingstones to professional nursing

FIFTH EDITION / *With 65 illustrations including 32 in full color*

THE C. V. MOSBY COMPANY

SAINT LOUIS 1971

Fifth edition

Previous editions copyrighted 1954, 1957, 1960, 1965

PRINTED IN THE UNITED STATES OF AMERICA

Standard Book Number 8016-0929-1

Library of Congress Catalog Card Number 76-158487

Distributed in Great Britain by Henry Kimpton, London

To today's students

who will be

TOMORROW'S NURSES

Preface

In basic views this fifth edition of *Steppingstones to Professional Nursing* does not deviate from the original and underlying principles proposed and developed in previous editions. The text still strives to help students grow and develop in professional effectiveness, to share with them a vision of the possibilities of a satisfying career in nursing, and to indicate some of the means of making those possibilities a reality.

This edition embodies some extensive changes from the old, the most obvious one being the new format. The organization of content in successive chapters replaces the previous system in which the material was integrated and arranged in units to parallel the levels of a nursing curriculum. This change expands the scope of the book, at no sacrifice of content, and makes the text more adaptable for use at any stage of the nursing curriculum and in all types of preservice education programs. This pattern of discrete chapters makes the content of the book adaptable for use as a basic text or as an adjunct and allows individual instructors more leeway to apply or adjust the material to their own school situation. The ways in which the information contained in this book can be utilized to the students' benefit will depend in large measure upon the manner in which the subject matter is presented and developed by the instructor for the particular group.

Steppingstones is based on the premise that there is a "core" of fundamental knowledge that should be extended to *all* students irrespective of the type of preservice education they may pursue.

For example, a graduate of any one of the various programs should be able to communicate effectively, understand the meaning and importance of professional and interpersonal relationships, have a good grounding in personal and professional ethics, and be aware of the legal responsibilities of a nurse practitioner. Basic to the appreciation of these marks of a true professional is knowledge of the facts that support them. In recognition of this fact, this edition presents a systematic statement of principles and accepted practice that underlie professional behavior and relationships, to be adapted to the needs of the students, the educational level of the program, and the objectives of the instructor.

The end-of-chapter worksheets have been redone so that they stress application of principles to problems in the particular educational situation and the personal experiences of the student. The exercises attempt not merely to ensure understanding of what was presented but also to direct some practice in developing powers that are essential in the professional life of the nurse.

Extensive revision of the majority of the chapters has been necessitated by the change in format. Many of the chapters have been completely rewritten, and some new ones added, to conform to the new pattern of presentation. The four initial chapters dealing with the historical foundations of nursing have been extended to include some of the developing trends in society and the emerging opportunities and responsibilities that can be anticipated for nurses in the years ahead. Chapter 5, a new chapter in this edition, contains essential information about the four existing types of preservice education programs, since we believe that all students need to be informed about other types of nursing preparation, in addition to their own programs. As future practicing members of the profession, graduates of all these programs will be working side by side in the performance of health care services in hospitals, clinics, physicians' offices, and other health agencies. Nurses must understand and work within the scope of their preparation and defined responsibility and be cognizant of the sphere of functioning of their co-workers if the total job of nursing is to be effectively accomplished.

Another innovation, introduced in Chapter 10, is the exposition of some of the common academic policies and scholastic requirements found in nursing programs and the reasons for them so that students will have a greater appreciation and insight into their responsibilities and obligations as learners. The fact that students are enrolled in a nursing program makes them partners with the school in the education venture. As partners, they should be fully acquainted with the conditions governing their acceptance and self-directing in the factors that control their continuance in the program. The role of counseling and how students may utilize counseling services available to them are treated in Chapter 12.

Individual chapters have been rewritten to provide beginning students with fundamental information about the context within which the nurse functions to assist in developing a conception of professional behavior and relationships. Other chapters are designed for advanced students about to enter the ranks of nursing to assist them in the transition from student to practitioner and to orient them to their professional responsibilities and obligations and the career opportunities open to them.

It is recognized that each year more and more men are entering the profession. The use of the feminine pronoun for referring to nurses in this book should in no way be considered a slight to male nurses but rather a means to circumvent involved sentence structure and awkward wording.

Many persons have helped us in the preparation of this fifth edition. Included in this group are our families, personal friends who have encouraged us to persevere, our co-workers on the faculties of the nursing departments of both Bakersfield College, Bakersfield, California, and Sinclair Community College, Dayton, Ohio, and our students throughout the years who have been our joy, our inspiration, and our challenge. To all we extend our sincere gratitude and appreciation.

We do, however, wish to acknowledge with special thanks the particular contributions of the following persons: Mr. William J. Heffernan, former Dean of Admissions and Records, Bakersfield College, for his meticulous review of content in Chapter 10 referring to the evaluation of academic achievement and grading systems; Mr. Maurice Katz, attorney-at-law, for reviewing the chapter on legal aspects of nursing; Miss Dorothy Luepp, executive secretary, Ohio State Board of Nursing Education and Nurse Registration; Captain Nancy Magel, Nurse Corps, U.S. Air Force; and Miss Rosalie Weinert, Ohio State Nurses' Association, for obtaining and sharing information used in the development of some chapters; Miss June Scarborough, for her personal interest and general assistance; Miss Jenny Sugarman, for her drawing of a medieval saint; a dear friend, known affectionately as "Plug," who helped in innumerable ways to achieve the compilation of this edition; Mr. Gilbert M. Martin, for his review and proofreading of part of the manuscript; and Mrs. Barbara Baker and Mrs. Sarah Taylor, for their final preparation of the manuscript.

Kathryn W. Cafferty
Leone K. Sugarman

Contents

1 Nursing's historical foundations, 1

2 The period of apprentice nursing, 8

3 The period of "educated" nursing, 25

4 The period of contemporary nursing, 42

5 Preservice nursing education programs, 47

6 Your first days in the nursing program, 59

7 Learning and working as a student in the nursing program, 77

8 Ethics for nursing, 99

9 Some interpretations of nursing, 105

10 Interpreting essential academic policies and requirements, 112

11 The National Student Nurses' Association, 123

12 The role of counseling in nursing programs, 128

13 Interpersonal relations, 134

14 Communication, 142

15 Communication skills and techniques, 155

16 Working in a team, 165

17 Legal aspects of nursing practice, 172

18 Basic considerations for spiritual health, 182

19 Looking ahead, 188

20 Building for economic security, 192

21 Keeping up to date, 205

22 Health and nursing legislation, 211

23 The graduate nurse's first job, 215

24 Opportunities for pursuing a career in nursing, 233

25 The official nursing organizations, 251

26 American Nurses' Association Position Paper, 269

Appendix

A Organizations and their addresses, 273

B Parliamentary procedures, 275

C Social etiquette: guide for use in correspondence, 283

Index, 289

Work sheets, 301

Steppingstones to professional nursing

CHAPTER 1

Nursing's historical foundations

Whoe'er excels in what we prize
Appears a hero in our eyes.

JONATHAN SWIFT

You have entered a school of nursing with one goal in mind—to become a nurse. How did nursing progress from the intuitive care that a cave-dwelling mother gave her child to the respected and exacting profession you are striving for? We hope to show you that the development of the modern nurse is part of the history of civilization. Modern nursing came into being as a reflection of the forces exerted from changes in social climate. These changes occurred because of the effects of religious ideologies; economic, social, and industrial revolutions; wars; crusades; improved educational opportunities and standards; and, most importantly, the emancipation of women with its correlated improved economic opportunity.

What is history? Yesterday is history today, and today is history tomorrow. History is not only the study of dates, conquests, discoveries, or research, it is also the yesterdays and todays of people who lived, who loved, who fought, and who died. Our era is the age of automation, space development, scientific discovery, and achievement. All of the things that we take for granted, whether they are good or bad, are the result of events that preceded us. Johann von Schiller, eighteenth century German poet-philosopher, said, "Die Welgeschichte ist das Weltgericht" ("History is one long day of judgment").

The general direction that nursing has taken is representative of the status of women throughout the ages. As women who are emancipated, free, and educated, you are able to embark upon any career you choose, to inherit property, and to control large business concerns. Since the beginning of biblical history, when God created Eve from the rib of Adam, the status of women has gone through many ups and downs; her role, however, has primarily been one of "Kuchen, Kinder, and Kirche"—cooking, children, and church. When prehistoric man left his cave to forage for food, his woman remained in their shelter to care for the children, the aged, and the infirm. In the twelfth century when the lord of the manor rode off to fight during the Crusades, his lady stayed in their manor estate. Until late in the nineteenth century marriages were arranged by parents, by elder brothers, or by the nearest male relative. There was no consideration given for the wishes or feelings of the lady in question. Even today this philosophy prevails in many parts of the world.

As we take a long look at history, we find that each generation, each change in the social and economic climate brought forth a leader, a reformer, a maverick. Abraham Lincoln may have remained a small-town lawyer instead of becoming president during the Civil War if there had not been a crying need for reform in the South. Without the United States' desire to achieve greatness in space Neil Armstrong and Edwin Aldren, Jr. may not have had the opportunity to be the first to walk on the moon. In the development of nursing the needs for reform and change called for by society's growth and development brought forth courageous leaders also. We will attempt to bring them into focus for you.

Nursing as we know it did not begin until the middle of the nineteenth century, when some formal education and preparation were introduced into the training of nurses. The many social forces, technological and scientific developments, and the recognition of the value of depth and breadth in educational background helped to create the modern nurse.

The evolution of the contemporary nurse can historically be divided into four great periods:

1. *Intuitive nursing.* This untaught nursing was instinctive. It dated from prehistoric times, was practiced among primitive tribes, and lasted through the early Christian era. It was performed out of a feeling of compassion for others, out of a desire to help, and out of a wish to "do good."
2. *Apprentice nursing.* This period could also be called the period of "on-the-job training." This historical period extends from the founding of religious nursing orders in the sixth century, through the Crusades which began in the eleventh century, to 1836, when the Deaconess School of Nursing at Kaiserswerth, Germany, was established by Pastor Fliedner and his wife.
3. *"Educated" nursing.* The period of educated nursing began in June 1860 when the Florence Nightingale School of Nursing opened at St. Thomas' Hospital in London. This school had the first program of formal education for the nurse. This period traces the growth of nursing in the United States and includes the social forces exerted and the trends resulting from wars, from an aroused social consciousness, from the emancipation of women, and from the increased educational opportunities offered to women.
4. *Contemporary nursing.* Contemporary nursing began at the end of World War II. This period includes scientific and technological developments, and many of the social changes occurring since 1945. This dynamic period, of which you are a part, introduces you to the profession of nursing in which you will be expected to practice.

INTUITIVE NURSING

The word *intuitive* means instinctive or untaught. We believe that woman is endowed biologically with a tender, compassionate nature that is readily adapted to her family's nursing care. Prehistoric man was a nomad. He traveled from place to place in search of food and shelter. Since the female of the tribe was probably less hardy, she was delegated the role of custodian and nurse. As Dr. William Osler has said: ". . . nursing as a practice originated in the dim past when some mother among the cave dwellers cooled the forehead of her sick child with water from the brook . . ."* The philosophy by which people in those early times lived was "the best for the most," or the law of self-preservation. Abandoning the aged and the infirm was not done as an act of cruelty but out of necessity, since food was scarce, travel was difficult, and the sick and the aged were fated to die soon anyway. Why waste time, effort, and meager supplies? Individuals did not count; it was the survival of the fittest! How much have our modern concepts changed? Instinct for self-preservation helped inspire prehistoric man in his search for knowledge. Does this same motivation lead us onto the paths of new research today?

Nursing among primitive cultures was also the function that belonged to women because of the place of the female in tribal society. The cause of illness, they believed, was the invasion of the victim's body by an evil spirit. This demon, sent either by an angered god or by a very powerful person, used black magic or voodoo to harm, and could only be driven out by using supernatural powers similar to the ones

*From Osler, W.: Aequanimitas and other addresses, Philadelphia, 1925, The Blakiston Company, p. 163.

that afflicted or invaded the victim. They believed that their medicine man, who was also called a *shaman* or *witch-doctor,* had the power to heal by using white magic—but he also had the ability to inflict greater harm through using black magic. Following a very strict code of therapy that had been handed down from generation to generation, the medicine man used hypnosis, charms, dances, incantations, purgatives, massage, fire, water, herbs or other vegetation, and even animals as means of driving the illness from the victim. Since the goal of therapy was directed toward driving the evil demon from the victim's body, if the methods listed above did not work, the medicine man was finally forced to resort to help this spirit leave by performing a trephine (drilling a hole in the skull with a rock or stone without benefit of anesthesia). The nurse's role among these people was instinctive —directed toward comforting, practicing midwifery, and being wet nurse to a child. These are normal, neighborly acts, performed without training or direction.

If you smile over these superstitious beliefs, think about your own behavior. Do you ever throw a pinch of salt over your shoulder for good luck? Do you avoid walking under ladders in order to preserve your good luck? Do you knock on wood for good luck? Or, are you like the student nurse who was late for her first class of the day so many times that her teacher (quite provoked) asked her the cause of this persistent tardiness. She answered: "I have to read my horoscope in the morning paper to see what sort of a day I am fated to have before I can actually begin. I want to be prepared for any eventuality." We really have not come as far from ancient superstitious belief as we would like to believe.

NURSING IN THE NEAR EAST

Man's mode of living changed from its nomadic beginnings to an agrarian society and then gradually developed into an urban community life. Man developed a means of communication and the beginnings of a body of scientific knowledge. With each changing social pattern, life became more complex, and this complexity brought with it an increase in health problems. Except in rare cases, however, nursing remained the duty of slaves, wives, sisters, or mothers. Ancient man did make progress in the practice of medicine, but nursing did not change. The care of the sick was still closely allied to religion, superstition, and magic. To their primitive medical therapeutics the ancients added astrology and numerology to assist in diagnosis and cure. Western civilization's roots emanated from a small area of the Near East, the birthplace of three great religious ideologies: Judaism, Christianity, and Mohammedism. Near Eastern culture was adopted by the Greeks and Romans, combined with the wonders of the Far East by returning Crusaders and explorers, improved upon and carried into Europe. In Europe during the Renaissance even more progress was made, thus creating an even greater body of knowledge. This accumulated knowledge was then brought to the New World by the early settlers.

In this tiny circumscribed area known as the birthplace of monotheism, situated between the Tigris and Euphrates Rivers in the Nile Valley, arose the cultures of Babylonia, Egypt, and the Hebrews. *Babylonia,* metropolis of the Near East, developed a highly complex, highly cultivated society. King Hammurabi, who ruled from 1945 B.C. to 1902 B.C., codified Babylonian laws that covered every facet of Babylonian life, including the practice of medicine. Harsh and cruel by our standards, the Code of Hammurabi is evidence of a government-controlled, well-regulated practice of medicine. The medical regulations established fees, discouraged experimentation, designated specific doctors for each disease, and gave each patient the right to choose between the use of charms, the use of medications, or a surgical procedure in the attempted cure of his disease. In this great code, excavated by archeologists in 1849, there is no mention of nurses or nursing.

Egypt, lying in the Valley of the Nile, made some remarkable medical advances 5,000 years ago, in spite of the people's lives being steeped in superstitious practice. The art of embalming enhanced their knowledge of human anatomy, but since all of this work was performed on the dead, they learned nothing of physiology. The Egyptians developed the ability to make keen clinical observations and left a record of 250 recognized diseases. Nursing is not mentioned in the Egyptian relics, however. It is assumed that, without hospitals and hospital personnel, the slaves and patients' families nursed the sick.

The history of the *Hebrew* people, written in the Five Books of Moses (the Old Testament), locates them in many areas of the Near East. In the Book of Genesis episodes are related that emphasize the teachings of Judaism regarding hospitality to the stranger and the acts of charity, which bring God's blessing. In Leviticus, the third book of the Old Testament, chapters 12 to 20 contain laws controlling the spread of communicable disease; laws governing cleanliness, the preparation of food, the purification of man and his food; the Judaic covenant with God directing the ritual of circumcision of the male child on the eighth day; and the establishment of the High Priest Aaron as physician of the people. All of these laws, which are practiced today by traditional Jews, have given to Moses the title "father of sanitation." Mosaic law is believed by some to be levitical, or purely religious, meant to keep the Hebrews pure so that they may enter the sanctuary without affronting God; others believe the laws were established as a means of survival—for health and hygienic reasons only. Reference to nurses, however, in these Five Books of Moses is as midwife, wet nurse, or child's nurse,* not to the nurse as we know her today. She performed her task instinctively and dutifully. Her acts can be described as compassionate and tender, the outpouring of the maternal instincts.

NURSING IN THE FAR EAST

Chinese culture was imbued with a belief in spirits and demons. So great was the influence of this belief on Chinese society that boy babies were given girl's names and dressed in girl's clothes to avoid evils befalling them. The practice of ancestor worship prohibited the dissection of the human body, thus thwarting scientific study. With all of these factors present to hamper advancement, China still gave the world knowledge of materia medica (pharmacology); quantities of classical literature; a prescribed method of treating wounds, infections, and muscular afflictions; and (although not directly concerned with medicine or nursing but certainly a great influence on all education) a method of making paper. In all of the Chinese writings no mention of nursing can be found, so we must assume that the care of the sick fell to the female members of the household.

In *India,* hampered by taboos resulting from the social structure and their practices of animal worship, men of medicine built hospitals, practiced an intuitive form of asepsis, and were proficient in the practice of medicine and surgery. It is here, for the first time in recorded history, that we find reference to the nurse's taking care of patients. In the writings of Sushurutu, written 200 or 300 years before Christ, can be found a list of the functions and qualifications of these nurses. These priest-nurses (probably the first lay brothers) were described as combination pharmacists, masseurs, physical therapists, and cooks. Medical practice, even though it was highly specialized, declined with the fall of Buddhism, the state religion. It was submerged in the morass created by the stress placed upon society by animal worship and the caste system.* The health of India became a major concern of England and the United States in the nineteenth and twentieth centuries.

NURSING IN ANCIENT GREECE

Greek culture made many contributions in the areas of astronomy, architecture, drama, poetry, philosophy, sculpture, esthetic arts, and

*In Exodus 2:7, Miriam asks Pharaoh's daughter, "Shall I go and call thee a nurse of the Hebrew women, that she may nurse the child for thee?"

*The caste system of India places each person in the social class in which he is born. It is impossible for any individual to rise above his birth level, no matter how hard he tries or what he accomplishes.

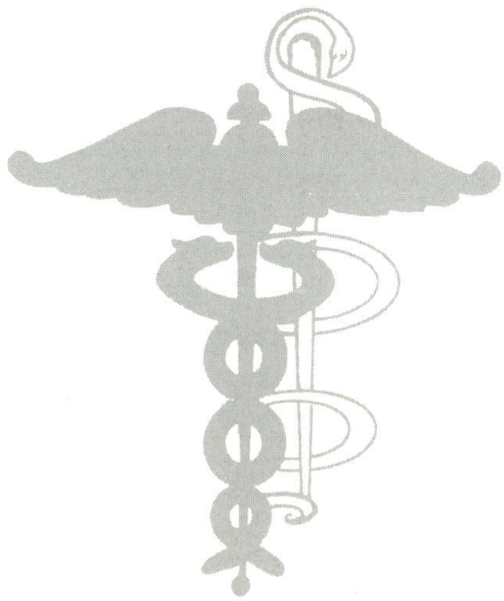

MEDICAL CADUCEUS.

clinical medicine, but nursing was the task of the untrained slave.

The caduceus, the insignia of the medical profession today, is one of the gifts from the Greeks. This symbol is associated with Aesculapius, the "father of medicine" in Greek mythology. A caduceus is composed of the staff of the traveler intertwined with two serpents, the symbol of Aesculapius and his healing power. At the apex of the staff are two wings of Hermes (Mercury) for speed.

The role women played in classical Greek society explained in part why they were not instructed in the art of nursing. Aristotle said:

> Again, as between the sexes, the male is by nature superior, and the female inferior, the male ruler, the female subject . . . . And since, as we saw, the science of household management has three divisions, one the relation of master to slave, one the paternal relation, and the third conjugal, it is a part of household science to rule over wife and children (over both as over freeman, yet not the same mode of government, but over the wife to exercise republican government and over children monarchial); for the male is better fitted to command than the female; except in some cases where their union had been formed contrary to nature.

I wonder what Aristotle would say if he were alive today, with much of the wealth of the financial world in the hands of women and women entering every profession. Hippocrates, the father of medicine, was born in Greece in 460 B.C. He developed a philosophy of medicine and practiced medical ethics that still seem modern. He rejected the belief that the origin of disease could be found in the supernatural. He developed a method of clinical observation through case-taking and recording of findings. Under his expert guidance ethical standards of medical practice reached a new high. But what did he recommend that the doctor do when his patient required nursing care?

> Let one of your pupils be left in charge, to carry instructions without unpleasantness, and to administer treatment. Choose out those who have been already admitted into the mysteries of the art, so as to add anything necessary and to give treatment with safety. He is there also to prevent those things escaping notice that might happen in the intervals between visits. Never put a layman in charge of anything, otherwise if a mischance occur the blame will fall on you.

As you read this quotation, you can readily see that even Hippocrates could not recognize the value of the care his patient would receive if there were qualified nurses available. He believed that only a medical student should remain with the patient.

TRANSITION FROM PAGAN TO CHRISTIAN PHILOSOPHY

Rome was master of the world from the first to the fourth centuries. Stoics, warriors, and materialists all had the same goal—pleasing themselves. The Romans attempted to maintain vigorous health, because illness was a sign of weakness. Care of those unfortunates who did become ill was left to the slaves or to Greek physicians; both groups were looked upon as inferior by Roman society. Contrast this egocentric attitude with Christ's teaching at the Last Supper: "A new commandment I give you, you also love one another. That as I have loved you, you also love one another" (John 13:34).

TRANSITION FROM PAGAN TO CHRISTIAN IDEALS*

PAGAN	CHRISTIAN
VIRTUES	
Personal asceticism	Ascetic mortification
Bravery as stoical endurance	Endurance of pain for love of God or nation
Charity—an economic gain (duty)	Charity—a privilege
Love of neighbor absent	Human brotherhood in Christ—goal of charity
IDEALS	
Perfection as:	Perfection through:
Physical beauty and	Dealing with moral nature of man through mortification
Athletic prowess—ends	Sanctification through personal asceticism
Sensual esthetic appreciations	Purity and love
Intellectual philosophizing	
GOALS	
Improvement of self for the State; civic betterment	Sanctification of self-following precepts of Christianity; love of one another for love of God
MEANS	
Ruthless suppression of all who in any way interfered with temporal goals	Works of charity based on counsels and precepts of Gospel

*From Sellew, G., and Ebel, Sr. E. M.: A history of nursing, ed. 3, St. Louis, 1955, The C. V. Mosby Co.

The contrast between the materialism of pagan society and the spirituality of the converted Christian can be seen in the story of the Roman matron, *Fabiola.* Taking sensual pleasure in the public baths, anointing her body with exotic oils, and adorning herself with fabulous jewels, beautiful Fabiola revelled in the pleasures of upper-class Roman society. Married young, Fabiola found life unbearable with her husband. He was a man so vile and vicious that life with him was pure torture. Fabiola obtained a divorce from this man, and shortly thereafter remarried. This second marriage, consummated while her first husband still lived, was evidently a happy one, since history tells us that she and her second husband remained together until his death. It was after she was widowed that Fabiola converted to Christianity, and it was after this conversion that she began a period of repentance. In a letter to Oceanus, St. Jerome writes:

> Yet it was then she put on sackcloth to make confession of her error. . . . in the presence of Rome . . . she stood in the ranks of the penitents and exposed before bishop, presbyters, and the people—all of whom wept when they saw her weep—her disheveled hair, pale features, soiled hands, and unwashed neck . . . that face by which she once had pleased her second husband she now smote with blows.

It is difficult for us in this enlightened age, with our knowledge of sanitation, to see that allowing one's self to become filthy could be a means of seeking forgiveness from the Almighty for sinful living. We are taught that cleanliness is next to godliness. Yet, for a person living in an age when the prime purpose in living was self-adornment, what better way to chastise, to humiliate, to pay penance for one's sins than to give up the status symbol of self-adornment. This concept is better described by St. Jerome: ". . . who is washed in the blood of Christ, needs not wash again. . . ."

Fabiola further humbled herself by giving service to less fortunate members of society. She literally dragged them into her home, which has been called the first hospital in the Christian world. She gave nursing care to the patients herself, regardless of their diagnosis. In a society that lived for satisfaction of selfish pleasures and used slave labor for even the most minute tasks (toil of any sort was abhorrent), her performance brought cries of derision from her selfish and pleasure-loving former friends, but praise from her brothers and sisters in Christ. Again we see neighbor caring for neighbor, but with this difference—neighbor cared for neighbor out of a love of God and as a means of gaining grace in the Kingdom of Heaven. This kind of care was motivated by Christ's words: "Believe me, when you did it to one of the least of my brethren here, you did it to me."*

*Matthew 25:40. Translated by Ronald Knox, New York: Sheed and Ward, Ltd., Publishers.

BIBLIOGRAPHY

Austin, A. L.: History of nursing source book, New York, 1957, G. P. Putnam's Sons, pp. 23-64.

Burows, M.: The Dead Sea Scrolls, New York, 1955, The Viking Press.

Caldwell, T.: Dear and glorious physician, New York, 1959, Doubleday, Doran & Co., Inc.

Chiera, E.: They wrote on clay: the Babylonian tablets speak today, Chicago, 1938, University of Chicago Press.

Dean, E.: All of the women of the Bible, New York, 1955, Harper & Brothers.

Dolan, J. A.: Goodnow's history of nursing, ed. 11., Philadelphia, 1963, W. B. Saunders Co., pp. 1-97.

Frank, Sister Charles Marie: Foundations of nursing, ed. 2, Philadelphia, 1959, W. B. Saunders Co., pp. 3-20.

Griffin, G. J., and Griffin, J. K.: Jensen's history and trends of professional nursing, ed. 6, St. Louis, 1969, The C. V. Mosby Co.

Haggard, H. W.: Mystery, magic and medicine, New York, 1933, Doubleday, Doran & Co., Inc.

Levine, E. B., and Levine, M. E.: Hippocrates, father of nursing too? American Journal of Nursing **65**:86, Dec. 1965.

Nutting, M. A., and Dock, L. L.: A history of nursing, 4 vols., New York, 1902, G. P. Putnam's Sons.

Robinson, V.: White caps, Philadelphia, 1946, J. B. Lippincott Co.

Sellew, G., and Ebel, Sr. M. E.: A history of nursing, ed. 3, St. Louis, 1955, The C. V. Mosby Co., pp. 25-35.

Shyrock, R. H.: The history of nursing, Philadelphia, 1957, W. B. Saunders Co.

COMPLETE WORK SHEET ON P. 303

CHAPTER 2

The period of apprentice nursing

Apprentice nursing is nursing care performed by people who are directed by more experienced nurses. Apprentice nursing is on-the-job training performed without any formal education. The profession of nursing must be eternally grateful to the religious orders of the Christian church for the early development of this kind of nursing. These orders built hospitals which were staffed by the religious who dedicated their lives to the care of the patients. The beginnings of organized nursing (apprentice type) can be found in the military, secular, and mendicant or begging orders.

THE CRUSADES

Pilgrimages to the Holy Land began almost immediately after the death of Christ and lasted until the eleventh century when the Turks captured Jerusalem and denied Christian pilgrims permission to visit the Holy Sepulcher. As a result of this "closed door" policy the Christian world united under papal leadership and conducted a series of Crusades, or wars, in an attempt to recapture this hallowed ground. From courses in history you know that religious fervor was only one of the motives for conducting these wars. Desire for economic gain, ambition for political power, and a craving for adventure were driving forces that motivated the crusaders in the holy wars. The military religious orders founded during the Crusades established hospitals and staffed them with men who served as nurses. Some of the earliest organized nursing, then, was most capably performed *by men.* The idea, which has been advanced since World War II, of increasing the number of men in nursing is not new.

The Knights of St. John of Jerusalem (Rhodes, Malta) and the Teutonic Knights fought first on the battlefield and when the fighting was over retired to nurse the wounded.

The Knights of St. Lazarus established their hospitals primarily for the nursing of lepers. Associated with each of these three military nursing orders were sisterhoods, but their impact on nursing was not as great as the orders of knights. Another monastic order, the Alexian Brothers, was founded in 1348. No discussion of nursing history would be complete without mentioning this order, which continues today in its service of the sick. For years the Alexian Brothers Hospital School of Nursing in Chicago was the largest school of nursing under religious auspices operated exclusively for men in the United States. The school, however, was closed in 1969.

RISE OF RELIGIOUS NURSING ORDERS

Rome fell in 476 A.D. Christian teaching gave equality to *all men,* but the value of woman was placed in her breeding power and in her ability to manage her home. Only by entering a convent could she follow a career, obtain an education, and perform the acts of charity that her faith taught would help her gain grace in Heaven. Many religious orders were founded by queens, princesses, and other ladies of royalty.

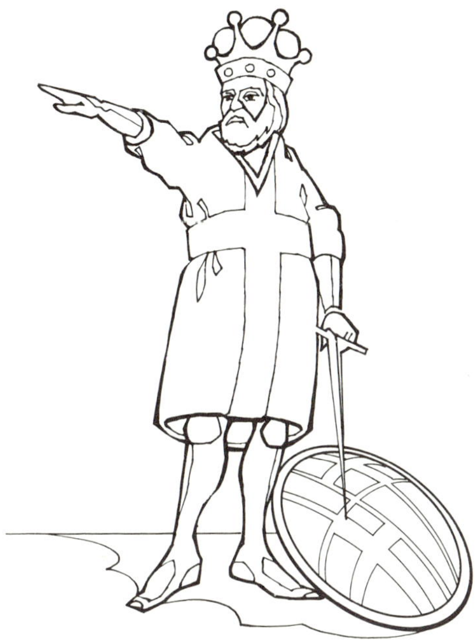

KNIGHT OF MALTA IN BATTLE DRESS.

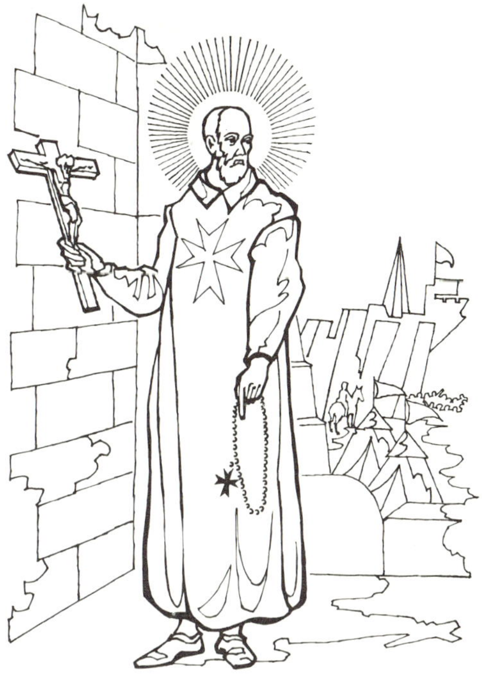

KNIGHT OF MALTA WITHIN HOSPITAL CONFINES.

Some of the secular orders founded before the Reformation, whose tasks included nursing, were the Augustinians, the Poor Clares (second order of St. Francis of Assisi), the Beguines, the Benedictines, the Ursulines, the tertiaries of St. Francis, and the tertiaries of St. Dominic. During the years these orders were being established some remarkable advances took place in medicine, but in nursing there were *none*.

The work of these nurses was complicated by religious taboos and the social restrictions of their culture and education. Also, the hospitals were poorly ventilated, and the beds had mattresses stuffed with straw that was cleaned about three times a year. Three or four patients (regardless of diagnosis or whether alive or dead) may have shared one bed. Facilities for keeping the area surrounding those clumsy beds clean and aseptic were practically nonexistent. The laundry was also done by the nurses.

Augustinian nuns nursed patients in the Hotel Dieu in Paris from its beginning in the seventh century. The older nuns prayed with and took care of patients, and the younger nuns took the soiled linen to the Seine River to wash it. They waded into the water, washing the linen by pounding and beating the material in the icy currents. The tide of the Seine was so treacherous that a man was placed on guard in a boat in the river near the wash area in order to rescue, by hooking her clothes, any nun unlucky enough to be caught in the tide. Today all we do is put soiled linen down a laundry chute, and automatic devices take over sorting, soaking, washing, drying, ironing, and folding.

NURSING SAINTS

The years between the twelfth and sixteenth centuries gave us many nursing saints, despite

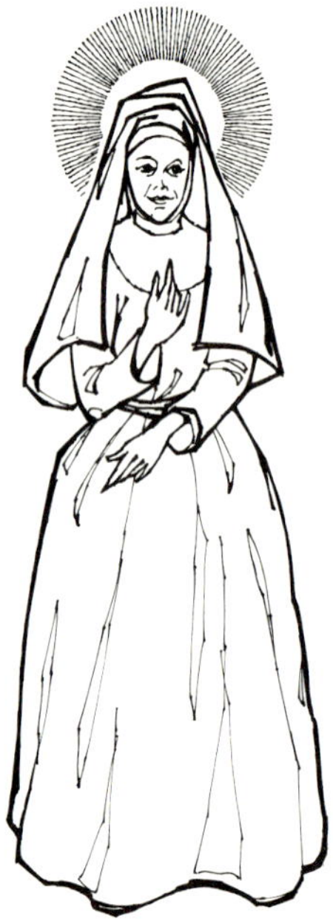

A NURSING SAINT.

the many obstacles these people faced. These devout men and women worked for God, and their lives were a continuous prayer to Him. Among them we find St. Clare (1194-1253), foundress of the second order of St. Francis of Assisi. These women, the Poor Clares, took vows of poverty, obedience, service, and chastity. In the Convent of San Damiano, St. Clare and her Sisters gave nursing care to all the people St. Francis and his followers sent to them. The Poor Clare order was the first of the many Franciscan orders that have followed in St. Clare's footsteps and that are still giving such a large share of the nursing care.

No history of nursing would be complete without mentioning St. Catherine of Siena, the first "lady with a lamp." Catherine (1347-1380) was the surviving twin from her mother's twenty-fifth delivery. Catherine dedicated her life to Christ at the age of seven years. When in her teens, Catherine became a tertiary of St. Dominic. One important task of the tertiaries is nursing. Tertiaries are religious who take vows of dedication and service but are not required to take vows of chastity and may live in the world uncloistered. Thus these dedicated people can engage in works of mercy among the sick and poor with considerable freedom. Catherine not only nursed patients in the hospital of Santa Maria della Scala, but also nursed in the homes of patients shunned by others. In an age when no woman, young or old, could safely travel outside her home unescorted, Catherine's lamp could be seen as she made rounds among her patients alone. In 1374 the bubonic plague wiped out a large percentage of the population of Siena. Catherine remained in the wards of the afflicted, refusing to leave. She organized other tertiaries of St. Dominic into teams of litter bearers so that they could bring those stricken with plague into the hospital for her care.

IMPACT OF SOCIAL REVOLUTIONS

The industrial and political revolutions and the Reformation in the sixteenth century left the world in the following situation:

1. The masses of people huddled in slums as a result of famine, wars, and the introduction of machinery.
2. Living in blighted slum areas, the people sank into a brutal and immoral way of life.
3. Ambition for power and the antagonism resulting from the attempts to achieve this power replaced human empathy.
4. Class lines could now be bypassed in some parts of the world, and people struggled against one another for power, wealth, and leisure.
5. Skepticism was the result of the political, intellectual, and ideologic revolutions; everything in life had to be based upon scientific fact, for nothing else was true.

Has the world changed? Do people really care enough about those less fortunate than themselves to do something about alleviating their suffering and want, or are the actions of the philanthropists mere soporifics to ease qualms of conscience?

RISE OF ORGANIZED CHARITY

In the sixteenth century hospitals were established for the care of the sick. In France, as in all of Europe, the hospitals were gloomy, cheerless, and airless. They were unsanitary according to the standards of the twentieth century, but were the best the world offered in the sixteenth century. People entered hospitals only under compulsion or as a last resort. What, then, of the poor and the hungry? There was little employment, and education was only for the rich and the titled. Begging, an organized profession in sixteenth century France, was not then, is not now, and never will be the answer—every man needs the satisfaction of personal accomplishment.

In the early part of the sixteenth century a French peasant was so farsighted and so aware of man's basic needs that he set up the first program of social service. His program even included the training and rehabilitation of these poor so that they could become self-sufficient. One Sunday two parishioners rushed to their pastor, Vincent de Paul, and asked him to make an appeal after Mass for the benefit of a needy family in their parish. He made the announcement. A few hours later Pastor Vincent called upon this needy family. As he walked toward their hut he met many of his parishioners returning from their visit to the family. On reaching the hut he found an overabundance of food. There was so much food, in fact, that much of it would spoil before it could be used. According to Vincent de Paul, there was much charity, but it had no direction. He established a plan to remedy this situation. He called a group of women together and presented them with a plan of social service that would be regulated so that there would not be feast one day and famine the next, and he named them "La Charité." To St. Vincent de Paul also goes the credit for organizing "The Community of the Sisters of Charity"—women who lived uncloistered who were dedicated to doing God's work in caring for the sick, the poor, the orphaned, and the widowed. The first superior and co-foundress was Louise de Gras (nee de Marillac).

THE REFORMATION AND NURSING

The period from the seventeenth to the nineteenth centuries has been labeled the "dark period of nursing." The practice of medicine during the Renaissance (which preceded and coincided with the Reformation) was in the hands of many capable physicians, but there were quacks as well. Surgery was done by barber-surgeons, as it was considered beneath the status of a physician to perform such a menial task. The practice of nursing was a different story. The building and the staffing of hospitals for centuries were handled by the Roman Catholic Church. These hospitals and their staffs were only as strong as the Church.

By the sixteenth century the Church had amassed not only great political power but also tremendous wealth. In protest there were factions within the Church striving to reform Church practices and policies. The revolt led by Martin Luther advocated reforms that separated his followers from the Church and resulted in his being excommunicated; the revolt led by Ignatius Loyola and his Society of Jesus exercised a potent influence in establishing reform within the Church. When these two factions succeeded in their respective moves, the institutions closely allied with the Church suffered or made gains with her as she prospered or fell. In those countries that permitted the Catholic Church to continue unmolested, nursing made no advances but it did not regress either. In Protestant countries, however, Church property was confiscated and religious personnel were homeless. Hunted and disbanded, they literally fled for their lives and there was no one to nurse the sick. Imagine what would happen today if the order were given to close all hospitals.

In sixteenth century England, for example, over one hundred hospitals were closed. The wealthy could be cared for in their homes, but no one thought to make any provision for the indigent sick. English women forced to earn their living turned to domestic service if their education did not permit them to obtain the position of governess. Homemaking and teaching were the only careers that a genteel woman could follow without losing face. Nursing, impossible for a "lady," became the work (drudgery) of the dregs of society. Those poor unfortunates, victims of circumstances beyond their control, took bribes from patients, stole the patient's food, and used alcohol as a tranquilizer. All of these things were done to make their miserable, depressing lives slightly more tolerable. They worked seven days a week with no relief, slept when they could in a cubbyhole near their hospital ward or patient, and ate scraps of food when they could find them. These people certainly were not nurses as we know them. They were uneducated, illiterate, and had no background for nursing, but they gave the best care they could.

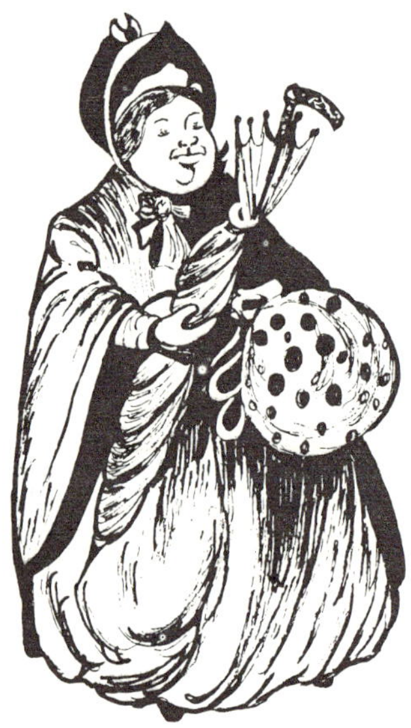

SAIREY, YOU INSPIRE ME*
CHERRY PARKER

"Many poems are written
To the Lady with a Lamp
But I feel the need to dedicate
An ode to Sairey Gamp.

"Sairey, you're real inspiring
To nurses, old and new.
How oft we mend our ways because
We'd hate to be like you."

*Parker, Cherry: Sairey, you inspire me, R.N. 17:34, May 1954 (illustration redrawn). Printed with permission.

Charles Dickens, reformer and novelist, gives an accurate description of seventeenth and eighteenth century English nursing in *Martin Chuzzlewit* (see also the accompanying illustrated poem). Dickens' description of Sairey Gamp follows:

> She was a fat old woman . . . with a husky voice and a moist eye, which she had a remarkable power of turning up and only showing the white of it. Having very little neck, it cost her some trouble to look over herself, if one may say so, at those to whom she talked. She wore a very rusty black gown, rather the worse for snuff, and a shawl and bonnet to correspond. . . . The face of Mrs. Gamp—the nose in particular—was somewhat red and swollen, and it was difficult to enjoy her society without becoming conscious of the smell of spirits. . . . 'If it wasn't for the nerve a little sip of liquor gives me . . ., I never could go through with what I sometimes has to do.' . . . I says 'leave the bottle on the chimley-piece and don't ask me to take none, but let me put my lips to it when I am so dispoged and then I will do what I'm engaged to do, according to the best of my ability.'

EFFECT OF THE SOCIAL REFORMS ON NURSING

The Old World was ripe for reform in the care of the mentally ill patients as well as those who were physically ill. At Bedlam (Bethlehem Hospital, London), the hospital for the insane, admission tickets were sold so that the public could watch the antics of the mentally ill. Can you imagine anything more inhumane? If those poor, unfortunate people were not mentally unbalanced before their incarceration, they most certainly became "mad" after they were confined. The inmates were unclad and chained or manacled to the wall. The conditions in this so-called hospital for people sick in mind were too horrible to imagine.

The situation in the prisons was equally bad. People of all ages were thrown into prison indiscriminately for the slightest misdemeanor (nonpayment of debt, for example). In nineteenth century England 250 crimes were punishable by death, and prisoners were often forced to live out the rest of their lives, sick or well, in jail. Appalled at what he had seen, John Howard (1726-1790), a hard working prison reformer, helped reduce the number of death penalties to three and improved the prison living conditions and gave prisoners renewed hope.

Nursing's need for reform was felt by philanthropists, writers, doctors, and clergymen. So convinced did some of the doctors become about the need for training for nurses, they even wrote a few textbooks for nursing practices. The books, however, were a wasted effort since most of the practicing nurses could not read. In an attempt to bring back into nursing the dedication of the early Christian era, Protestant and Catholic groups established nursing orders. In Ireland, for example, new Catholic orders included the Irish Sisters of Charity (1816) founded by Mother Mary Aikenhead and the Sisters of Mercy (1827) under the leadership of Mother Catherine M'Auley. Protestant religious nursing orders founded in an attempt to revitalize former dedication in nursing were the Protestant Sisters of Charity (later known as the Nursing Sisters) in 1840, the All Saints and St. Margaret's Sisterhoods, and the Cowlet Nursing Brothers. All of these women and men did their best to improve the nursing situation.

Germany, too, made many attempts to improve nursing care in this "dark period." The most successful and far-reaching of these nursing reforms was The Institution of Kaiserswerth on the Rhine for the Practical Training of Deaconesses. The school was established by Pastor Theodor Fliedner and his wife, Fredericke Münster Fliedner, in 1836; there were six students. This school of nursing could boast of two firsts:

1. A rotating three-year experience in cooking and housekeeping, laundry and linen, and nursing care in the women's and men's wards
2. A preliminary or probationary three-month period of trial and error for both school and student

These young women were from many social backgrounds but were treated equally. All were required to have a character reference from their

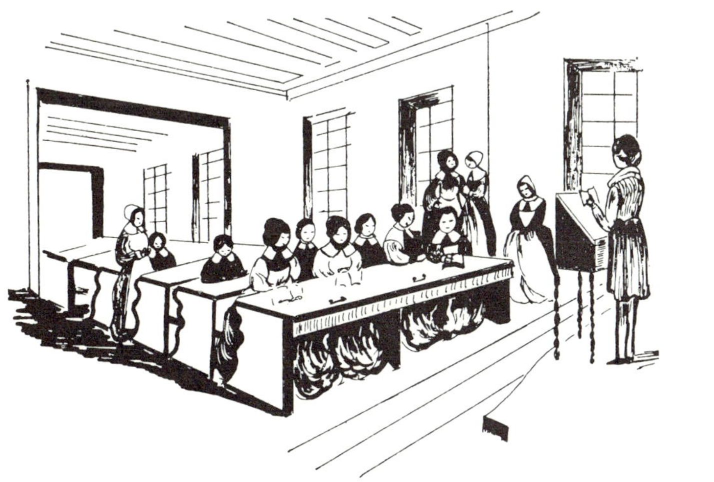

PASTOR FLIEDNER INSTRUCTING THE DEACONESSES OF KAISERSWERTH.

clergyman, a certificate of health from their physician, and permission from their nearest male relative before being admitted to the school. (How does this compare to the procedures you had to complete before you could enter your school of nursing?) The students received lectures in theory as illustrated in the accompanying drawing of a classroom setting. They were offered instruction at the bedside from a physician, were taught ethics and religious doctrine by Pastor Fliedner, and were introduced to the art and practice of nursing by Mrs. Fliedner. The Deaconess Hospitals, which emanated from this school, took the position that a nurse implicitly followed the doctor's orders; the doctor was therefore responsible for all of the nursing care. It was a requirement, also, that these deaconesses be treated as a member of the family and not as a servant when on private duty. What a difference between this treatment and that described by Dickens in *Martin Chuzzlewit!* The Deaconess School of Nursing at Kaiserswerth, then, can truly be called the first organized training school for nurses. Kaiserswerth left a significant influence on nursing. It was at Kaiserswerth that Florence Nightingale received some of her training and the inspiration for the establishment of her school of nursing.

NURSING IN THE NEW WORLD

The Crusades ended leaving the people with a desire for adventure, a desire for new conquests, and the need for new trade routes. These cravings for new worlds to conquer helped settle the North American continent. Living was hard in the wilderness, and fear was the settlers' constant companion—yet they came. Even hospitals were built in the wild country—one such hospital was a log cabin 24 feet by 60 feet. This building, pictured below, was divided into two wards, a kitchen, servants' quarters, and a room for the founder of the hospital, Mlle. Jeanne Mance.

At the age of 36 Mlle. Mance left her home in Langres, France, in the company of forty settlers and a governor. There were only three other women in their little band. In this wild country (now Montreal) Jeanne Mance founded the Hotel Dieu of Montreal in October of 1644. Her supplies had to be sent from France. In 1659 Jeanne, in need of reinforcements, returned to France. She returned to Montreal with three Sisters Hospitaliers of St. Joseph. Jeanne Mance, the first laywoman who worked as a nurse on the North American continent, died in 1673, but her work has been carried on by those Sisters Hos-

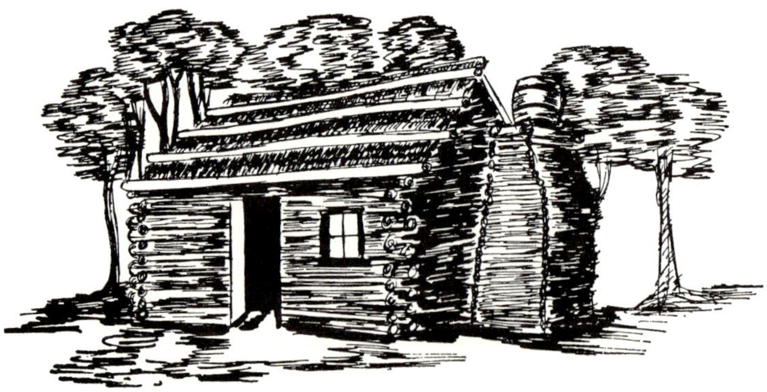

LOG CABIN HOSPITAL OF JEANNE MANCE.

pitaliers of St. Joseph, who celebrated their 300th anniversary in 1959.

PRE–CIVIL WAR NURSING

Nursing before the Civil War was carried on by religious orders, both Catholic and Protestant, in the United States and Canada. The Augustinian nuns established the Hotel Dieu in Quebec; the Ursuline Sisters staffed the St. John Hospital (now called Charity Hospital) in New Orleans; deaconesses of Kaiserswerth staffed many hospitals; Protestant Sisters of Charity, St. John's Sisterhood, Sisterhood of All Saints, St. Margaret's Sisterhood, and many other Catholic and Protestant sisterhoods helped found and staff hospitals and gave the nursing care during the Civil war.

Mrs. Elizabeth Seton, an American, founded the Sisters of Charity at Emmitsberg, Maryland, in 1809. This order, established primarily as a teaching order, branched into the field of nursing shortly thereafter. In 1823 these sisters opened a hospital in Baltimore, helped organize the nursing at Blockley in Philadelphia, and opened hospitals, schools, orphanages, and homes for unwed mothers in all parts of the country. In 1849, after the death of Mother Seton, the Emmitsberg Community affiliated and came under the same French Rule as the Daughters of Charity, Paris, France. The small group of sisters, however, who had come to Cincinnati to establish St. Joseph's Orphanage and Good Samaritan Hospital remained under the American regulations.

American reforms in nursing. To nineteenth century American society the word *hospital* brought with it a very different picture from what the word brings to mind today. Hospitals were pest houses; they were dirty and were considered a last resort. They had defective plumbing and lacked ventilation, and the staffs were unskilled in hygienic practices. Something had to be done. The nursing care in the United States prior to the Civil War was as inadequate as it was in the Old World. As had happened so many times in the long course of history, someone stepped forward and attempted to right the wrongs. Two of the reforms instituted to help resolve the dilemma in American nursing during the first half of the nineteenth century were the following:

1. The Nurse Society of Philadelphia organized a school of nursing under the direction of Dr. Joseph Warrington in 1839. Dr. Warrington was an obstetrician and he wanted his patients, both mother and child, to get better care. The nurses were trained on the job and attended some courses with the medical students at the Philadelphia Dispensary. Upon completing the course of instruction they were given a "Certificate of Approbation."
2. Women's Hospital in Philadelphia established a six-month course in nursing to increase the nurses' knowledge while they worked. The nurses were taught a minimum amount of medical and surgical nursing, materia medica, and dietetics in the hope that this would improve their nursing care. At the satisfactory completion of this combined program they were given a diploma.

NURSING DURING THE CIVIL WAR

When the Civil War erupted on April 12, 1861, there were no organizations of nurses to give care or any social service such as that provided by the Red Cross after 1900. The United States Sanitary Commission was appointed by the North in an attempt to bring some relief measures to prisoners and to the wounded, but the actual nursing of the injured was left to the religious sisterhoods and to volunteers. All of these nurses were under the direction of Dorothea Lynde Dix, who was not a nurse. She was appointed Superintendent of Female Nurses for the United States Government. Among the volunteer nurses can be found such illustrious names as Louisa May Alcott, author; Walt Whitman, poet; Clara Barton, founder of the American Red Cross; and Mary Ann Bickerdyke, humanitarian.

Mary Ann Bickerdyke, a widow, had answered the call that came to Galesburg, Illinois, from the camp at Cairo asking for help in nursing the wounded men there. She was herb doctor, hospital supervisor, and ministering angel to the thousands of her "boys" she cared for as a volunteer nurse. Mrs. Bickerdyke was called "Mother" by her "boys" and named "Cyclone in Calico" by Nina Baker in her book describing this remarkable woman's work during the Civil War. In her work she rode roughshod over officers, congressmen, and army rules and regulations. Her only goal was to give comfort to the men wounded in battle, and her only orders came from God. Anecdotes about her are legion.

When the troops rode in review before the President at the end of the Civil War, "Mother" Bickerdyke rode (in her calico dress and sunbonnet) beside General Logan. Mother Bickerdyke exemplifies those many courageous volunteers who did their best to nurse the wounded during the Civil War.

The end of the Civil War ushered in a period of tremendous growth in the United States. Immigration increased, cities grew, and the public became acutely aware that the health of the nation deserved better care. Some believed that well-trained nurses provided one of the answers. The American Medical Association, probably more aware that prepared nurses would be able to give their members greater assistance, appointed a committee to investigate, to make suggestions, and to make recommendations on the training of nurses to the association. The chairman of this committee, Dr. Samuel Gross, made the following report in 1869:*

> Nursing, in its more exalted sense is as much an art and a science as medicine . . . . It is a mistake to suppose . . . that every individual . . . is fitted for such an occupation, as if nursing, like poetry, were a gift of nature . . . . To afford the proper facilities for . . . providing adequate nursing service for all . . . every large and well organized hospital should have a school for the training of nurses, not only for the supply of its own necessities, but for private families, the teaching to be furnished by its own medical staff, assisted by the resident physicians.

At last doctors were able to realize the need and the advantage of having at their sides a well-prepared assistant—*a qualified nurse.*

*From Report of Committee on the Training of Nurses, Transactions of the American Medical Association, 1869, pp. 161-174.

BIBLIOGRAPHY

Alcott, L. M.: Hospital sketches, Boston, 1863, James Redpath. (Reprinted New York, 1957, Sagamore Press.)

Atherton, W. H.: The saintly life of Jeanne Mance, St. Louis, 1945, The Catholic Hospital Association of the United States.

Austin, A. L.: History of nursing source book, New York, 1957, G. P. Putnam's Sons, pp. 65-183.

Baker, N. B.: Cyclone in calico, Boston, 1952, Little, Brown and Co.

Bullough, B.: The origins of American nursing: the Civil War, Nurs. Forum II:12-27, Mar.-Apr. 1963.

Deutsch, A.: Dorothy Lynde Dix: apostle of the insane, American Journal of Nursing **36**:987, Oct. 1936.

DeWohl, L.: The last crusader, Philadelphia, 1956, J. B. Lippincott Co.

Dolan, J. A.: Goodnow's history of nursing, ed. 11., Philadelphia, 1963, W. B. Saunders Co., pp. 98-213.

Dyer, E. M.: A visit to Kaiserswerth, American Journal of Nursing **53**:562-563, May 1953.

Fishbein, M.: A history of the American Medical Association (1847-1947), Philadelphia, 1947, W. B. Saunders Co.

Frank, Sister Charles Marie: Foundations of nursing, ed. 2, Philadelphia, 1959, W. B. Saunders Co., pp. 43-64.

Guyot, Sister Henrietta: The nurse in Civil War literature, Nursing Outlook **10**:311-314, May 1962.

Griffin, G. J., and Griffin, J. K.: Jensen's history and trends of professional nursing, ed. 6, St. Louis, 1969, The C. V. Mosby Co.

Kernodle, P. B.: The Red Cross nurse in action, New York, 1949, Harper & Brothers.

Kossak, Z.: Blessed are the meek (translated by R. Langer), New York, 1944, Roy Publishers.

Lowenfels, W.: Walt Whitman's civil war, New York, 1961, Alfred A. Knopf, Inc.

Moses ben Maimon ben Joseph (Maimonides): The preservation of health, essays on health written in the 12th century (translated), New York, 1958, Philosophical Library, Inc.

Nutting, M. A., and Dock, L. L.: A history of nursing, vol. 2, New York, 1907, G. P. Putnam's Sons.

Roberts, M. M.: American nursing: history and interpretation, New York, 1954, The Macmillan Co., pp. 7-19.

Sellew, G., and Ebel, Sister M. Ethelreda: A history of nursing, ed. 3, St. Louis, 1955, The C. V. Mosby Co., pp. 155-165, 168-179.

Sister Henrietta: A famous New Orleans hospital, American Journal of Nursing **39**:249-256, Mar. 1939.

Thompson, M.: The cry and the covenant, New York, 1954, Doubleday, Doran & Co., Inc.

Williams, B.: Clara Barton, daughter of destiny, Philadelphia, 1941, J. B. Lippincott Co.

Wilson, F.: Crusader in crinoline, the life of Harriet Beecher Stowe, Philadelphia, 1941, J. B. Lippincott Co.

COMPLETE WORK SHEET ON PP. 305 AND 306

HISTORICAL EVENTS CONTRIBUTING TO THE FOUNDATION OF MEDICINE AND NURSING

HIPPOCRATES, 460-370 B.C., "FATHER OF MEDICINE" PRACTICING THE ART OF HEALING

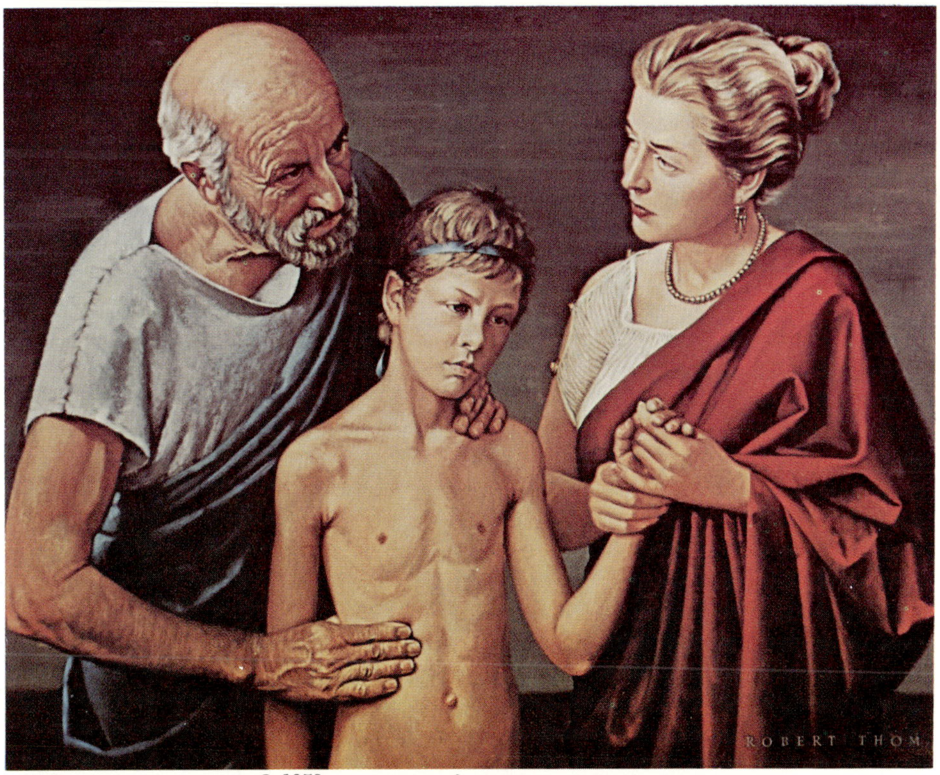

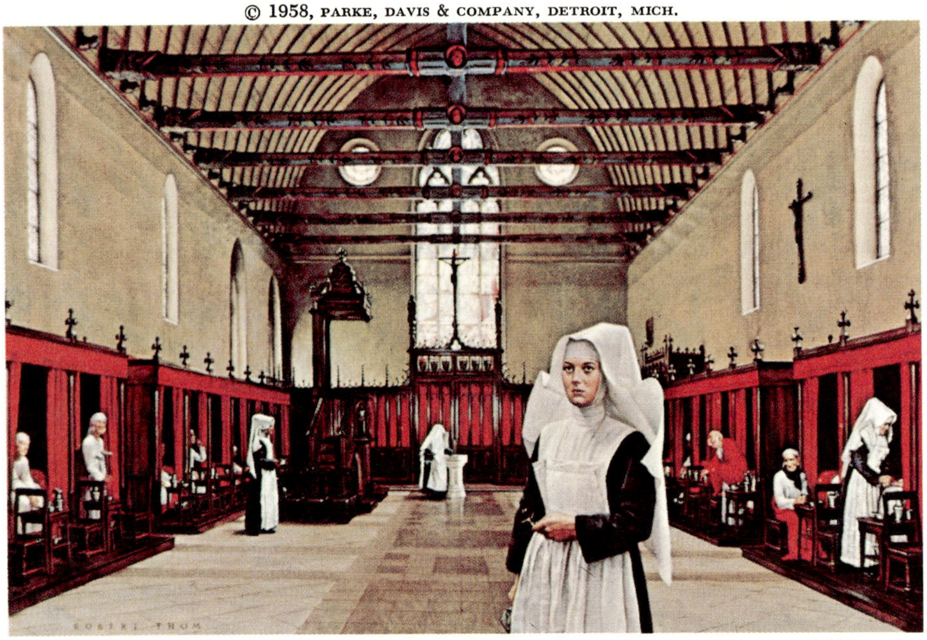

MEDIEVAL HOSPITAL, HOTEL DIEU OF BEAUNE, FRANCE, 1443;
SISTERS OF THE CONGREGATION OF SAINT MARTHE

LAENNEC, PARIS, 1816, BROKE THE "SOUND BARRIER" OF THE CHEST

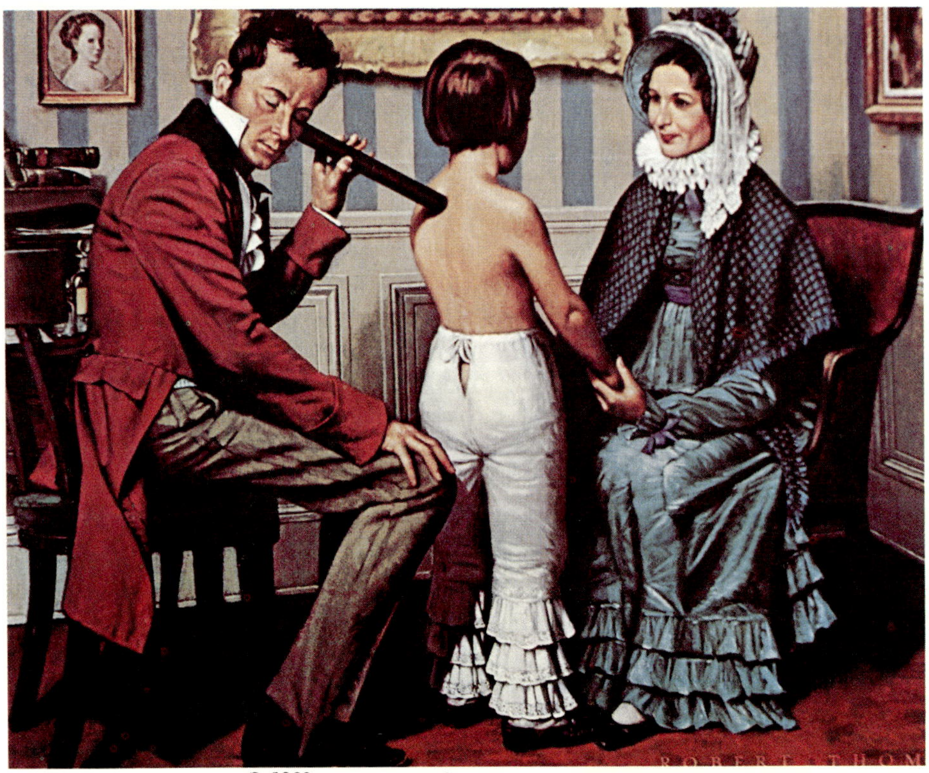

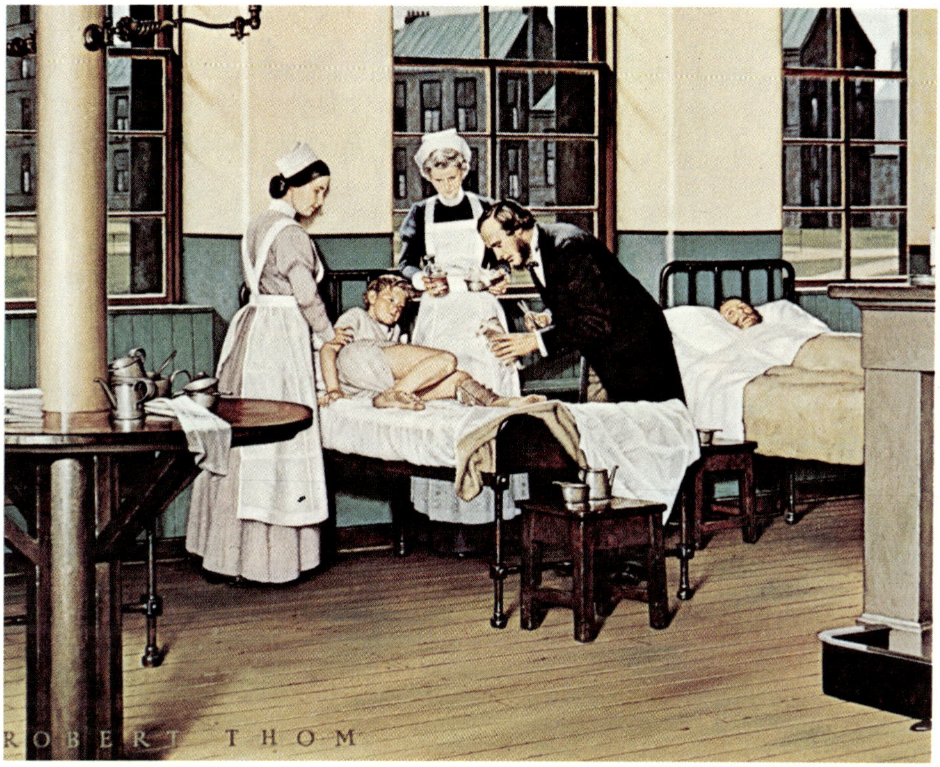

SURGEON, JOSEPH LISTER, GLASGOW, SCOTLAND, 1865; HOSPITALS WERE NO LONGER HOUSES OF HORROR

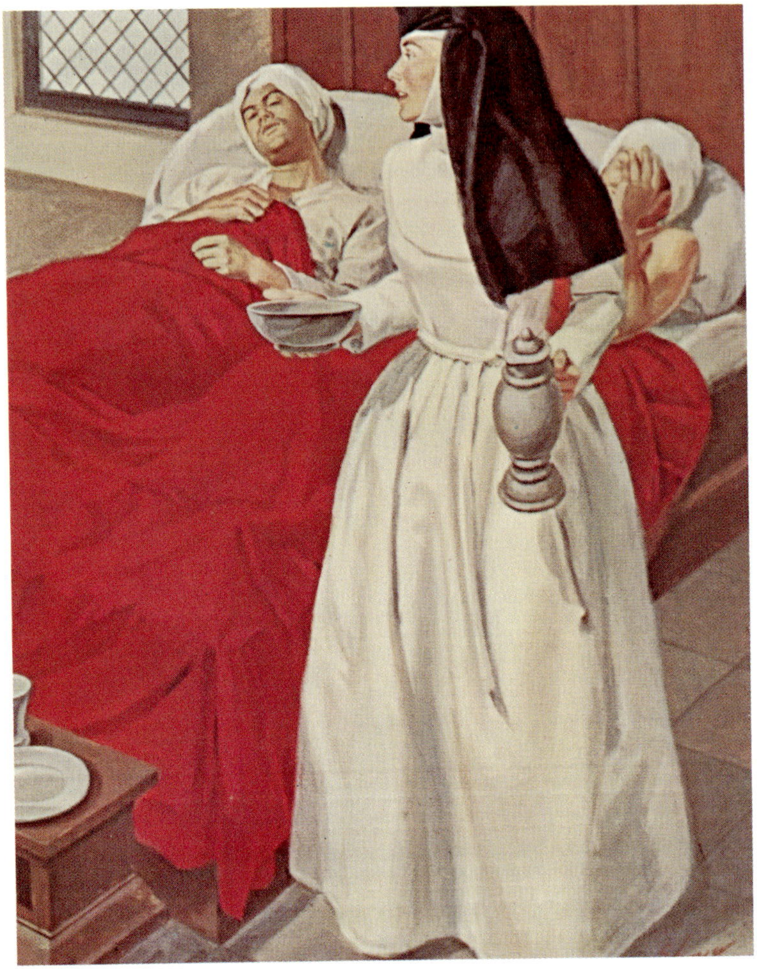

1242—HABIT OF THE CATHOLIC ORDER OF CANONESSES, BELIEVED TO BE ONE OF THE FIRST RELIGIOUS NURSING ORDERS

1540—THE ATTIRE OF A LAI ATTENDING THE SICK AT THE COURT OF HENRY VIII OF ENGLAND

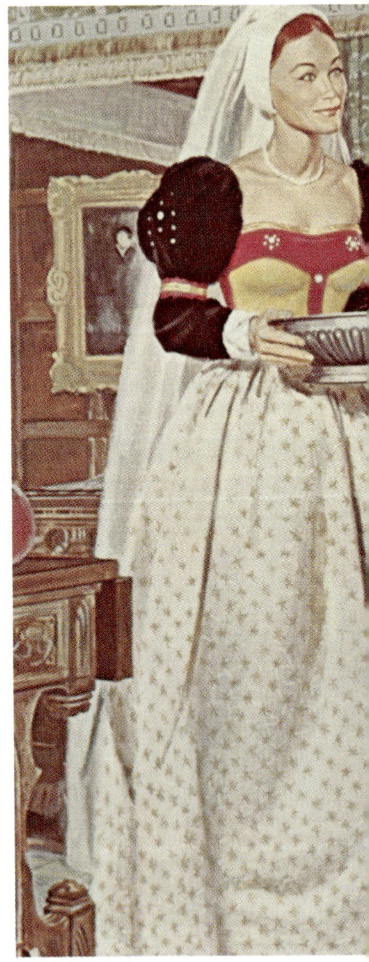

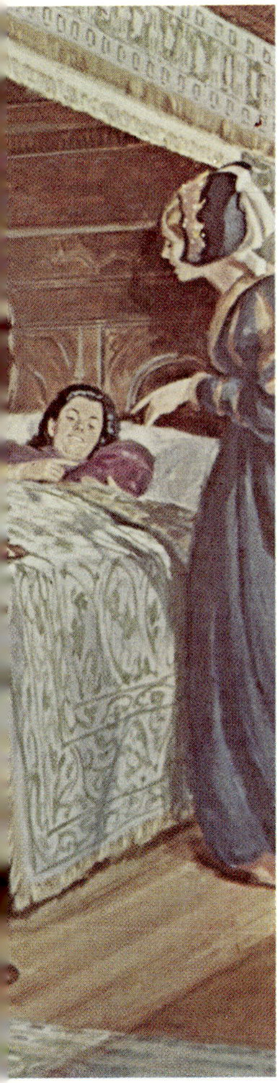

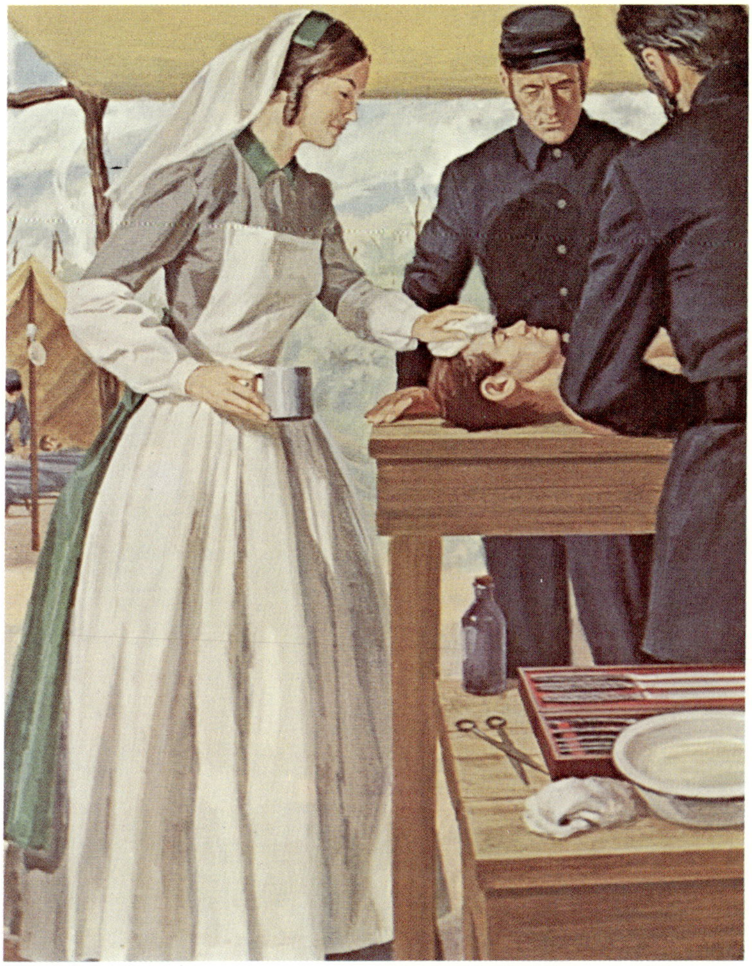

1863—A VOLUNTEER NURSE CARING FOR THE WOUNDED AT THE BATTLE OF GETTYSBURG

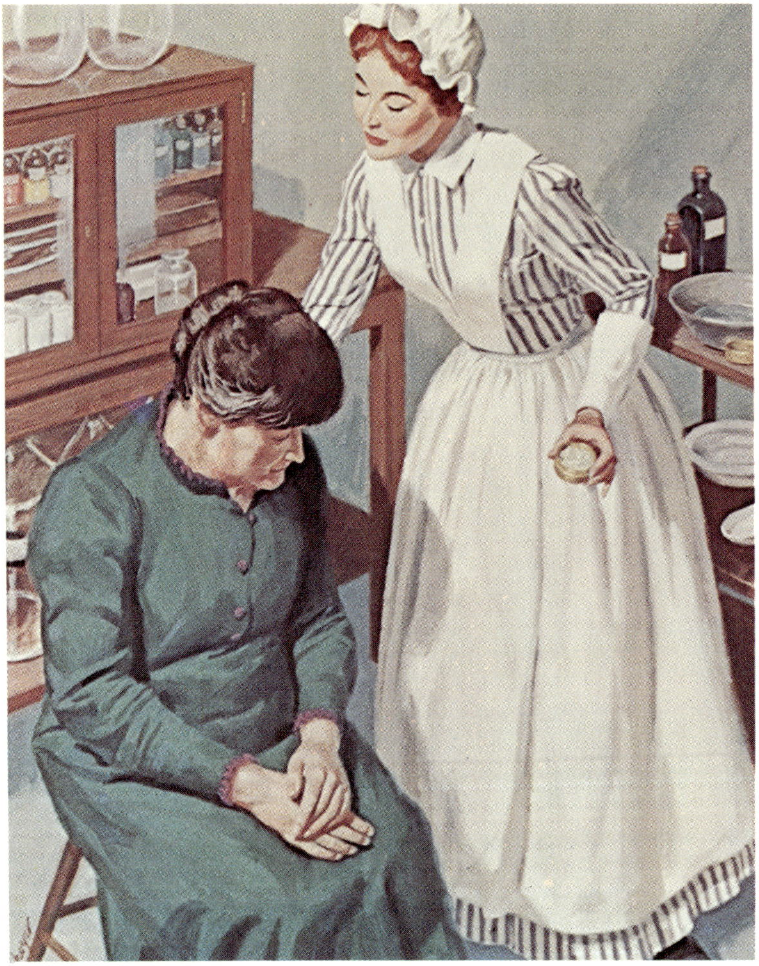

1880—AN EARLY MODEL OF THE NURSE'S UNIFORM

1898—AN AMERICAN NURSE
ON DUTY WITH
THE U. S. ARMY DURING
THE SPANISH-AMERICAN WAR

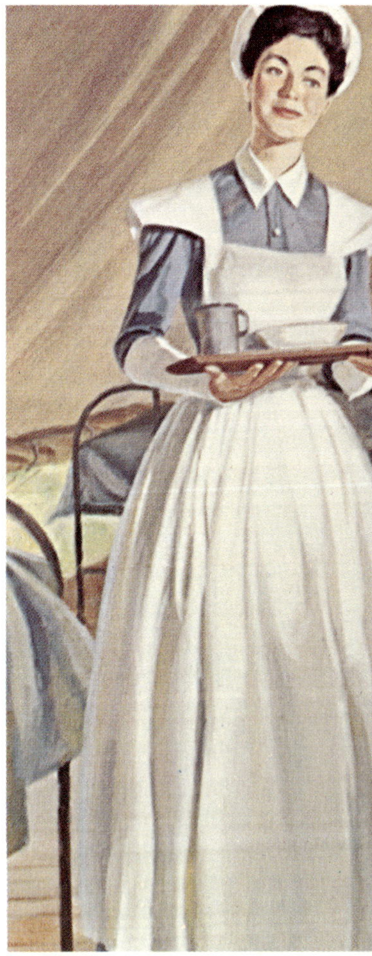

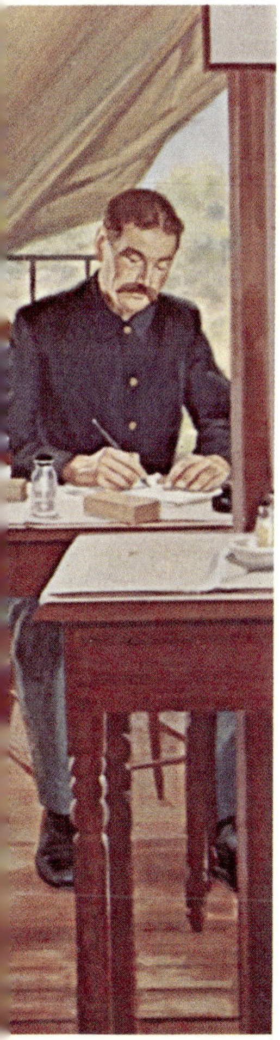

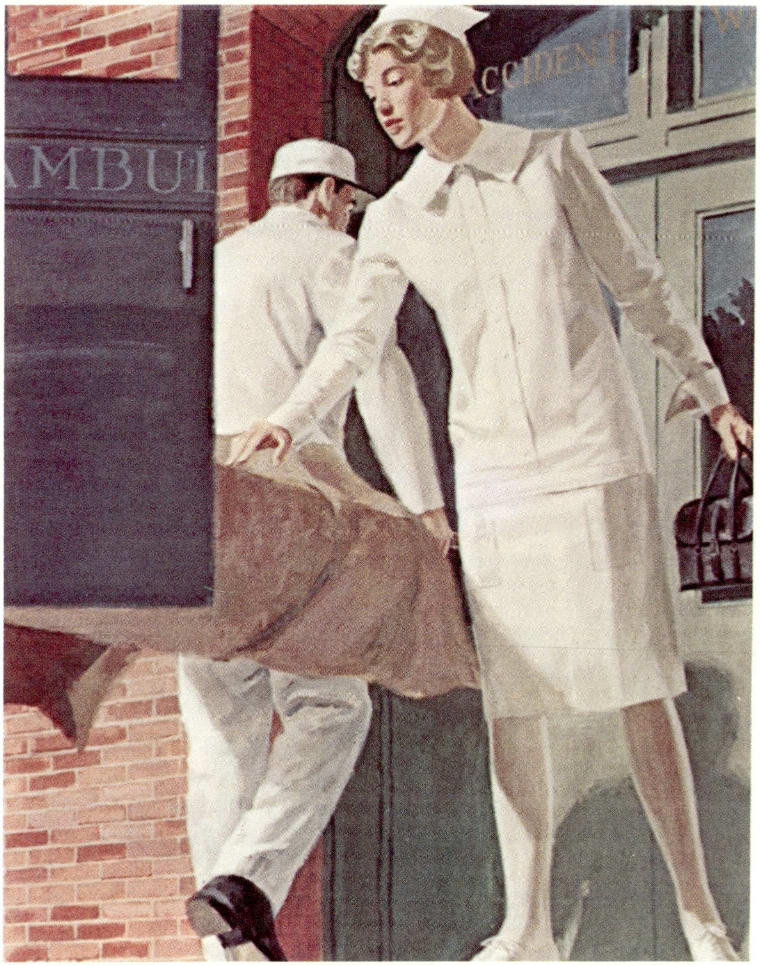

1925—THE "FLAPPER AGE" INFLUENCED THE DESIGN OF NURSES' UNIFORMS

COURTESY OF BARNES HOSPITAL, ST. LOUIS, MO.

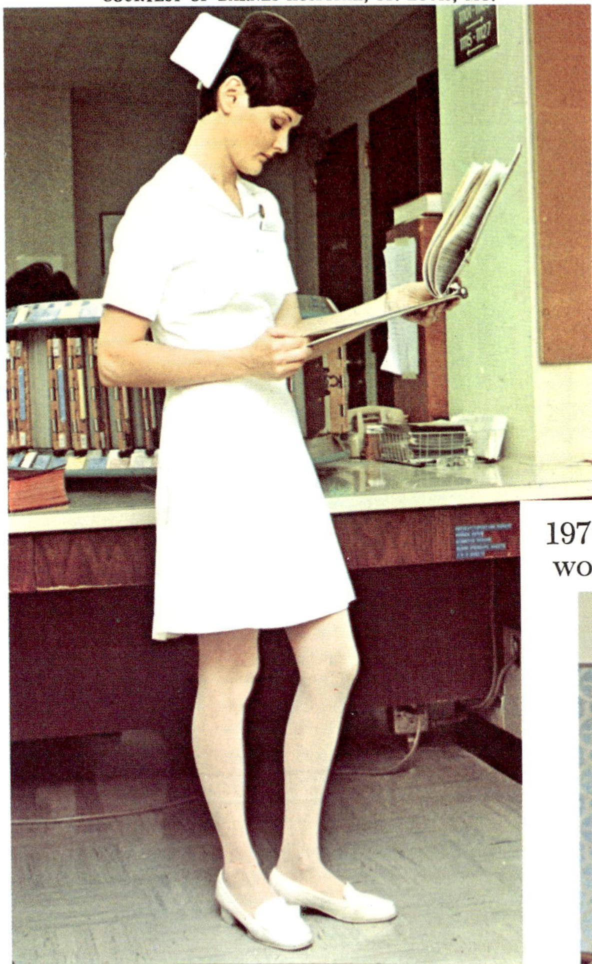

1971—THE UNIFORM OF TODAY'S NURSE REFLECTS TODAY'S STYLES JUST AS IT HAS DONE THROUGH THE YEARS

1971—THE MODERN HABIT AND THE DUTY UNIFORM WORN BY NURSE-SISTERS OF ONE RELIGIOUS ORDER

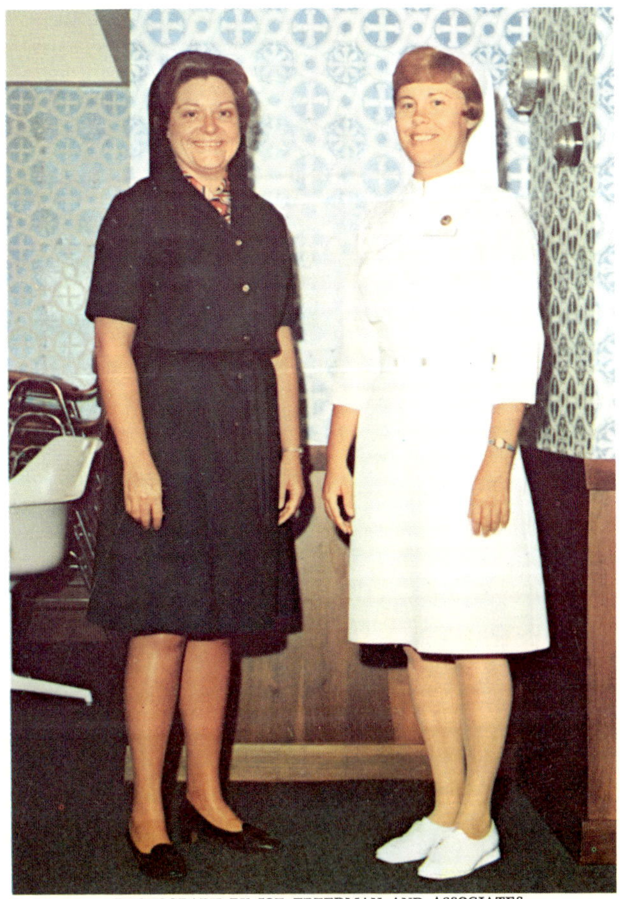

PHOTOGRAPH BY JOE FREEDMAN AND ASSOCIATES, PHOTOGRAPHERS, DAYTON, OHIO

CHAPTER 3

The period of "educated" nursing

FOUNDATION—THE NIGHTINGALE SYSTEM

June 15, 1860, is considered the day the cornerstone of nursing in England was laid. On that day fifteen probationers entered St. Thomas' Hospital in London to establish the Nightingale system of nursing. This system of nursing education, founded by Florence Nightingale, enabled young women from upperclass English society to enter the profession of nursing. It was based upon the assumption that the people of England would pay for the privilege of superior nursing care. The advent of this school began a separate history for nursing.

Florence Nightingale, born May 12, 1820, in Florence, Italy, was raised in an atmosphere of culture and affluence. Both she and her sister Parthenon were educated by their parents. They were taught languages, literature, and mathematics by their father, and the social graces by their mother. The two sisters rounded out their education in the usual manner for Victorian society by a continental tour when Florence (the younger of the two) was seventeen. At the completion of their tour in 1839, they were presented to Victorian society (probably at one of Queen Victoria's May Drawing-Rooms). It was the custom for a young Victorian lady to attend balls and parties and to perform small charitable acts until she married. How, then, did Florence Nightingale shake off the tight chains that social custom placed upon her in order to succeed in her self-appointed goal, to *change the profile of nursing?* It was not easy, and it did not happen overnight.

Florence Nightingale developed the habit at a very early age of keeping a journal of her observations as she traveled. During her continental tour she compiled notes of her visits to hospitals and her observations of the sanitation facilities (or lack of them, as the case might be). The neglected people of Europe living in filth and poverty were mentioned in her notes as well. She noted social problems of places visited, the need for preventive medicine, the need for good nursing care of those afflicted with the many diseases caused by want, and the lack of good hygienic practices. Even in England it was unsafe to walk down a street too close to a building lest the warning cry from above come too late to protect the person below from the slops that were unceremoniously thrown out of an upper story window. (It is no wonder that windows were kept closed; the odor must have been frightful.)

In spite of the restrictions placed upon young ladies of Queen Victoria's England, there were stirrings and rumblings of unrest among these women, and Florence Nightingale was one of those who minded the role the mores of England cast her in. She resented being a social butterfly. When she first approached her parents with the idea of entering a hospital for nurses' training, her family, especially her mother and sister, was aghast. At the age of 31, Miss Nightingale finally obtained the necessary parental permission to enter the Deaconess School at Kaiserswerth.

PREPARATION FOR NURSING

Miss Nightingale's educational background for her nursing positions in Crimea and St. Thomas' Hospital was meager by our standards. It included three months training at Kaiserswerth and working as superintendent of the "Establishment for Gentlewomen During Illness." She assumed the latter position in 1853 after working very hard to gain parental consent. Direction of this hospital for gentlewomen was in the hands of a committee of ladies. These women wanted to restrict patient admission to members of their own church, the Church of England. Displaying the tact that was to prove one of her greatest assets throughout her life, Miss Nightingale remained steadfast in her belief that this unchristian attitude was not compatible with health care. She finally received permission not only to admit patients of all faiths but also for clergymen of various faiths to visit the hospital patients, as long as she met the rabbi or priest at the door and escorted him to the patient's bedside.

THE CRIMEA

Florence Nightingale, however, had one desire that remained unfulfilled. She wanted to upgrade the practice of nursing and to make nursing an honorable profession for gentlewomen. Fate came to her aid in the form of Tsar Nicholas of Russia. The Tsar threatened the boundaries of Turkey, using his deep concern for the Greek Orthodox Church as an excuse. England, France, and Sardinia came to Turkey's aid. As in the Crusades, religious zeal was the expressed motive for invasion and threat, but power politics, trade rivalries, and territorial disputes were motives as well. The wars were not going well for the allies, and casualties mounted on both sides. Each country assumed responsibility for the care of its own wounded. William Howard Russell, reporter for the *London Times,* wrote about the almost barbaric nursing care the English wounded received. He described in detail the appalling filth, poor food, and the unsanitary conditions that existed in the medical barracks of the English fighting men. He asked, "Where were the Nursing Sisters? Where were the nurses like those who nursed the French wounded?"

After reading his reports, the English people, too, began to ask questions. Why was there such a lack of nursing personnel? Why were no women prepared to give nursing care at the front?

Sir Sidney Herbert, Minister of War in England, was afraid to defy English tradition so outrageously as to send genteel women to the battlefront. A letter from Florence Nightingale volunteering for this war service crossed the one from Sir Sidney asking her to assume charge of the nurses he would send to Crimea. Thirty-eight women (ten Roman Catholic Nursing Sisters, fourteen nurses from Protestant sisterhoods, and fourteen practical nurses) landed at Scutari in the Crimea on November 4, 1854. To speak of the hardships this brave little band faced would take pages. A long period of time elapsed before these nurses were even accepted and made welcome by medical officers and orderlies. Once recognized and asked to help, however, this group of nurses cleaned the area, thus reducing infection; cooked for the men, giving them much needed nourishment instead of the poor food they had been receiving; established a laundry close to the barracks which was staffed by soldiers' wives; provided some recreation for the men; and wrote letters to their families. The work of the Red Cross was in part inspired by the example of Miss Nightingale and her nurses. Miss Nightingale's title during this service was Superintendent of Female Nursing Establishment of English General Hospitals in Turkey.

During her long life Miss Nightingale continued her practice of recording all she saw and did. After the Crimean War ended, the Minister of War in England asked her to write a résumé of her experiences at the front. From her journals she compiled a thick book entitled *Notes on Matters Affecting the Health and Efficiency of the British Army.* This book had such tremendous impact that a commission, with Miss Nightingale's old friend Sir Sidney Herbert as chairman, was appointed in 1857 to investigate the medical service for the British Army. The work of this commission set up a program that safeguarded the health of the British Army at home and abroad.

NIGHTINGALE SCHOOL ESTABLISHED

Her years of experience had helped Miss Nightingale develop an entirely new concept of nursing education. She incorporated her own ideas with those she had observed in the religious nursing orders into the nursing plan that bears her name. She believed that schools of nursing should be self-supporting and not subject to the whims of the hospital board. This idea still has merit. She felt that schools of nursing should have decent living quarters for their students, that they should have paid nurse instructors (paid by both the school and the hospital), that the schools should correlate theory to practice, and that these students should be taught the "why," not just the "how," in nursing. (The correlation of theory to practice and teaching the "why" is part and parcel of nursing education of the 1970s.) Many tributes were paid to Florence Nightingale for her work in Crimea, but the most far-reaching was the fund given her by the English people (44,000 pounds sterling in all). This fund made it possible for her to realize her greatest dream—the opening of a school of nursing.

The Nightingale system of nursing began in St. Thomas' Hospital in London with the admission of two groups of students (regular and paying "lady probationers") in June of 1860. Since Miss Nightingale's health had suffered from her Crimean War experience, she appointed Mrs. Sarah Elizabeth Wardroper matron of the school. This first school that taught according to the "Nightingale System" spread theory of improved nursing practice to many parts of the world.

Posterity owes Miss Nightingale a debt of gratitude not only for the development of hospital and district nursing, but also for the suggested improvements in India, for sanitary reforms, and for the improved health care of English military men. All this she accomplished from her room. Because of the place of women in Victorian England, the very fact that she wasn't able to be out in society and could do her work behind the scenes was probably the difference between success and failure.

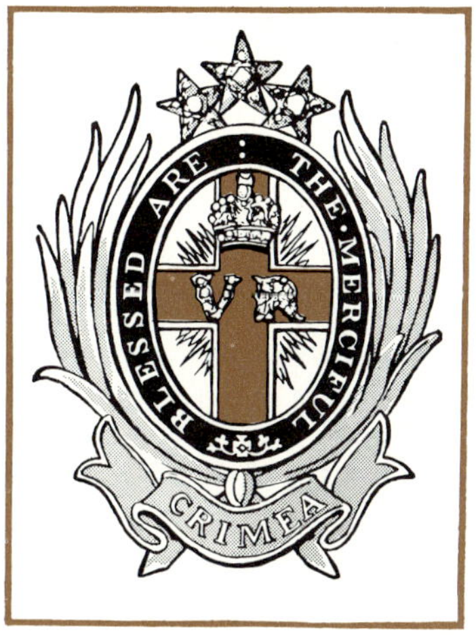

FLORENCE NIGHTINGALE BROOCH

A brooch inscribed: "To Miss Florence Nightingale, as a mark of esteem and gratitude for her devotion towards the Queen's brave soldiers from Victoria R. 1855." The pin, designed by Prince Albert, the Queen's husband, is a St. George's cross in red enamel surmounted by a diamond crown; it bears the words, "Crimea" and "Blessed are the merciful." (Courtesy Metropolitan Life Insurance Company.)

In focusing on her many successes, however, history has often overlooked the fact that Miss Nightingale did not always recognize and accept new scientific discoveries. She ignored bacteriologic research and placed no credence in the germ theory. She felt that disease could be eliminated by cleanliness. She definitely opposed a central registry for nurses. Miss Nightingale said that central registration would standardize nursing, and this standardization would in turn deter the progress of nursing. We have seen, however, that criteria setting and standardization for schools are necessary, and that nursing, instead of stagnating, has developed because of them. Nursing education continues to work diligently to eliminate social lag and attempts to meet the needs of society. The graduate nurse of today has more opportunities awaiting her than has any nurse in history.

Florence Nightingale died in 1910. In the ninety years she lived she saw her plan of nursing become the backbone of the profession in many countries. Two of her books on nursing and hospitals, *Notes on Nursing* and *Notes on Hospitals,* contain many timely portions, as applicable in the 1970s as they were in 1859. For example, at present the general public and nursing organizations are working to develop areas of nursing research and to promote continuing education for nurses. Miss Nightingale reminded her nurses more than one hundred years ago that any nurse who feels she is completely educated upon graduation is a conceited person. In Miss Nightingale's opinion a good nurse and a conceited nurse cannot be found in the same person. How do you feel about this?

Miss Nightingale's nurses helped establish district nursing in Liverpool, England; Army nursing in 1881 and Indian Army Nursing Service in 1888. In addition, because midwifery was included in this superior type of nursing, the practice of it was improved, also. By 1900 modern nursing and the care of people regardless of their diagnosis had a good start in England.

LAYING THE CORNERSTONE IN THE UNITED STATES

At the time that Florence Nightingale was opening her school in London, the United States was on the brink of the most costly war in her history, the Civil War. In the Reconstruction period that followed, the South was in a state of economic collapse. With family fortunes wiped out, proud Southern families were forced to earn their living without the help of slaves. They were forced to scratch a livelihood from the burned-out fields left in the wake of Sherman's march to Georgia and were further subjected to the indignities of an occupation by Northern carpetbaggers and scalawags. The North, although not afflicted with the tremendous economic losses of the South, lost many men and suffered the devastation that always follows war. However, even though the country was in a condition of chaos, nursing gained supporters from many quarters. It was the Volunteer Nurses, the untrained, civic-minded philanthropists who recognized, as a result of their war experiences, that programs to train nurses were needed. This group of volunteers received the staunch support of interested citizens.

On September 1, 1873, Linda Richards became the *first graduate nurse* in the United States. At the age of 32 Miss Richards completed her one-year course in nursing at the New England Hospital for Women and Children in Boston, Massachusetts. This course in nursing, the brainchild of Dr. Marie Zakrewska, was patterned after the Deaconess School of Kaiserswerth. Miss Richards received a few lectures by the doctors and some practical instruction in nursing from the women interns. The study of materia medica was omitted, however, since special precautions were taken to conceal the name of the drugs the physicians administered to patients. These drugs were ordered by number only, because the individual doctor was afraid to divulge the nature of his prescriptions lest someone steal his therapy. Miss Richards had no nursing textbooks as there were none written, and upon completing her training took no State Board examination. However, Linda Richards received the best training for nursing available anywhere in the United States in the year 1872 to 1873.

EARLY SCHOOLS OF NURSING

In 1873 three schools of nursing opened that were patterned after the Nightingale plan. The first of these was Bellevue Training School for Nurses in New York City. Bellevue was established as an almshouse, hospital, and prison in 1816, and by the 1870's the care was as bad as any seen in England during the "dark period." A group of women interested in doing charitable work had appointed Mrs. Joseph Hobson, a socialite, as their chairman. They decided that their work would be directed toward improving the lot of the sick and poor of New York. While making an observation tour of the hospital, Mrs. Hobson was appalled at the sight of the inmates, drunk or sober, giving their version of nursing care to other inmates. She was also dismayed at the smells and filth that confronted her. Mrs. Hobson became convinced that Bellevue and New York desperately needed a training school for nurses. She read all of the writings of Florence Nightingale she could find and became convinced that the Nightingale System of nurse education was the method that must be started at Bellevue. Dr. Gill Wylie, convinced that Mrs. Hobson's plan was a good one, paid his own way to England to enlist Florence Nightingale's help. Although it was not easy to see Miss Nightingale, Dr. Wylie brought back a letter from the "mother of nursing." This letter helped to inspire the good ladies of Mrs. Hobson's committee into even greater activity in order to achieve their goal. These zealous women, imbued with their desire to improve patient care, had to fight the prejudice of both the medical staff and the political machine before they could accomplish the monumental task they had set for themselves. The committee had the advantage of their wealth and social position to aid in their fight. On May 1, 1873, six of the hospital's wards were assigned to the experiment. Thus, the Bellevue system of nurse education, based upon the Nightingale plan, was born. The program was under the stern and capable direction of Sister Helen of the Episcopal Order of All Saints.

The training program for the Bellevue student nurses was planned with no regular lectures. The program was to last one year and was to include an additional year of experience. Graduates of the Bellevue Training School include many famous alumnae, such as Isabel Hampton (Robb), Lavinia Dock, and Jane Delano.

Other hospitals that opened schools of nursing in 1873 were the Connecticut Training School in New Haven and Massachusetts General Hospital in Boston. The Connecticut Training School began on October 1, 1873 with three probationers. The school opened at the insistence of its medical staff and received their complete cooperation. Massachusetts General, opening in November of that same year, had six probationers in the first class. This school was established with the aid of its women's committee, who had fought the prejudice of the medical staff in order to gain their objective. The Massachusetts General Nurses' Training program included a preliminary course, and for the first time the tasks of housekeeping were taken out of the hands of the nurses and delegated to attendants. The women's committee felt that long hours of work and the performing of these menial tasks reduced a nurse's efficiency.

The symbol of the nurse—her uniform. In 1873 nurses wore no distinctive uniform. They wore a housedress covered by a large apron for protection. The six students in Bellevue's first class wanted a uniform. They felt a uniform dress would be safer, cleaner, and more economical and would be a morale booster by helping them become less self conscious on the wards if they were all dressed alike. The uniform was patterned after a dress worn by Euphemia Van Rensselaer, a New York socialite, who was a member of this first class. The story is told that Euphemia went home one weekend and returned to the hospital dressed in blue and white striped seersucker, leg-o-mutton sleeves, trailing skirts and white apron, collar, cuffs, and cap. Girls being girls, it was not long before style-setter Miss Van Rensselaer saw all of her classmates wearing this same uniform.

The Bellevue cap, adopted at the same time, was patterned after the cap of the Nightingale nurses at St. Thomas' Hospital.

It is strange but true that what people wear on their heads can set them apart. The old Romans honored their champions with a laurel wreath; nations crown their kings and queens; and the taking of scholastic honors includes the wearing of a mortarboard with an appropriate tassel. Wreaths, crowns, and caps all carry their singular significance. They set their wearers apart as persons of distinction. The nurse's cap dates back to early times when a woman's humility and obedience were denoted by the veil she wore on her head. The ancient Hebrew woman covered her hair, considering this her crowning glory, from the sight of all save her espoused husband. Religious of the early Christian church covered their hair also. "The stiff white cap of the deaconess; the close fitting white linen caps of the nun which encircled the face and chin, with the variation of the fillet for the forehead, or perhaps the bib or maybe the veil of dark material, the fluted ruffle, or bows under the chin; all of these were forerunners of the present nurses' uniform cap."*

LATER SCHOOLS OF NURSING

Schools of nursing, both good and bad, mushroomed into existence all over the country. Even if a hospital opened a school as a means of acquiring cheap labor, these poorly trained nurses received a diploma. Between 1880 and 1900 hospitals, too, changed their modus operandi. They changed from a refuge for "down and outers" to a laboratory for the advances in medical care. Suddenly doctors could not get along without their handmaidens, the nurses. Programs of instruction, which began as one-year courses, became two-year courses, and finally three-year courses. The time came, however, when it was necessary to evaluate the many kinds of nursing programs offered. Nursing educators, on the basis of their evaluations and study, deduced that the length of the course was indicative of the quality of the nurse graduate. Her worth depended upon the caliber of education she received.

Johns Hopkins Hospital opened a school of nursing in 1889. Its first "principal," Isabel Hampton Robb was the person most influential in directing the development of nursing in the United States until her untimely death in 1910. Mrs. Robb, a graduate of Bellevue in 1883, had been superintendent of the Illinois Training School for Nurses (now Cook County Hospital) before coming to Baltimore to open the school of nursing at Johns Hopkins. She limited the day of the student nurse to twelve hours, allowing two hours per day for recreation. It is evident to anyone perusing the annals of nursing history in the years from 1883 to 1910 that Isabel Hampton Robb had a part in all progressive developments during that time. The paper she presented at the Chicago World's Fair in 1893 to the International Congress of Charities, Correction and Philanthropy, testifies to her ability to identify the problems of nursing education. She did not stop at identifying the problems, she sought resolution of them. She worked for state registration and standardization of nursing education programs and teacher preparation for instruction in schools of nursing. Through the efforts of this far-sighted, seemingly untiring woman and the members of the Society of Superintendents, classes at Teachers College, Columbia University began in 1899. This first course led to the establishment of the Department of Health at Teachers College, Columbia University.

Protection for those helping hands. Did you ever wonder where the idea for the wearing of rubber gloves as a protection originated? During the time Isabel Hampton Robb was the principal at Johns Hopkins, another Hampton, Caroline, also worked there. Caroline had graduated from the New York Hospital School of Nursing in 1888 and came to Baltimore as a head nurse in surgery when Johns Hopkins opened. The rivalry between the two Hamptons was quickly noted, but Dr. William Halstead brought the situation to a peaceable solution by appointing Caroline operating room supervisor. Caroline Hampton suffered from dermatitis. Because of this Dr. Halstead, a surgeon, took time out from his crowded schedule to go to New York to ask the Goodyear Rubber Company to make some rubber gauntlets to protect the hands of the extremely capable operating room nurse whom he did not want to lose. The order was filled, and Caroline's dermatitis cleared up after she began wearing these gloves.

"AWAKENING" OF NURSING

The last two decades of the nineteenth century may be called "the awakening" of the pro-

*Stimson, J. C.: The nurse's uniform, American Journal of Nursing 36:368, Apr. 1936.

fession of nursing. In 1893 the groundwork for the establishment of the two nursing organizations was laid. It was at the Chicago World's Fair in 1893 that the Associated Alumnae was begun, which in 1911 became The American Nurses' Association. The American Society of Superintendents of Training Schools for Nurses, which became the National League for Nursing Education in 1912, also began. Isabel Hampton Robb helped to organize and develop both of these groups.

SPANISH-AMERICAN WAR

From April 12, to August 12, 1898 the United States was at war with Spain. When the United States entered the war there was no organized Army Nurse Corps; therefore, no system had been established for providing nursing care to the military services. The Surgeon General had received an appropriation from Congress to engage the services of graduate nurses under contract. He was approached by Dr. Anita Newcomb McGee to permit the Daughters of the American Revolution to serve as a recruitment agency for these needed nurses. Nursing during the Spanish-American War was concerned as much with the care of wounded as with the care to those attacked by the fevers that raged through the regions in which the war took place. Malaria and yellow fever were the two greatest offenders. Still not convinced of the necessity of having nurses at the front, the Surgeon General finally gave his consent to Dr. McGee's plan, and 1,600 graduate nurses served under contract.

One of the 1,600 was Clara Louise Maas of East Orange, New Jersey. In the House of Representatives on February 5, 1964, the Honorable Joseph G. Minish, Democrat from New Jersey, called the attention of his Congressional colleagues to a Resolution which he introduced on that date. Representative Minish's remarks, in part, were the following:

MR. SPEAKER: I have introduced in the House of Representatives today a resolution authorizing and directing the Postmaster General to issue a special postage stamp in memory of Nurse Clara Louise Maas, who, in 1901 gave her life for the advancement of medical science in the search to control yellow fever. The heroic young woman who made the supreme sacrifice for humanity is a shining example of the dedication and selflessness that mark the members of the noble nursing profession. Issuance of a commemorative stamp would be a most fitting tribute to her superb services to mankind and would honor the values which guided her life.

Nurse Maas was born in East Orange, New Jersey in 1876, and died in Cuba at the age of 25, gallant and unafraid. The City Council of her native city recently adopted a Resolution in honor of the young humanitarian whose brief life is an inspiration to all people. The Resolution follows:

WHEREAS Nurse Clara Louise Maas in the service of humanity and all mankind sacrificed her life August 24, 1901, while engaged in medical research on yellow fever; and WHEREAS after completing nurse's training in 1895 at Newark German Hospital, which is now called Clara Maas Memorial Hospital, she served as an Army nurse in Cuba and in the Philippines during and following the Spanish-American War; and WHEREAS Nurse Maas volunteered to participate in experiments conducted in Cuba by Dr. Walter Reed, Dr. William C. Gorgas and Dr. Carlos Finlay to prove that yellow fever was transmitted solely by the Stegomyia Mosquito; and WHEREAS, through her death, methods of controlling yellow fever were developed and countless thousands of lives were saved; and WHEREAS the interest among the citizens of East Orange has been mobilized and articulated by Reverend Arthur Herbert, Pastor of Holy Trinity Church of East Orange, who has sought, in behalf of the citizens and residents of the city, as the place of her birth in 1876, to achieve recognition of her service to mankind through means of a commemorative stamp to be issued by the United States honoring Miss Maas. NOW THEREFORE, be it RESOLVED, that the City Council for itself, the mayor, the city officials and employees, and all residents of the city of East Orange do hereby petition the Postmaster General of the United States to authorize the issuance of a commemorative postage stamp honoring Nurse Clara Louise Maas and her contribution to humanity; and be it further resolved that copies of this resolution be distributed to appropriate State and Federal Officials that they assist in favoring our endeavors.*

As a result of the work of Miss Maas and the many other self-sacrificing nurses who served during the Spanish-American War the Army continued to employ nurses. They were employed, however, without benefit of rank. When the idea of contracted nursing service was first presented to them, medical officers and their medical aides could not see the necessity for such a move; they could not imagine what they

*Excerpts from the Congressional Record, February 5, 1964.

would do with these women. After the war, however, in looking back over the period of the war and the service these brave women had given, they wondered how they would have managed without their help.

TWENTIETH CENTURY
FIRST DECADE

Nursing service between 1900 and 1912 developed not only in hospital service, but also in other fields. Private duty, settlement house nursing (the forerunner of public health nursing), school nursing, government service, and prenatal and maternal health nursing also advanced. All of these opportunities for nursing practice came about as a result of the general public and the profession's growing awareness of the need for preventive measures that could be used to maintain the health of the nation. The age of the rugged individualist in America was over, and the age of social awareness and man's responsibility for his fellow man had dawned. The heavy demands placed upon nurses in these new nursing services came at a time when nurses were really not prepared to meet these challenges. As a result, hospitals literally mushroomed into existence, each with its own school. There were no uniform educational standards. The basic principle followed in the curriculum of these schools of nursing—a principle nurtured by the medical profession and traditionalists in nursing practice—was to develop in each nurse a deep and unquestioning loyalty to the physician. Instructors taught the "how" but did not teach the "why" in nursing practice as had been recommended by Florence Nightingale.

In rural areas there was an almost desperate shortage of nurses because graduate nurses remained in the large cities believing there were better opportunities, better pay, and more lucrative rewards in the nursing of the wealthy.

AGE OF SPECIALIZATION

Nursing leaders of this first decade of the twentieth century realized that the physicians were beginning to specialize and that hospitals would no doubt follow the same pattern. They made plans for schools of nursing to offer students experience in the nursing care of patients in all of the specialized fields. They believed that unless graduate nurses had some introduction to all disease conditions, they were only half trained. By 1910 these leaders in nursing were faced with some puzzling problems. As one looks at these problems, they have a familiar ring. These problems included: Under whose direction should the organization and administration of nursing education come? How could nursing education be directed to meet the myriad needs of society? What should be the realistic objectives of a *good* school of nursing? Proposals for solutions to these problems in 1910 were:

1. Affiliations for those experiences that the home hospital did not have the facilities to include
2. The opportunity for postgraduate experience (not collegiate education, but experience in specialized areas of nursing such as the operating room and anesthesia)
3. The opening of collegiate programs in nursing education

STANDARDS ARE SET

Between 1913 and 1937 guidelines were established out of necessity. A standard curriculum for schools of nursing was prepared by the National League for Nursing Education, and the so-called practice of nursing was gradually infiltrated with educational objectives. The financial cost of nursing programs, the control of administration, and the advisability of transferring emphasis from the hospital's responsibilities to care for the patient to the school's responsibilities to educate the student for nursing were among problems to be analyzed during these twenty years.

During the years that immediately preceded the United States' entry into World War I (1913-1917) nursing educators attempted to change and improve nursing care through revision of the nursing curriculum. These dedicated women in nursing, working anywhere from twelve to twenty-four hours a day, still took the time to write textbooks for schools of nursing, to alter educational methods, and to set up a committee to prepare and publish the first of a series of curriculum guides for schools of nursing. In the attempt to set definite standards, they also evaluated the product of these schools, the graduate nurse. The National League for Nursing Education, the nursing organization that made these attempts to establish sound patterns of nursing education, was hampered in that it could only suggest revision; it did not have the power to enforce change. Part of the reason was the dependent position of women in society. It took World War I to help ratify the Nineteenth Amendment to the Constitution, which legalized some of the rights of women. Hospitals were under the direction of men, the physicians, whose greatest fear was that nursing leaders were attempting to "overeducate" the nurse. Many doctors believed that nurses would become so educated that they would forget their places—forget they were nurses. Nursing during the 1920s still did not answer the question "why"; only the question "how" to care for a patient was included in nursing curriculum.

In spite of the often expressed objection of Florence Nightingale and the objection of physicians, American nursing leaders believed in the ultimate worth of central registries under the control of nurses. Prior to the establishment of professional registries for employment, graduate nurses were tied to their home school for work (mostly in private duty nursing), since doctors and patients were accustomed to call the hospitals when they were in need of a nurse.

WORLD WAR I

While in the United States schools of nursing were feeling the growing pains described above, Europe was in the throes of a bloody holocaust. On Sunday, June 28, 1914, in Sarajevo, the capitol of Austria, Archduke Francis Ferdinand, heir to the throne of Austria-Hungary, and his wife Sophie were assassinated. The assassination of the Archduke and Archduchess triggered a series of events that soon involved most of Europe, and eventually the world, in what is now called World War I.

The nursing in World War I was ably assisted by the International Red Cross. Many nurses accomplished monumental tasks and their names should certainly be written for all to see. Space, however, does not permit a discussion of all these nurses, so we have elected to tell the story of just one of these women—Edith Cavell. She was called Mata Hari (spy) by the enemy, and martyr and patriot by her allies. Edith Cavell was the daughter of the Vicar of Swardston (England). She had been a governess and teacher, and finally become a nurse at the age of 31. She was small, quiet, reserved, and possessed no sense of humor. Upon meeting this serious woman, people always envied her indomitable spirit. From her earliest years, Miss Cavell's reply when asked what she would like to do with her life was that she would like to do something for people, something to ease their hurts, erase their sorrows, and in some way help them because most people were so helpless. While Miss Cavell was serving as governess to the François family in Brussels, Belgium, she was called home by the death of her father. In 1896 Edith entered London Hospital to learn nursing. During her years there no one seemed to become closely acquainted with her. She kept to herself and never seemed to participate in any of the good times her classmates indulged in.

At this time, Dr. DePage of Brussels was very unhappy with the caliber of nursing offered in Belgian hospitals. He had heard much of the wonderful nursing care given by English nurses trained by the Nightingale system and went looking for an English nurse who could speak French. Edith Cavell's good friends, the François, suggested her name to Dr. DePage. On October 1, 1907, Miss Cavell left England to open her school of nursing at l'Ecole Belge d'Infermieres Diplômeés. Working round the clock in her usual serious manner, Edith Cavell trained Belgian and Dutch girls after the English pattern. On vacation in England in 1914 Edith cut her journey short when she began to see ominous reports of threats of war against

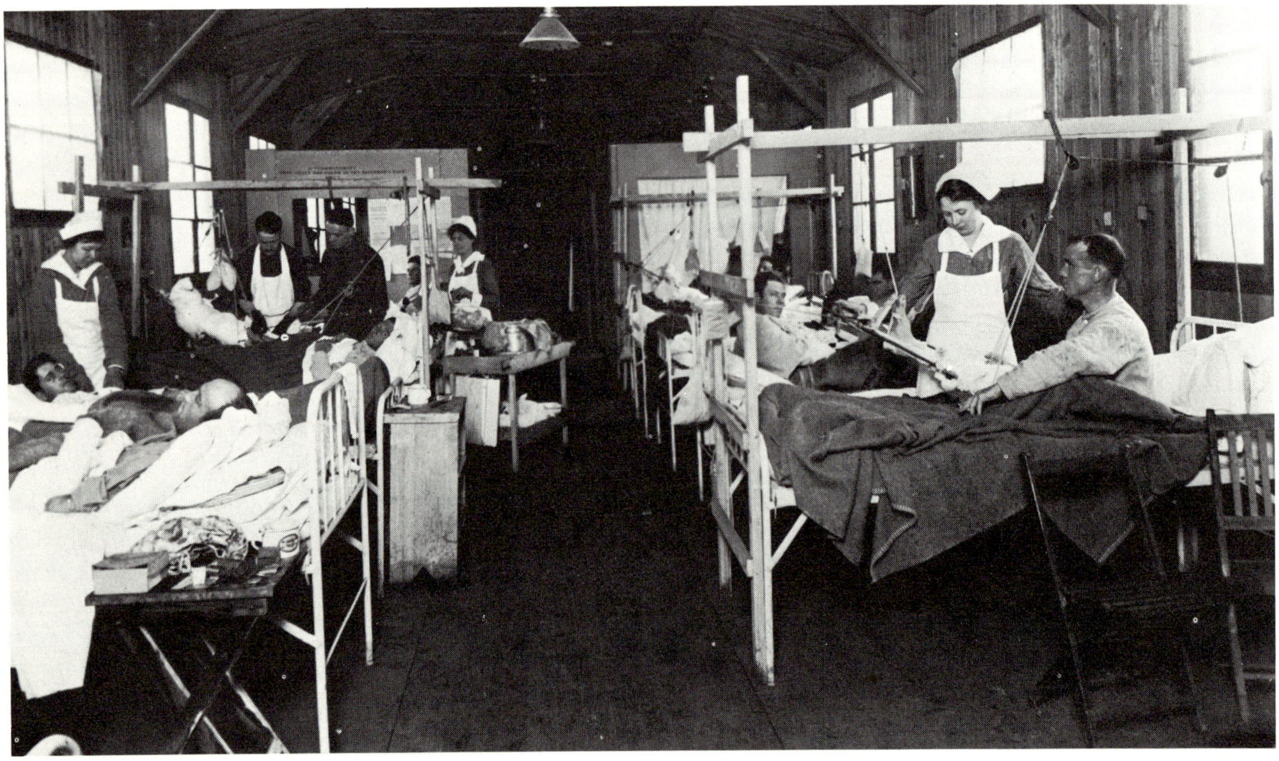

FRONTLINE NURSING IN WORLD WAR I

Haute Marne, France, 1917—General view of Ward 1, Base Hospital No. 52, includes Capt. Frank Bird dressing a patient and nurses Miss L. Rodskapp, Miss Margaret Dell, and Miss Ruth Edmunds. (Courtesy The American National Red Cross.)

Belgium. She believed she should be back on the job as the head of her school of nursing if this dreaded threat were to materialize.

In 1914 the Germans occupied Belgium. Miss Cavell continued to nurse whether her patient was a German or one of the Allies, and saw that her nurses did likewise. However, many allied soldiers were trapped in Belgium. Edith Cavell helped these men escape so that they could return to their own countries. It is for this reason that the Germans labeled her a spy and the allies called her heroine and martyr. Humanitarian and martyred nurse, Edith Cavell was shot as a spy by the Germans on the morning of October 12, 1915.

At Charing Cross Road in London stands a statue of Edith Cavell. On the base of this statue are inscribed the last words she uttered: "Patriotism is not enough. I must have no hatred or bitterness for anyone."

UNITED STATES ENTERS WORLD WAR I

The United States officially entered the war in 1917 after repeated provocations. Many doctors and nurses were already serving overseas with units from various American hospitals. In the accompanying photograph nurses are seen assisting in the care of wounded in a base hospital. In April of 1917, 400 nurses were enrolled in the Army Nurse Corps. This number increased to about 22,000 and approximately 10,000 of them served overseas before the war ended. These patriotic nurses served without the benefits that accompany military rank, but they lived under the same military restrictions as did the rest of the military. Julia Stimson, the first woman to hold the rank of Major (1920), was appointed director of the American Expeditionary Force of nurses. The American Nursing Service of the Red Cross, founded in 1917 under the direction of Miss Jane Delano, acted as recruitment and procurement agency for the Army and Navy Nurse Corps.

As a result of the tremendous public enthusiasm for the training of an increased number of nurses to serve at home and abroad, two schools of nursing were opened:

1. The Army School of Nursing opened in 1918 with Miss Annie W. Goodrich as director. A three year training program was established in army hospitals, with affiliations planned in areas such as pediatrics, obstetrics, and public health. The Army School of Nursing graduated 500 nurses in 1921. Enrollment, however, dwindled until this school closed in 1932.
2. Vassar Training Camp at Vassar College answered the appeal for the help of college women in World War I. Four-hundred-thirty young women from 115 colleges in forty-one states enrolled in this program. These nurses spent twelve weeks in a preclinical period followed by a two-year nursing course. The Armistice was signed before these women graduated, but these graduates are important to the history of nursing because some of them acted as disciples in advancing the educational programs in schools of nursing during the postwar period.

Bearing the brunt of the hospital load of patient care in hospitals on the home front were the student nurses. They coped with the usual nursing problems and with the influenza epidemic as well. These nurses, even though many were poorly trained and deprived of proper supervision, worked a twelve-hour day or more. One nurse tells of entering a school of nursing in October of 1917; the very first day she was sent to the Emergency Room to help care for accident victims who had just been admitted. Traumatic as the experience may have been, these young women believed they were doing their patriotic duty.

THE ARMISTICE PERIOD

The Armistice was signed on November 11, 1918, with the hope that war would never again take place. Public health work truly began in earnest after the war, not just in the United States, but throughout Europe as well. Nurses had to deal with the aftermath of war, with malnutrition, tuberculosis, the influenza epidemic, and the rehabilitation of those disabled in war. The work of the public health nurse was planned as a service to the community and was based on community needs. The public health nurses, then as now, brought health education, rehabilitation, and nursing services to all members of the community.

Between World Wars I and II many changes occurred as a result of scientific research, scientific developments, changes in the status of women, increased educational opportunities for all and the many additional educational programs offered in colleges and universities. All of the changes in the social environment, as well as the United States' position as a world power, were reflected in nursing's growth and development.

After World War I ended, Congress failed to approve either the Treaty of Versailles (based on President Wilson's Fourteen Points) or the covenant of the League of Nations. During the 1920s American foreign policy became more conservative and more isolationist. Americans closed their eyes to the plight of unfortunates abroad. Their philosophy was to stay out of foreign entanglements: charity begins at home. Their attitude was to live for themselves, and live they did! The 1920s saw ten years of stock market spiralling and speculation, ten years of fantastic spending, and ten years of real estate booms even in remote areas of the United States. It was ten years of jazz music, marathon dancing, corrupt politics, growth of new industries such as radio, and firsts such as Charles A. Lindbergh's solo flight in the *Spirit of St. Louis* across the Atlantic Ocean in 1927. This Jazz Age also brought with it ten years of revolt against the Volstead Act.*

In 1920 with the ratification of the Nineteenth Amendment† to the Constitution women could vote. American women had already manifested their rebellion against puritanical or Victorian restrictions by bobbing their hair, wearing obvious make-up, shortening their skirts, wearing rolled stockings, and smoking cigarettes. This picture is only the surface view of American womanhood from 1920 to 1929. Women still believed in the sanctity of the home and in their personal responsibility for their neighbors' welfare. Present on the American scene from 1920 to 1929 were a group of nursing leaders, who were energetic, uncompromising, and constantly warring against hospital dirt, immorality, irresponsibility, and political corruption. This group of women evaluated nursing and nursing education. They were dedicated, stern, severe, and steadfast; sometimes they were called "tough martinets." Nurses of the National League for Nursing Education, The American Nurses' Association, and the National Organization of Public Health Nurses, with representation from the American Medical Association, American Hospital Association, and the American Public Health Association, collaborated in an evaluation of nursing and schools of nursing in 1925. This committee made three reports:

(1) *Nurses, Patients, and Pocketbooks* by Dr. May Ayres Burgess in 1928; (2) *An Activity Analysis of Nursing* by Ethel Johns and Blanche Pfefferkorn in 1934, and (3) *Nursing Schools Today and Tomorrow* in 1934. The recommendations of this committee laid the foundation for the development of the accrediting program still being conducted by the National League for Nursing.

THE GREAT DEPRESSION

Because you are accustomed to hearing about the critical need for nurses, it will be hard to imagine a time when this situation did not exist. In the 1930s nurses were in tremendous oversupply. The swing of the economic pendulum affected every person.

October 29, 1929 (Black Friday), marked the beginning of a financial crisis in these United States, which affected the American people in every city, town, and village across the nation. The stock market collapsed, businesses closed, and people were jobless and in utter despair. They were unable to furnish their families with even the barest necessities of life. Some were so despondent they committed suicide. Hardier people joined forces, and families united under one roof. Bread lines formed and the unemployed sold apples on street corners. How did this financial crisis affect nurses? At graduation exercises from schools of nursing in 1928, the young graduates were congratulated on being launched into a life of economic security; but, by 1930 the situation had changed drastically. A Registrar wrote in *The American Journal of Nursing* what a typical telephone call to her might be. "Nurse

*Volstead Act: 18th Amendment: Proposed December, 1917, declared ratified January 29, 1919. "After one year from the ratification of this article the manufacture, sale, or transportation of intoxicating liquors within, the importation thereof into, or the exportation thereof from the U.S. and all territory subject to the jurisdiction thereof for beverage purposes is hereby prohibited.

"The Congress and the several States shall have concurrent power to enforce this article by appropriate legislation.

"This article shall be inoperative unless it shall have been ratified as an amendment to the Constitution by the legislatures of the several States, as provided in the Constitution within seven years from the date of the submission hereof to the States by the Congress."

†19th Amendment of the Constitution of the United States: Proposed June 4, 1919, declared ratified August 26, 1920. "The right of the citizens of the United States to vote shall not be denied or abridged by the United States or any States on account of sex. The Congress shall have the power, by appropriate legislation, to enforce the provisions of this article."

X calls the Registry and asks 'Please, tell me, what number on the list am I? When am I going to work? If you don't give me something I don't know what I'll do. I am down to my last dollar'."* Added to the work shortage was that new American plan: buy now and pay later. Everything was on the installment plan.

By 1932 most nurses, especially those doing private duty, were unemployed. Some graduate nurses, desperately in need of a place to live and food to eat, nursed two or three days a week to earn their board and room. Many hospitals, unable to take the strain of the patient shortage, had to close their doors. (After all, the American parent overlooked his own illness and certainly did not enter the private hospitals, because each small piece of change was needed to feed his youngsters.) Free and part-pay clinics, however, did a booming business, and the charity wards of hospitals were full. Everyone was afraid.

In his inaugural address in 1933, President Franklin D. Roosevelt said: "The only thing we have to fear is fear itself." His New Deal policy was instituted to calm these fears, with measures directed toward immediate relief of the economic collapse and the introduction of measures that would ensure the American people against another depression. The Federal Emergency Relief Administration† and the Civilian Conservation Corps‡ were two agencies established for this relief. In 1935 these agencies developed into the Works Progress Administration (WPA).

Nurses were employed under the Nursing and Public Health Program of the WPA. They provided free bedside care to underprivileged families. The program employed 2,606 professional nurses at its peak. In an *American Journal of Nursing* report in 1937, thirty registries reported that 180 nurses gave 440 days of gratuitous nursing service.

*The trials of a registrar, American Journal of Nursing **30**:153, Feb. 1930.

†The Federal Emergency Relief Administration under Harry L. Hopkins paid out about $3,000,000 for relief and public work wages.

‡The Civilian Conservation Corps (CCC) was an agency that employed young men in forestry work, road building, and flood control.

An example of the difference in the cost of living can be seen in the advertisement in the *American Journal of Nursing* of hotel accommodations for the 1937 American Nurses' Convention held in Kansas City.

For single room—$1.50 to $4.00

For double rooms—$2.00 to $8.00

Schools of nursing between 1929 and 1937, in an attempt to keep alive, reduced their enrollment and only took in one class a year. Many schools, accustomed to giving their student nurses a monthly stipend, eliminated this practice. It was a period of continuous austerity. Admission policies for nursing became even more rigid, and minority groups met with quota systems restricting their admission to nursing. Rules for dormitory living were strict and standards were high. Students were dropped at the slightest infraction and the least drop in grades. It was truly a period of survival of the fittest. Young people, because of the economic strain on families, married later. As a result of these late marriages and the crowded living quarters, they produced smaller families.

FINANCIAL REHABILITATION

From 1935 to 1937 Congress passed a series of Social Security laws concerning unemployment insurance, old age pensions, and dependency allotments. As a result of the strain placed upon the economics of the country by the enactment of these laws, it was necessary for Congress to pass a new income tax law in 1937. The first change in this law was put into effect in 1964 (Medicare). Because of the financial relief from the 1937 Social Security laws and the many hospital insurance plans, hospital utilization increased and a nursing shortage was created in the 1940s, which, to this day, has not been alleviated.

PREPARATION FOR WAR

The first peacetime selective service law was passed on September 16, 1940, which drafted all young men between the ages of 18 and 35 into the Armed Services of the United States. The sudden increase in military manpower led to the call from the American Red Cross Nursing Service for more nurses to care for these recruits. Many nurses had not waited for this call. They enlisted without coercion and certainly without the enticement of greater financial gains. Because more people were being hospitalized and there was already a shortage of nurses the situation became increasingly acute as nurses left civilian life for the military.

National nursing organization leaders, anticipating that an even greater need for nurses would soon be felt at home and abroad, believed that the country's potential nursing personnel should be evaluated. Isabel Stewart, professor of Nursing Education at Teacher's College, Columbia University, wrote to Miss Stella Goostray (President of the NLNE) asking her help in setting up an official nursing commission. As a result of Miss Stewart's letter, a meeting was held in New York on July 29, 1940, with representatives of all nursing organizations present.* This far-sighted group of nursing leaders established the Nursing Council for National Defense. The purpose of this Council was to coordinate the defense activities of all nursing organizations for better utilization of nursing manpower.

Since neither the nation nor the nursing leaders had any knowledge of the nursing potential in the United States, a questionnaire was compiled and sent to all Registered Nurses by the United States Public Health Service. When replies from almost 300,000 active nurses (75% return) were analyzed, the result showed that almost 100,000 of these nurses were eligible for military duty (they were unmarried and under 40 years of age), and 25,000 of the inactive nurses could be available for full-time services.

The Nursing Council of National Defense found one solution to the problem, but a still greater problem faced them. Enrollment in schools of nursing was rapidly declining. Added to the fact that there were fewer potential nurses (because families were smaller during the depression years) were the complications of increased wartime factory employment, more women entering the military services, and increased opportunities in the business world. Also, the schools themselves were handicapped by a dearth of nurse instructors. The Council appointed a subcommittee, the Committee on Education Policies and Resources, which recommended that the government give Federal Aid for nursing education. The result of this recommendation was the Bolton Bill (HR4926), which became Public Law Number 146 on July 1, 1941. This law, sponsored by Representative Frances Payne Bolton of Cleveland, Ohio, provided public funds for:

1. Postgraduate preparation
2. Refresher courses for nurses no longer in active nursing
3. Financial aid to more than 200 schools
4. The stimulation of recruitment programs for schools of nursing

All of these maneuvers helped, but the nursing shortage was not resolved. By January 1942 there were 10,000 nurses in the Army and Navy, and it was estimated that 10,000 more would be needed before July. In 1943 the Army issued a call for a corps of 35,000 nurses. Simultaneously, a survey revealed that approximately 17,000 nurses were needed in civilian hospitals. Where would they come from? Even with the increase in nursing school enrollment, these needs couldn't possibly be met. Again, Representative Bolton came to the rescue, and on July 1, 1943, The Nurse Training Act became Public Law Number 74, which created the United States Cadet Nurse Corps. After the bill became law Surgeon General Parran sent telegrams to the nation's schools of nursing, which read: "Both Houses of Congress have approved funds to operate Bolton Nurse Training Law. Students enrolled after December, 1940 in schools with accelerated courses and otherwise eligible to participate may become members of the United States Cadet Corps, receiving tuition, fees, uniforms, $15 monthly for first 9 months training, $20 monthly for next 15 to 21 months, if they agree to make their services available in nursing for duration of war. Also schools will be paid

*See Appendix A of United States Cadet Nurse Corps, 1943–1948, Federal Security Agency, Public Health Service, Washington, D.C., 1950, U. S. Government Printing Office.

for maintenance of student during first 9 months of course. I hope for participation of all eligible schools and immediate intensive recruitment of large fall classes."*

The United States Cadet Nurse Corps became the Student War Nursing Reserve and was administered by Surgeon General Parran, with Lucille Petry (Leone) as Director and Eugenia Spalding as Associate Director.

Miss Petry reviewed the purposes of the Nurse Training Act to the Advisory Committee of the Division of Nursing Education of the United States Public Health Service on June 25, 1943. She stated that the purpose was directed toward increasing the number of nurses available for both military and civilian needs. This the program did, but it accomplished even more. Even though the criteria of the Corps did not standardize the educational programs in the affiliated schools, it upgraded these schools, provided better housing and educational facilities, and helped lay the groundwork for a unified accrediting program and registration by endorsement for graduate nurses between the states.

Clad in their dress uniforms of soft dark grey wool, reefer topcoat, and Montgomery beret, and displaying the insignia on their upper left sleeve of a Maltese Cross in silver against a dark red background, 170,000 nurses had joined the United States Cadet Corps before the termination of this program on October 15, 1945.

Lucille Petry Leone was Chief of the Division of Nurse Education of the United States Public Health Service and Director of the Cadet Nurse Corps. Mrs. Leone, a graduate of Johns Hopkins Hospital School of Nursing, received a Bachelor of Arts degree from the University of Delaware and a Master of Arts degree from Teacher's College, Columbia University. As the director of the Cadet Nurse Corps she acquired a comprehensive knowledge of nursing and nursing education. Mrs. Leone has served on the boards of the national nursing organizations. Eight universities have granted her honorary doctoral degrees, and after World War II she served as Nurse Advisor to the first (1948) and ninth (1956) assemblies of the World Health Organization and continues to serve as a member of the WHO panel of experts. Mrs. Leone has the distinction of being the first woman to serve as Assistant Surgeon General of the United States Public Health Service.

*Reprinted in U. S. Cadet Nurse Corps., 1943-1948, Federal Security Agency, Public Health Service, Washington, D. C., 1950, U. S. Government Printing Office, p. 18.

THOSE WHO ALSO SERVED

Another nurse corps was the general duty nurse staff in civilian hospitals. They received no special honors, no Purple Hearts, no Distinguished Service Crosses, and no Congressional medals, but they served patriotically and zealously. A hospital aide leaves for war work, another nurse enters the Armed Forces, and the nurse on duty at home must stretch herself a bit farther. They worked quietly, efficiently, swiftly. Without the loyal, selfless service of these soldiers behind the lines and of these unsung heroes on the home front we truly could not have won the war. Retired nurses took refresher courses, and volunteer gray ladies, pink ladies, and men's groups gave of themselves unstintingly.

NURSES IN THE ARMED FORCES

There were several differences between nursing in World War I and World War II. To begin with nurses were inducted with an officer's rating, and there were nurses stationed at various Army and Navy installations prior to Dec. 7, 1941. The greatest difference, however, was that wherever the Army, Navy, or Air Force was sent, nurses went with the troops. They served in front line aid stations as well as behind the lines.* Different, too, was the orientation the nurse corps received in preparation for their service, since everywhere was the "front" because of aerial warfare.

*For a description of nursing under fire in World War II, read Lt. Juanita Redmond's *I Served on Bataan,* Philadelphia, 1943, J. B. Lippincott Co.

A thumbnail description of the preparation of registered nurses for their responsibilities in combat would read as follows. After passing her physical examination, the nurse took her oath of office.* She was now a Second Lieutenant, and she went through two months (or more) of basic training. In basic training the nurse was oriented to camp life, took daily exercise, learned to use a gas mask (in case of gas warfare), and gave some nursing care at the base hospital. She was then ready for maneuvers. For two or more months she hiked under combat conditions (sometimes with live ammunition overhead), learned to dig and use a foxhole, took six mile hikes wearing fatigues, learned to set up an aid station under battle conditions, learned to pitch a tent, went through obstacle courses, and climbed down a Jacob's ladder simulating a beachhead landing. None of this training was wasted, because the nurses went wherever the Armed Forces went.

SERVICE BEYOND THE CALL OF DUTY

Sixty-six nurses were captured with the United States Army and were interned in the Philippines by the Japanese. Nurses served in capacities far beyond that called for in the line of duty. While they were prisoners, they gave nursing care to other inmates with meager supplies until they were liberated by the United States Forces. Alice Clarke describes this liberation:

> As we watched from the window wondering what was happening, there came the rumbling and clanking of tanks. . . . As the tanks lumbered down . . . to Santo Tomas, the smell of American gasoline thrilled us. . . . Those American soldiers looked like angels despite the fact that their language did not originate in heaven and their wings were tanks."

What they had suffered at the hands of their captors in the thirty-seven months they were held prisoner is another story.

It is no wonder, then, that a suitable commemoration of these brave nurses was sought. The plaque in the nurses' quarters at Finney General Hospital in Thomasville, Georgia, best describes the public feeling:

> Wherever our fighting forces plant their banners, there go the nurses who serve so courageously. Only the brave of heart, the great of soul, the free of spirit, can wear the uniform that wins the reverent salute from all our embattled nations.

JAPANESE SURRENDER

On September 2, 1945 the Japanese surrendered. On the deck of the battleship *Missouri* Japanese diplomats signed the papers of surrender, which brought 1,351 days of horrible war to a close. At the end of the war the American people, for the third time in one hundred years, were faced with the "three R's":

1. *Reconversion* to a peacetime economy without lowering the standard of living.
2. *Reconstruction* of lives disrupted by the call to "service" and of business called to wartime production.
3. *Restoration* of normal social relationships of millions of displaced persons still homeless, and of 12,000,000 servicemen and women into civilian life.

*"As an Army nurse, I accept the responsibility of an officer in the Army Nurse Corps. I shall give faithful care to the men who fight for the freedom of this country and to the women who stand behind them. I shall bring to the American soldier, wherever he may be, the best of my knowledge and professional skill. I shall approach him cheerfully at all times under any conditions I may find. I shall endeavor to maintain the highest nursing standards possible in the performance of my duties. I shall appear fearless in the presence of danger and quiet the fears of others to the best of my ability. My only criticism shall be constructive. The reputation and good name of the Army Nurse Corps and of the nursing profession shall be uppermost in my thoughts, second only to the care of my patients. I shall endeavor to be a credit to my country and the uniform I wear."

*Clarke, A. R.: Thirty-seven months as prisoner of war, American Journal of Nursing **45**:345, May 1943. Reprinted with permission.

BIBLIOGRAPHY

Browne, H. E.: A tribute to Mary Breckenridge, Nursing Outlook **14**:54-55, May 1966.

Carrying on for Jane Delano, American Journal of Nursing 37:737-740, July 1937.

Clark, A. R.: Thirty-seven months as a prisoner of war, American Journal of Nursing, **45**:345, May 1945.

Cope, Sir Zachary: Florence Nightingale and the doctors, Philadelphia, 1958, J. B. Lippincott Co.

Davis, M. D.: I was a student nurse over fifty years ago, Nursing Outlook **9**:221-222, April 1961.

DeKruif, P.: Microbe hunters, New York, 1926, Harcourt, Brace and Co.

Draper, W. F.: The national health program and the nurse, American Journal of Nursing **39**:471-479, May 1939.

Fife, G. L.: The nurse as an anesthetist, American Journal of Nursing **47**:308-309, May 1947.

Filmore, A.: Scene U.S.A. 1900, American Journal of Nursing **41**:913-915, Aug. 1941.

Sister Henrietta: A famous New Orleans hospital, American Journal of Nursing **39**:249-256, Mar. 1939.

Jensen, D. M.: History and trends of professional nursing, ed. 4, St. Louis, 1959, The C. V. Mosby Co., pp. 108-134.

Judson, H.: Edith Cavell, New York, 1941, The Macmillan Co.

Kandel, P. M.: Postgraduate training for nurses, its affect on hospital administration, Trained Nurse and Hospital Review **LXLIV**:60-65, Jan. 1965.

Koch, H. B.: Militant angel, New York, 1951, The Macmillan Co.

Kruesi, W.: The Social Security Act and the nurse, American Journal of Nursing **42**:524-527, May 1942.

Longfellow, H. W.: Santo Filomena (a tribute to Florence Nightingale). In The Children's Hour, book 15, Chicago, 1954, Spencer Press, Inc., pp. 244-245.

Morison, S. E., and Commanger, H. S.: The growth of the American republic, 2 vols., ed. 4, New York, 1960, Oxford University Press, pp. 653-662.

McIver, P.: Registered nurse in the United States, American Journal of Nursing **42**:769, July 1942.

Nightingale, F.: Notes on nursing; what it is and what it is not. Reprinted by J. B. Lippincott Co., 1946.

O'Malley, I. B.: Florence Nightingale after the Crimea (1856-1861), Trained Nurse and Hospital Review **LXLIV**(5):401-407, May 1935.

Owen, M. A.: Lest we forget, Trained Nurse and Hospital Review **LXLV**(5):415-420, Nov. 1935.

Poole, E.: Nurses on horseback, New York, 1932, The Macmillan Co.

Redmond, Lt. J.: I served in Bataan, Philadelphia, 1943, J. B. Lippincott Co.

Roberts, M. M.: American nursing—history and interpretation, New York, 1954, The Macmillan Co.

Roberts, M. M.: Lavinia Lloyd Dock—nurse, feminist, internationalist, American Journal of Nursing **56**:176-178, Feb. 1956.

Seymer, L. R.: The Nightingale jewel, American Journal of Nursing **55**:549, May 1955.

Stewart, I. M.: Isabel M. Stewart recalls the early years, American Journal of Nursing **60**:1426-1430, Oct. 1960.

Stimson, J. C.: The nurse's uniform, American Journal of Nursing **36**:368, Apr. 1936.

United States Cadet Nurse Corps 1943-1948, Federal Security Agency Public Health Service, Washington, D. C., 1950, U. S. Government Printing Office.

Wald, L.: House on Henry Street, New York, 1938, Henry Holt and Co.

Woodham-Smith, C.: Florence Nightingale, 1820-1910, London, 1950, Constable Publishing Co.

COMPLETE WORK SHEET ON PP. 307 AND 308

CHAPTER 4

The period of contemporary nursing

WORLD WAR II ENDS

By the end of World War II two strong political forces, Western democracy and Soviet communism, had emerged. Nations that had once been powerful were bankrupt, while many small countries were striving to establish their independence. Scientific, technical, and social developments forced leaders to realize that manpower alone could not protect any country from aggression. Protective weapons and strategy backed by great wealth were only part of the answer, however. Leaders saw the need for an international organization based upon the sovereign equality of all nations. From August 27 to October 7, 1944, representatives of the United States, England, Soviet Union, and China met at Dumbarton Oaks, Washington, D. C. These representatives wrote the *Dumbarton Oaks proposal,* which became the basis for the United Nations Charter.

UNITED NATIONS

Fifty-one nations signed the Charter creating a United Nations in San Francisco, California, in 1945; by 1969 the member nations totaled 126. The two-fold purpose of this body is international peace and international security. Written into the Charter are provisions for equal justice, machinery for peaceful settlement of disputes, and provision for assuring human rights, social justice, and economic progress. Each member nation, regardless of size or wealth, has equal status according to Charter provisions. Councils established by the Charter to promote and implement its purpose are the *General Assembly,* in which all nations are represented with equal right to speak and vote; the *Security Council,* the executive branch, which acts as the decision-making body; the *Economic and Social Council,* whose function is to research and recommend improvements for all nations; the *Trusteeship Council,* which is authorized to supervise, visit, review internal affairs, examine petitions, and make recommendations to the General Assembly concerning any trustee territory; the *World Court,* also called the International Council of Justice, which serves as the main judicial body of the United Nations; and the *Secretariat,* which directs the activities of the General Assembly.

In the hope of creating a climate of peaceful coexistence, the United Nations sponsors many special agencies whose members work diligently attempting to bring knowledge to all parts of the world. The *World Health Organization* (WHO) is such an agency. Established in Geneva, Switzerland in 1948, this agency was formed to assist in fighting disease by providing health information and improving the nutrition, living standards, and environmental conditions for all people. Associated with its public health program, every aspect of maternal and child health receives special emphasis. Since the beginning of WHO, American nurses have been actively involved in its organization and implementation, and they have served as members of the WHO Expert Committee for Nursing. In the December, 1963 issue of *World Health Magazine* the functions of involved nursing personnel as defined by the WHO Expert Committee for

Nursing are listed. These functions are still appropriate to nurses and include the following:

"Carrying out the therapeutic program as designed by physicians for sick patients which should include hygiene and comfort measures.

"Maintaining a physical and psychological climate conducive to recovery and to health.

"Engaging the patient and his family in his recovery and rehabilitation.

"Health teaching (both sick and well) to promote physical and mental health in a positive sense.

"Carrying out measures for disease prevention.

"Coordinating nursing with the efforts of the other members of the health team and other community groups."

SCIENTIFIC AND TECHNICAL RESEARCH

Scientific and technical research since the end of World War II has developed at such an accelerated rate that many therapeutics used in the 1950s and 1960s are now obsolete. The results of research affect all people whether they are sick or well. Each new development means there must be a corresponding change in the practice of nursing. The knowledge and skills of nursing must reflect the progress made in disease prevention and health care. Among the many developments influencing nursing are atomic energy, computers, discriminating diagnostic and therapeutic agents, and space exploration.

ATOMIC ENERGY

Atomic energy was first used as a weapon of war, but it has many potential uses. It can be used as an inexhaustible source of energy to replace coal, gas, and oil thus reducing air pollution (by reducing the amount of sulfur-containing compounds and carbon monoxide in the air). Fission (atomic) reactors produce neutrons and gamma rays, which are important in the production of isotopes used for medical diagnosis and treatment. For example, radioactive cobalt and gamma rays are used to treat cancer, and iodine 131 is used both diagnostically and therapeutically. The potential for peaceful utilization of atomic energy is difficult to imagine, but you will see many more situations for its advantageous and life-saving use.

COMPUTERS

Computers are used for collecting data, teaching, obtaining information, establishing a diagnosis, maintaining a perpetual inventory, making up payrolls and paychecks, record keeping, and billing. Some experimentation with patient charting and the processing of physician's orders has been tried also. Whenever a new device is placed on the market, someone must be taught to use it. Acceptance of its purposes is the first step in the meaningful utilization of computers. Because industry, research centers, hospitals, and other facilities have begun using computers, many individuals have had to learn both computer language and the "how" and "why" of computer use. Other people have been taught to build, to repair, to program, and to teach others to utilize the computer to its best advantage. A device is only of value if it is used correctly.

Physicians are investigating ways to use computers both as time-savers and as a means of increasing efficiency in patient care. One group of physicians is developing a plan to establish a computerized bank of patients' records, placing this programmed information on a satellite system for storage and distribution. The plan includes a code number for patient and country. Anyone becoming ill, even 5,000 or more miles from home base, could have his case history in the hands of an attending physician in a very few minutes.

It is wise to remember, however, that the computer is only as good as the information programmed into it. *Input* (information placed in the program) is subject to human error, and the *output* (information forthcoming) will only include that which is programmed. Do not lose sight, also, of the fact that machines cannot take the place of a nurse who *listens* and puts what she has heard into action for the patient's benefit. No machine can replace you, but it *can* increase your accuracy and your efficiency. A machine is only an aid to the intelligent human using it.

DIAGNOSTIC AND THERAPEUTIC AGENTS

More sophisticated equipment for diagnosis and therapy has been developed in the past twenty-five years than in any other comparable period. Some of these developments include isotopes, heart-lung machines, the use of prostheses to replace defective tissues, transplantation of living tissues and organs, hemodialysis, pacemakers for heart muscle, pacemakers to assist paraplegics to become moderately self-sufficient, monitoring equipment, and the many chemotherapeutic agents.

Any innovation developed for patient care means that the nurse must be willing to *continually learn* so that she will be knowledgeable enough to develop the skills necessary to help her meet the needs of the patients under her care. Since information about the latest developments in treatment and therapy is reported in the mass media, the American public is an informed one. Your patient is likely to know what treatments he is receiving and why, whether they are being given on time and spaced properly, what the correct dosage of a drug should be, what precautions he should take, what side effects may occur, and whether his therapy is having the desired effect. This knowledgeable person is your patient. Can you afford to be less aware than he?

SPACE MEDICINE

Any mention of scientific and technologic achievements in the years between 1945 and 1970 must include the first ventures into space and certainly the Moon landing July 20, 1969. It soon became evident to a few far-sighted people in the space program that there was a need for qualified and prepared nurses. Colonel Pearl E. Tucker, Air Force Nurse, developed a comprehensive one-year course for qualified nurses. On July 1, 1965 two nurses enrolled in the first class at the School for Aerospace Nursing at Cape Kennedy. The day may soon come when the United States will have hospital satellites in space. Wherever the military goes, the American nurse goes, and nurses will be needed for these hospitals. Colonel Tucker's pioneering efforts have been duly rewarded. In May, 1970 she received an Honorary Doctor of Humane Letters Degree from Capital University in Columbus, Ohio. Her work continues, and more and more nurses are being involved in this preparation. The future of space nursing is challenging and exciting.

SOCIAL FORCES AFFECTING NURSING

The work done by the nurses during World War II has continued in both civilian and military life. Nurses still serve at home, at the front, behind the lines at base hospitals, or on planes evacuating the wounded to another hospital for specific treatment. Wherever the patient requires emergency care, intensive care, or rehabilitative care, the American nurse is on duty.

However, as you have seen in preceding chapters, the present world is the outcome of the past and only the beginning of what the future holds. The social structure of American society has changed drastically during the past twenty-five years, and in order to meet the needs of society, the practice of nursing cannot retain its traditional pattern. The Code for Professional Nurses states that it is nursing's responsibility "to conserve life and promote health." For nursing to assume its responsibility in its fullest sense requires that with each scientific or technical development or change in the social structure there be a corresponding change in the practice of nursing. With such changes it becomes necessary to make more and more decisions.

LEGISLATION

Equal opportunity laws were enacted in an attempt to eliminate all second-class citizenship and to finally put teeth into the Civil Rights Acts. These laws give every person the right to an equal opportunity to live in a healthy environment, to receive the necessary education, to obtain employment based on merit and not on privilege, and to earn the salary commensurate with ability, regardless of sex, religion, race, or national origin. Implementation of the Civil Rights Acts is still not resolved. As the 1970s begin unrest and disagreements as to their interpretation are like a plague upon this great land. The machinery for implementation of equal opportunity is written into the Constitution and into the law; understanding and amicable resolution of disagreements will come.

Legislation affecting health care includes several amendments to the Social Security Act of 1935. In 1950 nurses were finally included under old age Social Security plans and the United States Public Health Service was placed in the Department of Health, Education and Welfare. Activities of the Public Health Service include nursing in public health service hospitals, the Indian Service hospitals and clinics (1956), and the National Institutes of Health Clinic Center (1953) in Bethesda, Maryland. The expanding role of public health nursing involves participation in research, control programs, and consultation services.

PREPAID HEALTH CARE

In 1966 Medicare was enacted into law. This law makes it possible for everyone over age 65 to receive free hospital benefits and medical benefits at low cost. Although the more affluent citizens have been able to carry private health and accident insurance, older citizens often could not afford this protection. Medicare, because it has aided in disease prevention and detection, is helping to lengthen the life-span.

However, Medicare and Social Security laws have created some hardships. Although the senior citizen is provided with health care benefits and the probability of living longer, he is being forced to retire at age 65 regardless of his physical or mental condition. Because he is confronted with leisure time he is not emotionally prepared for, the senior citizen suddenly finds himself a noncontributing member of society. This change of image only increases his anxiety and compounds his health problems, both of which increase his frustrations.

Because the number of aged is increasing, more health care and more bed space in hospitals are needed at a time when both are in short supply. The need for additional extended care facilities has become very evident, as has the need for more qualified nurses.

NURSING INVOLVEMENT WITH MINORITY GROUPS

For over one hundred years nurses have overtly demonstrated their concern for their neighbor and have been the community's partner in the fight for health and welfare. Today's nurses manifest even greater concern. Besides their activities in hospitals, clinics, and public health agencies, they are also involved in assisting the underprivileged and in aiding in minority group issues. Their involvement extends to such programs as VISTA, Ship Hope, Medico, Appalachia, Migratory Worker Camps, and WHO. Nurses have also become involved in economic security programs for themselves.

TECHNOLOGIC EFFICIENCY

Because disposable, pre-packaged, and pre-prepared hospital equipment can now be supplied at a reasonable cost, the nurse has been relieved of many tedious tasks. Pre-preparation ensures that supplies are of uniform quality and sterility, which is an additional safety factor for the patient. Although pre-packaging is a time-saving factor for the nurse, it has not resulted in increased leisure time for her. The nurse is constantly assuming responsibilities of patient care that were formerly the sole prerogative of the physician.

Nursing will continue to develop flexibly in order to meet the health care needs of society completely and safely. There will be many obstacles that must be overcome, but remember that the history of nursing does not end on this page. Your achievement in the practice of nursing will be the history of nursing tomorrow. As

Shakespeare said: ". . . some are born great, some achieve greatness, and some have greatness thrust upon them."* What will be your role?

*Twelfth Night, Act II, Scene 5.

BIBLIOGRAPHY

American Nursing Association defines role of nurses; American Nursing Association sees "no major objections," RN, Apr. 1969, p. 60.

Andreoli, K. G., and Stead, E. A., Jr.: Training physicians' assistants at Duke, American Journal of Nursing **67**:1442-1443, July 1967.

Burgess, A., and Lazare, A.: Dual therapy by nurse and psychiatrist, American Journal of Nursing **70**:1292-1298, June 1970.

Donnelly, A.: The extended care facility as a clinical laboratory, Nursing Outlook **16**:32-35, Feb. 1968.

Drury, A.: Advice and consent, New York, 1961, Popular Library Eagle Books (paperback), Doubleday & Co., Inc.

Drury, A.: A shade of difference, New York, 1963, Popular Library Eagle Books (paperback), Doubleday & Co., Inc.

Drury, A.: Capable of honor, New York, 1966, Dell Publishing Co. (paperback).

Drury, A.: Preserve and protect, New York, 1968, Popular Library Eagle Books (paperback), Doubleday & Co., Inc.

Edelstein, R. R.: Automation: its effect on the nurse, American Journal of Nursing **66**:2194-2198, Oct. 1966.

Evans, F. C.: The role of the nurse in community mental health, New York, 1968, The Macmillan Co.

Fagin, C. M.: The clinical specialist as supervision, Nursing Outlook **15**:34, Jan. 1967.

George, J. H.: Electronic monitoring of vital signs, American Journal of Nursing **65**:68, Feb. 1965.

Hershey, N.: Standard care for mental patients, American Journal of Nursing **65**:99-101, Jan. 1965.

Kramer, M.: The new graduate speaks, American Journal of Nursing **66**:2420-2424, Nov. 1966.

Mattson, H. W.: Future hospitals, International Science and Technology, Aug. 1966, pp. 30-37.

Mereness, D.: Expanding role of the nurse, Nursing Outlook **18**:30-33, May 1970.

Mereness, D.: Freedom and responsibility for nursing students, American Journal of Nursing **67**:69-71, Jan. 1967.

Moore, M. L.: Nursing *is* making progress, RN, Apr. 1969, pp. 56-59.

Novotny, D. R.: Suited for space life, American Journal of Nursing **67**:1655-1657, Aug. 1967.

Olson, E. V.: Education—for what? American Journal of Nursing **70**:1292-1298, June 1970.

Olson, E. V.: Health manpower—needed: a shake-up in the status quo, American Journal of Nursing **68**:1491-1495, July 1968.

Palmiere, D.: Medicare's effects on medical care, Public Health Reports **83**:705-708, Sept. 1968.

Pope, I.: Medicare—impetus for change, Nursing Outlook **16**:34, Jan. 1968.

Pratt, H.: The doctor's view of the changing nurse-physician relationship, Journal Medical Education **40**:767-777, Aug. 1967.

Public health at the crossroads, Medical World News, Aug. 14, 1964, pp. 42-43.

Rosenberg, M., and Carriter, D.: Automating nurse's notes, American Journal of Nursing **66**:1021-1023, May 1966.

Rowan, R. L.: Automation: its effect on the hospital, American Journal of Nursing **66**:2199, Oct. 1966.

Sugar, S. R.: Some reflections on being a student again, RN, Mar. 1964.

Tarrant, B. J.: Automation: its effect on the patient, American Journal of Nursing **66**:2190-2193, Oct. 1966.

West, W. L.: Occupational therapy philosophy and preparation, American Journal of Nursing, **68**:1708, Aug. 1968.

Wooley, A. S.: The "now" generation in nursing, Nursing Outlook **16**:26, Mar. 1968.

COMPLETE WORK SHEET ON PP. 309 AND 310

CHAPTER 5

Preservice nursing education programs

EARLY DEVELOPMENT OF NURSING SCHOOLS

The first nursing schools in this country were operated by hospitals and offered what we call today on-the-job training or apprentice-type learning. Occasionally you will hear some of the older graduates refer to their "training school" or to events that occurred when they were "in training."

In these early hospital-affiliated schools of nursing the students performed nearly all services required on the hospital wards. This was regarded as repayment for the cost of their training. A school of nursing virtually ensured the sponsoring hospital of a readily available nursing service for its patients. Because students were the primary source of manpower, a staff of paid hospital employees such as we have today was unknown. Except for the graduates who functioned as private duty nurses, the students provided all the patient care and essential nursing services. There were no graduate nurses except for the head nurse. There were no practical nurses, nurse aides, technicians, ward aides, or other ancillary personnel to staff the operating room, delivery room, central supply service, cast room, diet kitchens, and housekeeping services.

As late as the 1930s, students were often expected to work a sixty-hour week, including class hours. Schedules were based upon a "split shift," which meant that the students worked from 7:00 A.M. to 7:00 P.M. with formal classes held during their three hours off in the afternoon. A class would often meet after 7:00 P.M. when the students got off duty. Students were on night duty, which was a twelve-hour shift, for as long as two months at a time. However, night duty and days off did not excuse students from attending a scheduled class. During their senior year students were frequently assigned as charge nurses on the hospital wards.

The established period for a nurse's training was three years. This is the historical basis for the diploma program as it is known today. In order to graduate and receive her diploma, the student had to fulfill a stated time requirement, whether it was calculated as 36 months, 156 weeks, or 1,095 days.

Before the first national studies of nursing and nursing education were made in 1920s, there were no standards to regulate either the number and kind of classes or the number of hours of practical experience given in these three years. Many hospitals established schools of nursing for purely economic reasons. Training programs were organized to meet their staffing needs rather than the educational requirements of the students. Many of these hospitals did not have segregated services, and because there were no established standards for nursing education, it was possible for students to graduate from a school of nursing with little or no experience in essential clinical areas. This was especially true in the areas of pediatrics, obstetrics, and communicable diseases, since these services were provided in segregated units distinct from the medical-surgical units. Graduates of these programs were penalized by the poverty of their training. Graduates were often unable to register in another state without making up the deficiencies in their basic preparation.

Some of the problems that plagued the system of nursing education in the past still confront nursing today. A case in point is the controversy over the status of nursing as a *profession.* Since the time of the early schools, the term "professional" has been used indiscriminately, with little regard given to the differences among the various types of educational programs. Regardless of background, all graduates have been considered "professionals."

Not all of the early schools of nursing were like the ones described above. Some hospitals did conduct schools that offered their students effective preparation and sound instruction. The success of these schools was due, in part, to the excellent clinical facilities of the hospitals and to the fact that their directors were prepared to teach and carry out the tasks necessary to the administration of a nursing program.

It is anticipated that the nurse instructors in your program will provide opportunities throughout your nursing courses to study and discuss in some detail the efforts of those early leaders who charted the way and laid the groundwork for improving the education of future students.

TYPES OF EDUCATIONAL PROGRAMS

At the present time there are four types of preservice educational programs to prepare the student for a career either as a registered nurse or as a practical/vocational nurse. Although these programs differ in length, nature and organization of content, and clinical experiences, all of them have a common goal: the education of people qualified to administer direct nursing care and service to patients. The graduates of all four types of programs are eligible for licensure and, after passing a state board examination, may use the legal title of Registered Nurse (RN), Licensed Practical Nurse (LPN), or Licensed Vocational Nurse (LVN), whichever applies. Nurses may practice within the state in which they are licensed.

The educational programs that prepare students for beginning practice in nursing are referred to as *basic* or *preservice* programs to differentiate them from programs for advanced professional study. These programs are offered in a variety of institutions including hospital schools, technologic institutes, junior or community colleges, and four-year colleges and universities. For purposes of recognition these various programs are commonly identified according to the credential awarded by the sponsoring institution; that is, diploma program, certificate program, associate degree program, or baccalaureate degree program.

State board approval is mandatory for all schools conducting recognized programs of nursing education in the United States and its territories. Before any school of nursing can be recognized and operate as a school, the state board of nursing (the administrative agency created by the licensing law of a given state to regulate nursing education and nursing practice) is legally responsible for determining whether or not the nursing program meets the minimum requirements of that state. Only graduates of state board–approved or accredited nursing programs are eligible to take the state board examination, which is a prerequisite to obtaining the necessary license to practice nursing.

In 1961 the National League for Nursing, in assembled convention, approved a statement entitled *Opportunities for Education in Nursing,* which was later revised for publication purposes to *Nursing Education Programs Today.* This document states that "the system of present day nursing education as a whole is a continuing developmental process. Through improvement and reorganization of some types of programs and additions of others, it has evolved from nursing education of the past. The need for continuity and constant expansion and improvement of nursing services vital to the public welfare makes it essential that there should be no break in this progress."*

This statement goes on to say that there are certain characteristics associated with each pro-

*National League for Nursing: Nursing education programs today, New York, 1961, The League, p. 5.

Basic (preservice) Nursing Education Programs →	Credential Awarded →	Legal Recognition →	Careers in Nursing →	Identification in Nursing Profession
Baccalaureate (4 years)	B.S-B.A.		Beginning positions (staff) in hospitals—clinics—public health agency Nursing Care Team Leader (following experience) Head nurse (following experience) Beginning teacher (following experience) Eligible for admission to advanced degree program	Professional Nurse
Associate Degree (2 years)	A.A.-A.S.	State Board Exam (R.N.)	Beginning positions (staff) in hospitals—clinics—doctors office—private practice at side of patient Eligible for admission to baccalaureate program	Nurse Technician
Hospital School (2-3 years)	Diploma		Beginning positions (staff) in hospitals—clinics—doctors office—private practice at side of patient Eligible for admission to baccalaureate program	Nurse Technician
Practical/Vocational (1 year, generally)	Certificate or Diploma	State Board Exam (L.P.N./L.V.N.)	Selected clinical practice (under supervision of M.D. or R.N.)	Assisting Nurse Technician

FOUR TYPES OF PRESERVICE EDUCATIONAL PROGRAMS TO PREPARE FOR CAREERS IN NURSING.

gram and certain characteristics that are common to all. These common characteristics include the following:

Each type, within its own scope, is concerned with the best development of the potentials of individual students as persons, citizens and competent practitioners.

Each includes, in due proportion to its scope and purposes, foundations in theoretical learning, including actual experience in the nursing care of patients.

In each program, a qualified faculty or instructional staff in nursing—in cooperation with appropriate colleagues—develops, implements, and controls the curriculum within the framework of standards for that type of program and the administrative and educational policies of the institution offering it.

In each case, the institution offering the program provides for the educational resources or facilities that are needed.*

Because of the opportunity to select among the various nursing education programs, students are encouraged to be realistic and practical in evaluating their potential as they consider their immediate and their future goals. Hopefully, each student enrolled in a preservice program in nursing education has chosen the program that best meets both his personal needs and his professional goals. It is hoped, also, that each nursing program will provide a challenge to

*National League for Nursing: Nursing education programs today, New York, 1961, The League, p. 8.

learn and the incentive to make use of every opportunity for extending and expanding skills and interest within the scope and goals of the particular program.

THE HOSPITAL SCHOOL (DIPLOMA PROGRAM)

Purpose. The diploma program is designed to prepare students for the practice of nursing as it applies in the direct care of patients. A published statement of the purpose for which a hospital conducts a basic or preservice program is a requirement for accreditation of the program and is published in the school's brochure.

The diploma program is a terminal-type occupational program. It is *not* a preparatory course for a baccalaureate degree.

A terminal program, by definition, is one that prepares its graduates for a given function or occupation upon completion of the course. The phrase "terminal program" used in this context does not mean the "end of the line" for progression in one's career. Indeed, the graduates of a diploma program can continue their education and receive baccalaureate and graduate degrees.

Graduates of a diploma program who plan further formal education must qualify for admission to the baccalaureate program of their choice and must meet entrance requirements of the college or university to which they apply. Collegiate educational programs will be discussed later.

Upon graduation the student receives a diploma, not an academic degree. The diploma attests to the student's successful completion of the nursing education program offered by the hospital. It entitles the graduate to apply for admission to the state board examination for licensure and, upon passing the examinations, to practice as a registered nurse.

Requirements for admission. Each hospital school establishes its own requirements for the selection of students. These requirements are developed by the faculty and reflect the program's philosophy and objectives. Admission requirements include such items as age range for acceptance, evidence of the applicant's academic preparation and scholastic achievement in high school courses, health records, and reports on the scores in the school's pre-entrance examinations. All records and forms must be submitted before an individual's application can be evaluated and acted upon.

Finances. Students in nursing, in common with students in other kinds of educational programs, are expected to underwrite the costs of their education. Tuition fees, the cost of uniforms, textbooks and supplies, and other known expenses are reported in the school's brochure, together with the school's policy for their payment. Hospitals no longer provide room, board, and laundering for the student, and few hospitals today grant monthly stipends to students. Most schools have administrative policies requiring health and hospitalization insurance for students that are outlined in the school brochure.

Information about scholarships, grants in aid, loan funds, and the conditions under which they are available may be reported in the brochure or discussed with the director of the nursing program. Financial assistance is usually readily available to students who have demonstrated their ability to pursue their educational goals. This topic is discussed in Chapter 20.

Residence. In general, hospitals conducting nursing programs maintain a students' residence, which provides space for living quarters, recreational activities, social gatherings, and educational facilities such as classrooms, laboratories, faculty offices, study areas, and a library.

Design of curriculum. The nursing curriculum for diploma programs is designed to educate students in accordance with a stated purpose.

Length of course. Traditionally the diploma program was thirty-six months in length, hence the name "three-year program." However, in recent years many hospitals have shortened the program, in some instances to twenty-two or twenty-four months, as a result of a reorganization of the basic curriculum. By 1965 51 percent of the diploma programs had been shortened to less than the traditional three years. Current thinking holds that the *quality* of a school's educational program is more important than *the length of time* required to complete the program. Today emphasis is on planning a curriculum that provides for careful correlation of theory and practice under the guidance and supervision of qualified clinical instructors to prepare skilled, professionally oriented nurses.

Formal classes and clinical laboratory. Hours of formal classes and clinical practice are scheduled in the diploma curriculum according to an established ratio. The program of study includes courses in the areas of the behavioral, physical, and biologic sciences and courses that contribute to the student's personal and professional development. Clinical practice is scheduled in a given subject area together with formal class instruction in order to achieve a correlation of theory and practice. Maternity nursing classes, for example, are scheduled during the period in which students are assigned to the maternity division for their clinical experiences.

Some programs augment their curriculum through affiliation with other institutions for certain types of instruction and clinical experience, such as nursing care of the mentally ill, pediatric nursing, or maternity nursing.

There should be a formal rotation pattern established for assigning students to the various clinical areas for planned learning experiences. This pattern, the diagram of each student's clinical laboratory assignments, is a vital part of the hospital's school curriculum. It should be drawn up for each class group and should cover the duration of the program of study. No doubt you who are enrolled in a diploma program are familiar with the diagrammed rotation pattern offered by your hospital school, or it will be discussed with you as part of your orientation program.

Purchased courses. In addition to the classes taught by the nursing faculty, many hospital schools "purchase" course instruction from local colleges to meet their curriculum requirements. Arrangements for teaching such classes are generally made with individual college instructors. In many instances these classes are taught in the school of nursing, not on the college campus. These courses carry college credit and the final grade is incorporated as part of the student's academic record for the diploma program. Students generally pay for this instruction. Purchased courses include chemistry, sociology, psychology, ethics, and courses in the humanities.

Faculty. Hospital schools employ their own faculty. These faculty members are responsible for developing, coordinating, and implementing the curriculum of the school.

What graduates are prepared to do. Graduates of a diploma program are technically prepared to give efficient and skillful care either as general duty staff nurses in a hospital, clinic, or physician's office or as nurses in private practice. They are able to apply the scientific principles upon which their nursing skills are based. They are expected to recognize the symptoms of diseases and disabilities and to participate with other health personnel in meeting the patient's need for supportive and therapeutic care. As they develop nursing skills and nursing judgment, they may, with guidance and assistance, qualify to serve as leaders of nursing care teams in the clinical divisions of the hospitals where they are employed.

THE COLLEGIATE SCHOOL (BACCALAUREATE PROGRAM)

There are some students whose career goal in nursing includes a college education and a bachelor of science degree. These students will select a college or university that offers a degree in nursing. Students electing this type of program obtain a bachelor's degree and preparation for nursing at the same time. Graduates of these programs like graduates of other preservice programs take the state examination for licensure to practice as registered nurses.

Historical overview. The first university school of nursing was established in 1909 at the University of Minnesota. Since that time other universities and colleges throughout the country have developed nursing programs. In 1968 there were a total of 235 baccalaureate programs of nursing in the United States and territories. This number represented about 27.7 percent of the total preservice programs preparing graduates for practice as registered nurses.

A milestone in baccalaureate nursing education was reached in 1953 with the publication of a report based on a study of existing patterns of education in the United States for which the baccalaureate degree in nursing was awarded. Dr. Margaret Bridgman, Dean of Instruction at Skidmore College in New York, studied the baccalaureate nursing programs offered by eighty senior college institutions. This study revealed diversities in the curriculum patterns of nursing education and in the administrative policies of senior collegiate institutions conducting these programs. A positive outcome of Bridgman's research was that university and college administrators and educators, together with nursing leaders and nurse educators, looked critically at the structure and operation of existing collegiate nursing programs. As a result of this study some changes were made to preserve the integrity of the degree itself and to strengthen the nursing program. Another outcome was the development of criteria to assist in evaluating the purposes and objectives of existing programs and in establishing and developing new programs that would maintain a consistent standard in course design and content. This concerted effort has resulted in the emergence of strong preservice nursing programs functioning in accordance with sound academic policies that benefit the student, the college or university, and the community.

At present the baccalaureate nursing program is recognized as being authentically collegiate. The university or college administration is responsible for creating the major in nursing and for planning the classes and various clinical learning assignments. The faculty of the nursing department have status and position similar to faculty in other departments. Standards and educational policies for the nursing department are the same as those in effect for all other programs in the university or college. Academic credits for courses in the nursing major are assigned on the same basis as credits for all other academic courses offered by the institution.

Students in collegiate nursing programs have responsibilities and opportunities similar to those of students in other academic areas. They are expected to perform and achieve on a level required of other students in the college. They are expected to benefit from the courses in general education and to utilize course content of subjects in related fields that will strengthen and deepen their understanding.

Purpose. A preservice collegiate program is generally designed as a four-year course. Its overall objective is to prepare nurse practitioners for potential leadership assignments. Graduates of the program must meet the requirement of the state's board of nursing for admission to the examination for a registered nurse license.

Structure and organization. The baccalaureate program is structured to provide a range of academic study that is impossible to include in less comprehensive preservice nursing programs. It is the initial step toward the advanced degrees required in specialized areas of nursing. Nursing content includes formal instruction and clinical practice in medical, surgical, maternity, pediatric, and psychiatric nursing. Most programs also include instruction and supervised practice in public health nursing. Graduates of baccalaureate programs possess resources in various areas of nursing intended to prepare them to identify numerous problems related to nursing care and to devise effective ways of solving them.

Nursing faculty in collegiate nursing programs are responsible to the college administration for the students' instruction in clinical nursing subjects and for the supervision of students' clinical practice. Use of hospital areas and related clinical facilities is based on written agreements between the college or university and each agency used as a teaching laboratory. Nursing faculty select the learning experiences in patient care on the clinical areas to which students are assigned. They cooperate with head nurses on the nursing units in arranging for student assignments within the overall time schedule. They are responsible for assignments and for supervising the administration of nursing care given by students.

Requirements for admission. Students who plan to earn a baccalaureate degree in nursing may do so in one of two ways. They may qualify for admission directly to the senior college or university offering a nursing program, or they may enroll for one to two years of academic study in a community junior college or college of liberal arts for the purpose of completing lower division courses required by the senior institution's nursing program. In the latter instance, admission to the baccalaureate program may then be sought on the basis of transfer to the college or university from which the student hopes to graduate.

Students in collegiate programs are expected to meet the college or university's general admission requirements as well as the requirements of their departmental major. Students are responsible for meeting their class obligations and maintaining the scholastic standards that ensure successful achievement and promotion.

Design of curriculum. Students take general courses including behavioral, physical, and biologic sciences, communication, and humanities, in addition to courses in nursing. Students are expected to acquire knowledge and skills, develop understanding and judgment, and recognize their own responsibility to provide competent, professional nursing care.

What graduates are prepared to do. Nurses graduating from baccalaureate programs are prepared, following licensure, for beginning assignments in nursing practice in all clinical areas and, generally, in public health nursing. As beginners they are entitled to an orientation in the working world of nursing and they are urged to avail themselves of this experience. It should be noted, however, that since these graduates have had a broader educational background and some familiarity with the techniques involving leadership skills, it is expected that progression to beginning supervisory and teaching functions will occur fairly quickly. One nurse educator notes that the knowledge and the competence of graduates of baccalaureate programs need to be recognized and used effectively. She states, "Only when these nurses have had an opportunity to realize their potentialities as practitioners can the value of their competence be fully estimated."*

The nursing profession needs many more qualified nurses than are currently available for placement in assignments of nursing service supervision and administration, teaching in schools of nursing, directing public health nursing services, and administering nursing education programs. Those whose preservice preparation is based on a baccalaureate degree are academically prepared to take the next step—graduate work for advancement within the profession. (See figure on page 49.)

THE COMMUNITY OR JUNIOR COLLEGE (ASSOCIATE DEGREE PROGRAM)

Historical overview. The associate degree program is the newest type of preservice program to prepare students for the direct nursing care of patients. It is sometimes referred to as the "two-year program" because of its identification with the junior college system and to distinguish it, in terms of time, from the diploma and baccalaureate programs. However, this differentiation on the basis of time no longer holds true since many diploma programs are based on two years of study.

The associate degree program was envisioned in 1951 following publication of a study by Dr. Mildred L. Montag of Teachers College, Columbia University. Dr. Montag's study, *The Education of Nursing Technicians,* identified society's immediate and long-term needs for increasingly large numbers of nurses prepared to carry out the technical functions associated with patient-centered nursing care. Montag also recognized that existing preservice diploma and baccalaureate nursing programs were not attracting the numbers of applicants needed to meet the increasing demands for quality nursing care. The establishment of a program to prepare nurses within the community or junior college could tap a new resource of potential nurse personnel. Community colleges as educational institutions exist to meet the community's needs, and the willingness of college administrators to participate in programs to prepare qualified nurses to meet essential health needs of the community justified the inauguration of this new pattern of education.

Associate degree programs were not estab-

*Johnson, D.: Competence in practice: technical and professional, Nursing Outlook **14**:33, Oct. 1966.

lished in order to do away with existing programs. The need for more nurses was given priority by leaders in the profession. The establishment of the program under educational auspices provided for experimentation with various curriculum patterns, for designing new patterns of curricula, and for scheduling the rotation of students through experiences centered on learning nursing care. The program also provided for the development of clinical facilities that were separate from those used by currently existing curriculum patterns. Inauguration of the associate degree program provided opportunities for educational institutions to attempt new approaches for the solution of a serious nursing problem—providing for increased numbers of prepared personnel able to meet the nursing care needs of the community.

In 1952 the first two programs were begun at Orange County Community College in New York and at Fairleigh Dickinson College, New Jersey. The number of programs in the United States and its territories had increased to 330 by 1968. Each year there has been a corresponding increase in the number of graduates of these programs. In 1957, 276 nurses were graduated and eleven years later the number of graduates had risen to 6,213. This latter figure represented approximately 15 percent of the total number of registered nurses graduated from all preservice programs in that year.

Purpose. The community or junior college is legally authorized to provide programs of study including instruction and guided learning experiences at the thirteenth and fourteenth grade levels and to award the associate degree for successful compliance with stated graduation requirements.

Nursing education programs in community colleges teach the fundamental knowledge and techniques of nursing that a registered nurse must have to administer direct care to patients. The emphasis is on students learning those skills basic to effective administration of direct nursing care and the development of these skills under instructional supervision to ensure technical competence. Stated another way, one purpose of the nursing program in a community college is to prepare a person to become skilled in the technicalities of nursing for practice primarily at the side of the patient.

Another purpose of this program is to prepare, in a short period of time, a greater number of nurses who are able to give competent nursing care and who can plan with other health care personnel for more effective care of groups of patients.

A third purpose relates specifically to the individual needs and interests of students. Some students choose the associate degree program because they could not qualify for admission to a university or senior college, or they cannot devote four years to acquiring a preservice education. Other students do not choose to apply for admission to a hospital school. Many students who are interested in nursing seek admission to a program conducted by an institution offering education on a college level that can be completed in two years and that has stature equal to collegiate programs in other fields that award an associate degree.

This type of program has particular appeal for young students who want to live at home for personal or financial reasons, married students whose family responsibilities require their presence at home, and older students who have never attended college or whose education was interrupted. Indeed, many older women whose families are grown and who now have both the time and the desire to develop their potential find that this program offers a real challenge. Many women have reported that they wanted to enter the nursing profession when they were young but were unable to do so. Others had been in nursing schools for a time but married before graduation and had to withdraw from the program. For this latter group, the opportunity for a second chance is a motivating factor contributing to their success as students and to their dedication to nursing following graduation.

Requirements for admission. Applicants selected for admission to the associate degree program are expected to meet the general entrance requirements of the college and the specific requirements of the nursing program. These requirements are listed in the school's brochure or catalogue. In addition, it is expected that students have demonstrated ability to meet scholastic requirements at the college level.

Structure and organization. The associate degree program in nursing is developed as one of the curricular offerings of the community or junior college of which it is a part. It is controlled and administered by the college. Its identity and status within the overall organization is similar to that of other programs in the college. All faculty members associated with the program are appointed by, and accountable to, the college administration. They, through the nurse administrator, are responsible to the college for instruction and supervision of students throughout the entire program.

Students are enrolled as regular students in the college and must meet the general college requirements as well as the requirements of the nursing major. Laboratory practice in the nursing care of patients is obtained in local hospitals and other clinical agencies in accordance with the students' learning needs. Clinical laboratory practice is scheduled and supervised by the nurse faculty of the college working in cooperation with the nursing service personnel and administrators of the agency.

Design of curriculum. The curriculum reveals a balance between general education and nursing courses that meets the policy requirements of the college. In addition, the provisions for correlation of content, the ratio of nursing classes to clinical practice laboratory hours, and the pattern for the rotation of students through required clinical experiences must be approved by the state's nursing board.

The curriculum is designed to operate within the structure of the college calendar and to comply with regulations in force for the academic school year. Nursing faculty members are assigned to teach and supervise all nursing content identified as part of the students' program of study. The use of hospital clinical facilities as laboratories for nursing practice is assured through written agreement by the college and the agency, but the hospital or agency assumes no responsibility for the students or for their education.

The curriculum devised for these nursing programs provides two years of post–high school general education integrated with nursing education. Montag identifies this curriculum as being "based upon the principle that education prepares the student for earning a living and for living."* Students must meet the college's graduation requirements to be awarded the associate degree. Following graduation the nurse is eligible to apply for admission to the state's examination for registered nurse licensure.

The associate degree program in the junior college curriculum, like the diploma program in the hospital school, is a terminal-type program. It exists in its own right and for its own purpose. It should be understood that the associate degree program in nursing is *not* a preparatory program for the baccalaureate program in a senior college or university. Students wishing to continue their education and earn a bachelor of science degree must qualify for admission and meet the entrance requirements of the college or university program to which they apply.

What graduates are prepared to do. Graduates of associate degree programs are technically competent and knowledgeable as beginning practitioners in the administration of direct nursing care to all types of patients. They are qualified to accept employment as beginning general duty staff nurses in hospitals, clinics and related health facilities, physicians' offices, or as private practice nurses. As beginning practitioners they are expected to participate in, and benefit from, planned inservice instruction and orientation programs offered by their employers to assure their adjustment to their jobs as new employees and to become effective members of the institutional team. As skill and competence are developed in the administration of quality patient-centered nursing care they may, with guidance and supervision, serve as leaders of selected nursing care teams in the clinical areas to which they are assigned.

• • •

Graduates of *all types* of preservice nursing programs should recognize the distinct difference between the administration of quality pa-

*Montag, M. L.: The education of nursing technicians, New York, 1951, G. P. Putnam's Sons.

tient care and the administration of nursing services. Their educational programs prepare them as beginning practitioners in nursing. The skills and techniques of management as well as the responsibilities for planning activities of other workers require additional education in administration. Hopefully, beginning registered nurse practitioners from each type of basic preservice program will be assigned to the care of patients as their first priority and will be permitted to develop their potential as nurse practitioners before they are encouraged or pressured to take the step into administrative activities for which they lack preparation.

PRACTICAL/VOCATIONAL NURSING PROGRAM

Historical overview. The term "vocational nurse" is the legal title used by Texas and California to identify the persons who are legally recognized elsewhere as practical nurses. All other states and territories of this country use the designation practical nurse, and to avoid confusion, the term practical nurse will be used in this section.

Practical nursing did not develop as a distinct career area until World War II. Its basic elements were the domestic skills and activities used by women in the course of managing their homes, raising families, and in helping to care for sick friends and neighbors. These skills and abilities of the "born nurse" were passed from mother to daughter and shared with other relatives and friends. Family doctors often taught certain basic procedures to women who were willing to learn them and who had earned the confidence of family and neighbors as they applied these skills.

One skill basic to practical nursing was some ability to maintain a household on an even keel in periods of lingering illness or during the extended convalescence of a family member. Early practical nurses demonstrated an understanding of the need to help others in time of sickness and family crisis. They showed compassion and patience in ministering to their charges and, as a result, the community called upon them for the nursing services they could provide.

In time, however, it became evident that some plan of formal training was needed to prepare people to care for the sick as well as to arrange some form of security and compensation for women who undertook the tasks of nursing others in everyday situations. The early schools for practical nurses were established through financial assistance from individual citizens, and the course of training was usually directed by private agencies. One school established in 1897 in New York City under the auspices of the Young Women's Christian Association received its funds from a Miss Ballard. The Ballard School for practical nurses provided three months' instruction and practice. Later the program was extended to nine months.

Other schools identified with the early development of formal practical nursing preparation include the Thompson School for Practical Nursing Attendants in Brattleboro, Vermont, and the Household Nursing Association, Inc., of Boston, Massachusetts (now known as the Shephard-Gill School of Practical Nursing). These two schools are still in operation today, functioning in accordance with present-day requirements.

After World War II it became apparent that more specific standards were required for the activities of practical nurses and for the educational preparation needed for their development. In 1944 the Smith-Hughes Act had made federal funds available to directors of education in the various states. It was felt that training for practical nurses could be improved and extended if these funds were spent on educational programs organized under the auspices of a state pattern for vocational education.

Consequently, a study was made of practical nursing as an occupation and in 1947 a report entitled *Practical Nursing and Analysis of the Practical Nurse Occupation with Suggestions for the Organization of Training Programs* was published by the United States Office of Education. This study pointed up the need for a curriculum guide. The guide, which was developed by a committee and published in 1950 by the United

States Office of Education, was entitled *Practical Nursing Curriculum—Suggestions for Developing a Program for Instruction Based Upon the Analysis of the Practical Nurse Occupation.* These two reports have been basic resources in the development of practical nursing programs.

No one questions the need for practical nurses to assist in meeting the demands for nursing care. As early as 1923 the Goldmark Report, which was concerned with educational standards of hospital schools, recommended that auxiliary nursing personnel be trained in courses of eight to nine months' duration "to help care for the less seriously ill and chronically ill patients." By 1968 there were 1,191 approved practical nurse programs in operation. The number of graduates from these programs for the same year totaled 30,833. It is reasonable to assume that the need for prepared practical nurses will continue to increase in the foreseeable future because of the burgeoning number of hospitals, clinics, and long-term care and convalescent units required for a complete spectrum of quality health care.

Purpose. Practical nursing programs prepare students to give direct nursing care to patients within specified limitations. Legally, practical nurses must carry out their nursing assignments under the direct supervision of a registered nurse or a physician. If the patient's condition requires complex care and attention to details beyond the practical nurse's scope and area of responsibility, she may serve as an assistant to the registered nurse, working with her and under her guidance. The practical nurse must always keep in mind her responsibility for functioning within the legal definition of practical nurse practice.

The preservice program to prepare practical nurses has both identity and stature. It appeals to students who do not wish or who could not plan to enroll in programs of longer duration. It prepares students for a career and gives them an opportunity to serve within a range of knowledge and skills identified broadly as basic nursing care activities. It provides both men and women within a broad age range the opportunity of becoming involved as valued team members in an area of service that offers deep personal satisfaction and a respected place in both the health care field and the community at large.

Requirements for admission. Requirements for admission to a practical nursing program are usually outlined in the school's brochure. These include the minimum education requirements established for acceptance into the program, the age range, evidences of good personal health based on a physician's physical examination, completion of a battery of pre-entrance tests with acceptable scores, and a personal interview.

Structure and organization. Approved practical nursing programs are now conducted by hospitals, by vocational-technical trade schools and institutes under the state's system of public education, by community or junior colleges, and by other approved community agencies. The length of the programs vary from one year to eighteen months, depending on the curriculum approved by each state's nursing board. Like the other preservice educational programs, the practical nurse program is complete for its purpose. It is approved by the state's licensing board as an accredited program. The graduate earns a diploma or certificate of completion and is then eligible to take the state examination for licensure in order to practice as a licensed practical/vocational nurse (LPN/LVN).

Design of curriculum. The practical nurse curriculum focuses on the preparation of students, through carefully planned classes and coordinated clinical learning assignments, to become proficient in the administration of direct basic care to patients.

The purposes of the curriculum are stated, developed, and implemented by the faculty assigned to the program. The pattern of instruction and the supervision of students assigned to clinical practice areas are the primary responsibilities of the faculty. Students are expected to demonstrate ability for learning and applying those concepts of behavioral and biologic sciences that specifically relate to ther practice of nursing as they develop their knowledge and skills.

What practical nurses are prepared to do. Graduates of practical nurse programs are prepared to administer specific types of direct nursing care to selected patients. Practical nurses carry out many functions and assignments under the supervision of a registered nurse or a physician. They may also be members of nursing care teams assisting the registered nurse in caring for critically ill patients where their combined efforts center on improving the patient's welfare (see figure on page 49). Practical nurses should participate in inservice and orientation instruction offered by their employers.

Licensed practical nurses have an important contribution to make in the care of patients and are especially needed in convalescent hospitals, long-term nursing care units, and some types of rehabilitation centers. Reorganization of patient care services in hospitals and medical centers, expansion of state and local planning for long-term facilities, and increased federal and state services for medical care to the chronically ill and the aging citizen will require adjustments in our present methods of providing nursing care. Providing services with skill, patience, and compassion for those in need of nursing care offers a real challenge to the talents and the dedication of the practical nurse.

The broad variety of functions required in nursing today and the attempts to prepare individuals to meet these requirements through a variety of educational programs stem from the needs of a dynamic society. But we must make certain that the overriding goal to which all nursing education is oriented is the preparation of practitioners to give quality nursing care. It is hoped that every student in nursing has selected the program that most effectively challenges and stimulates his or her desire to learn and to contribute constructively.

Today's students, regardless of the type of nursing program in which they are enrolled, are tomorrow's nurse practitioners. Cooperation and mutual respect within the nursing profession are obligations for all. The challenge of nursing and the quality of its contribution to individual and community well-being depends upon the individual practitioner's willingness to function as a member of a team and to apply formal preparation and continued learning for the welfare of others.

BIBLIOGRAPHY

American Nurses' Association: Facts about nursing, New York, 1969, The Association.

Barnard, J.: Beginning or the end for three year nursing education? RN **29**:43-49, Oct. 1966.

Bridgman, M.: Collegiate education for nursing, New York, 1953, Russell Sage Foundation.

Bullough, V. L., and Bullough, B.: The emergence of modern nursing, ed. 2, New York, 1969, The Macmillan Co.

Cafferty, K. W.: The role of the administrator of the nursing program in the community-junior college, New York, 1960, National League of Nursing (The League Exchange No. 51).

Dineen, M. A.: Current trends in collegiate nursing education, Nursing Outlook **17**:22-26, Aug. 1969.

DeYoung, L.: The foundations of nursing, St. Louis, 1966, The C. V. Mosby Co.

Educational preparation for nursing—1968, Nursing Outlook **17**:9, Sept. 1969.

Fitch, G. E.: The role and responsibility of the practical nurse, New York, 1969, The Macmillan Co.

Johnson, D.: Competence in practice: technical and professional, Nursing Outlook **14**:33, Oct. 1966.

Kelly, C. W.: Dimensions of professional nursing, ed. 2, New York, 1968, The Macmillan Co.

Montag, M. L.: The education of nursing technicians, New York, 1951, G. P. Putnam's Sons.

National League for Nursing: Nursing education programs today, New York, 1961, The League.

Roberts, M. M.: American nursing, history and interpretation, New York, 1954, The Macmillan Co.

COMPLETE WORK SHEET ON PP. 311 AND 312

CHAPTER 6

Your first days in the nursing program

ENTERING A NEW WORLD

The start of your nursing program should be an exciting experience. Now you and your classmates are taking a giant step into your future. You are meeting new people, making new friends, and enjoying new experiences.

After you were notified of your acceptance, you probably received information about your school's orientation program for new students. Many schools have a printed sheet or handbook that includes information to help make your entrance into your new world orderly and easy. It is the first of many guides and pointers you will receive as a nursing student.

An important part of getting settled involves living accommodations. This is particularly important to students and their parents whose home is at some distance from the community in which the school is located. The residence established in conjunction with the nursing school is supervised by a residence director or housemother who will help to maintain and direct the services and programs associated with your off-duty hours. Upper classmen, "big sisters," or the officers of the student government organization can help you to become acquainted with the activities and programs of the residence.

The welcome for those of you living in a school-sponsored residence probably included assignments to rooms and mailboxes, help with baggage, and other small services that new students need to feel at home. A welcome party may have been scheduled to greet you and help you become acquainted with the other students. If you share a room, plans were probably made to introduce you to your new roommate as soon as you arrived at the residence. If students are permitted to live off campus, assistance in locating suitable quarters is often available.

Each school of nursing is concerned about its students' welfare, and the administration and faculty want to convey the feeling that each of you is truly part of the program. Provisions have been made to help you and the members of your class to understand the routines associated with group living and group assignments, including introductions to your teachers, advisors, administrative personnel, and the supervisors with whom you will be working and learning. The school also provides tours of all its educational facilities and visits to the clinical areas in the hospital where you will have your nursing experience. You will probably want to explore the community's shopping centers, parks, museums, churches, libraries, and recreational and cultural centers. In addition, you may visit agencies concerned with community health, safety, and welfare. Maps, transportation routes, bus schedules, local newspapers, and descriptive brochures from the city's Chamber of Commerce are basic references. You are urged to take advantage of all community resources that interest you so that you can truly become a part of this new environment and educational experience. Your cooperation and active participation will help to make this program truly rewarding.

Whenever a group of people live and work together, some general rules are needed for harmony within the group and for the welfare of all members. Orientation may well involve learning rules and regulations for:

1. The use of living facilities shared in common, such as lounges, kitchenettes, recreation, and laundry areas
2. The occupancy of students' living (sleeping) quarters
3. Use of equipment such as radios, TV, record players, and musical instruments
4. Use of the telephone, mail services, dining areas, and other group-shared facilities
5. "Noise" control within the residential and classroom areas
6. Policies for vehicle parking, storage facilities, and use of, and liability for, special equipment
7. Policies regarding individual and group safety and procedures in the event of fire, bodily injury, or property damage
8. Policies for reporting your whereabouts in case of emergency

It would be safe to assume that similar rules are a part of your own home life and they are equally important in your new home. Regulations similar to the above are often established by the landlords who rent rooms and apartments to student tenants. You can appreciate the need of basic regulations when persons live in proximity and function together in groups. Without a plan for cooperation confusion and chaos would result.

PERSONAL ADJUSTMENTS

Students in a nursing program are expected to develop and display the courtesies and social graces that identify the well-mannered person. People who are thoughtful and considerate of others naturally find it much easier to enter new surroundings and new group situations. Your first weeks in the program with new friends and classmates give you a good opportunity to "brush up" your social graces and acquire greater ease in social situations.

Becoming familiar with the regulations established for residence or dormitory life is part of your learning assignment in your new social environment, and you are expected to accept these basic rules and help to make them work. Consider your entrance into the world of nursing as a challenge to your ability to make adjustments to the new experiences that are a part of your life as a student nurse. Your adjustment to this new environment is a first step in growing to meet the demands that the nursing program and your chosen profession will make later on. You will need to be flexible in considering the needs of those with whom you are living and working. Although you may encounter some difficulties, remember that others are facing the same situation and that this give-and-take is part of the process of becoming a mature, responsible person.

Because you have chosen to be a part of the nursing program, your instructors and supervisors expect that you will use every opportunity for developing your character, your personality, and your known, as well as your hidden or potential, talents. Through this exciting time of learning and growing, you can become the person, the nurse, the citizen you want to be. You will find yourself becoming a poised, confident, and responsible young person both professionally and in your private life.

The student-learner. One of the fundamental adjustments any student needs to make is to accept her role as a learner. In your nursing program you are a student-learner whose educational experience will require close attention to the demands of the classroom, the laboratory, the hospital, and related areas used for planned clinical assignments. You were accepted into this program because you gave evidence of your ability to do well, and your primary responsibility is to develop this ability. In order to do this you must believe in yourself and proceed with confidence that you can learn and that you can measure up. Of course, you will have time to learn. Being a student nurse is work and it is demanding. In order to do your best, you must participate actively. Your instructors and supervisors are available to guide and help you and challenge you to put forth your best efforts. After you have learned the fundamentals of your program, you will have the opportunity to apply this knowledge in your practice of nursing.

The many teachers you will have are interested in your development. They expect achievement and you will have to carefully plan your time for adequate study and class preparation. Demanding instructors, advisors, and supervisors should be counted among the best friends a student has, although some students frequently misinterpret the demands of a strict teacher, and consequently deprive themselves of a stimulating and cooperative relationship that could mean much to them. When you accept the responsibility of doing your best by taking time to learn and *think* about what you are learning, you demonstrate that you have respect for yourself and your ability. So use your capacity for learning to increase your knowledge and skills. Give yourself a chance to realize your full potential.

You will soon find that you have acquired a new identity and a new loyalty. You are now a student nurse. Your family and friends think of you as being "in nursing." You are a part of your program, your class, and your school.

Your classmates are a group of new acquaintances; some of them may become life-long friends. To become part of this group you may need to take the first step in making friendly overtures. Everyone in your class is experiencing the feeling of "newness," so try to overcome your own shyness and hesitation. Your courtesy and friendliness will break the barriers of reserve and establish those first important contacts. An informal exchange of introductions, a helping hand offered to assist a classmate in some way, or a friendly chat about items of mutual interest, may be the first step. The rest is easy.

Walking to classes in a group, joining others in the cafeteria or student lounge, getting together at a coffee break, or making impromptu plans with a few classmates for a trip to town are all good ways of getting better acquainted. Visiting with classmates in their rooms at the residence or getting together to study or listen to records are other pleasant ways of getting to know others and letting them get to know you. Whether "getting together" is informal and spontaneous or part of a planned activity, the important thing for you is to be friendly and sociable yourself and to do your part to bring a shy person into the circle. As you learn to know your classmates and expand your round of activities, remember that it is up to you to go half-way in developing and deepening relationships. To earn another's friendship you must also be a friend.

In the excitement of this new experience, don't forget to keep in touch with your family. If you are living away from home it is important that you keep in touch frequently through letters, postcards, or an occasional telephone call to let them know how you are getting along. Share with them the things that have made your days important and exciting and make them a part of your new life. It is natural for you to miss your family and friends at home, but your decision to leave home to prepare yourself for future responsibility is part of the process of growing up and becoming mature. Your family and friends want you to succeed and they have confidence in your ability to meet your new challenges. Keeping in touch will reassure them and help you to overcome your loneliness. They will be looking forward to your weekend visits or regular vacation periods just as much as you.

"SECOND THOUGHTS" ABOUT YOUR CAREER CHOICE

You may also want to think about another aspect of the world of nursing. Is nursing really the best career for you? If you are having second thoughts about nursing as a career, or if you are worried about your ability to meet the demands of nursing, you may find it helpful to discuss your feelings with your counselor or the director of your program. For your own peace of mind you should act without delay. Request an appointment for a conference. Make an honest and careful review of the problems that are causing you to wonder whether you have made the right choice. In the course of such a conference you may be surprised to learn that you are trying too hard and that you expect results too rapidly. You may need to give yourself a chance to adjust to your new world by literally meeting each day as it comes. By taking things in stride and by doing your best in each assignment, the pieces of your puzzle will fit into place. When you are able to achieve perspective it is easier to proceed with less doubt and difficulty in accomplishing your goals.

Discussing problems of this nature with an advisor who is able to see the entire picture can give you the help you need. You should not feel that advisors will try to keep you in a nursing program against your will. Hopefully an advisor can assist you to objectively consider all the facts so that you can make the decision that is best.

There are students who apply for admission to nursing programs with a sincere intention of making nursing their career. Sometimes students discover they simply cannot accept or meet the demands nursing makes upon them. Nursing may not be what they expected, and for these students nursing is clearly not the best career. If a student does her best but is unable to accomplish her work with any degree of satisfaction, she should not consider herself a failure. She should realistically and honestly face her situation as a fact of life. It is important that students realize that there are other career areas which may be better suited to their own personalities, goals, and abilities.

Nursing, like every other profession, needs people who are happy in their jobs. People who know that, for them, nursing is the best career are likely to feel a sense of achievement, security, and general satisfaction with living. These people bring enthusiasm and concern to their work. A nurse who is unhappy because she feels "trapped" in nursing and is unhappy in performing the tasks of nursing naturally will not be very successful in her work. This unhappiness is reflected in the reactions and relationships of co-workers, and it affects the atmosphere in which nursing services are performed. Nursing is a demanding profession and student nurses must recognize this fact.

If you find the demands of a nursing career physically, intellectually, or emotionally unacceptable, you should face up to this fact honestly and choose another career. Furthermore, a student who makes this decision should not feel guilty, ashamed, or inadequate. *A student's first responsibility is to herself.* She must choose the way in which she will derive the greatest personal and professional satisfaction, for she, more than anyone else, has to live with herself. If a student were to remain in nursing in spite of dissatisfaction or unhappiness, she would be failing herself in a very basic way. Each year a number of students accepted into nursing leave within a few days or months following admission. This fact is verified by reports from schools of nursing throughout the country. While the great need for nurses makes this regrettable, it is nonetheless a reality that must be faced for the good of the individual and the profession.

But what about the students who remain? What is in store for you as you proceed with your education? First, you should know that your school considers you an important person. You have successfully met standards for admission to a program that offers you the chance to test and develop your capacity for learning.

Your school is responsible to you for providing an educational program based on clearly defined objectives. It has met standards for accreditation and has a qualified faculty and other personnel who will teach you and guide your progress throughout your educational program, challenging you to put forth your best efforts. You will be expected to think, to learn, and use your knowledge in order to complete your academic program. At the same time your school will be achieving its own purpose of educating competent practitioners by helping *you* to become such a nurse.

Look in your school catalogue for the sequence of courses and the pattern used for scheduling subject matter throughout your total program of studies. Review also the description of every course included in your program. These descriptions report what material will be presented and what type of clinical learning assignments will be scheduled by the instructor teaching each course. Every course description is, in effect, an evidence of your school's compact with you. Each course makes a particular contribution to your education and each course will serve as a basis for additional information during your formal training and during your practice of nursing.

Learning and applying principles to your clinical practice will not be without incident. There will be times when everything seems to go wrong. You will have moments of frustration, discouragement, and anxiety. This is part of living and learning and *it happens to everyone.* Being overanxious or afraid that you are not doing everything perfectly the first time you do it or that you cannot remember everything you have been told the first time you hear it is being unfair to yourself. *Remember that you are learning, and making mistakes is part of the learning process.* Do not permit a temporary snag in your day to discourage you. Think about things as you study them or practice them in clinical situations. Let your sense of humor and your self-confidence come to your rescue.

Victor Hugo said, "Have courage for the great sorrows of life and patience for the small ones. And when you have finished your daily task, go to sleep in peace. God is awake." Tomorrow is a new day, and with it comes new energy and the opportunity to get in tune again with the world about you. Keep in mind that nursing requires day-to-day persistence because it makes extraordinary demands. You will grow as you learn to identify and then meet these demands. If you do your part and have faith, you will experience success and the satisfaction of knowing that your efforts have not been in vain.

If you follow these suggestions you will do much to speed your progress as a student in laying the foundations for continued growth.

1. Use time to your advantage.
2. Remember that twenty-four hours are available each day for work, rest, and relaxation.
3. Remember that learning and understanding your new knowledge is the most important job at hand.
4. Listen attentively, think constructively, and observe carefully.
5. Develop your sense of wonder and your appreciation of life's blessing.
6. Be true to yourself and your ideals.
7. Practice self-discipline.
8. Take time to think about yourself, your goals and dreams, and about your plans for shaping your future.
9. Be a friend to others.
10. Be kind.

TAKE A GOOD LOOK AT YOURSELF

As you begin your study of nursing, consider again your new role and your potential for success in a nursing career. Do not forget that you are an individual with a unique identity and innate dignity and that you are a part of human society. You bring to your chosen career the character and the personality that identifies *you.* Standards of personal conduct, characteristics identifying your personality, and impressions made on others by the pattern of your daily living all contribute to your identity as a nurse.

CHARACTER

The word "character" has many meanings, but it has particular importance when we think about the identity of an individual. In this context character refers to the moral values and beliefs that are used as guides for personal behavior and actions.

A person's character is shaped in part by the moral values to which he subscribes and by his definition of right and wrong. It has been stated that character is what a person is *inside.* Character develops in proportion to emotional and intellectual growth and involves the degree to which you understand, direct, and channel your feelings. Every aspect of your daily life not only reveals your character, but should also encourage you to develop your beliefs and values as they relate both to your present circumstances, and to those that will be encountered in the future.

The desire to help others and to give support and skilled assistance to patients helps a nurse focus on doing good for others. Nursing is

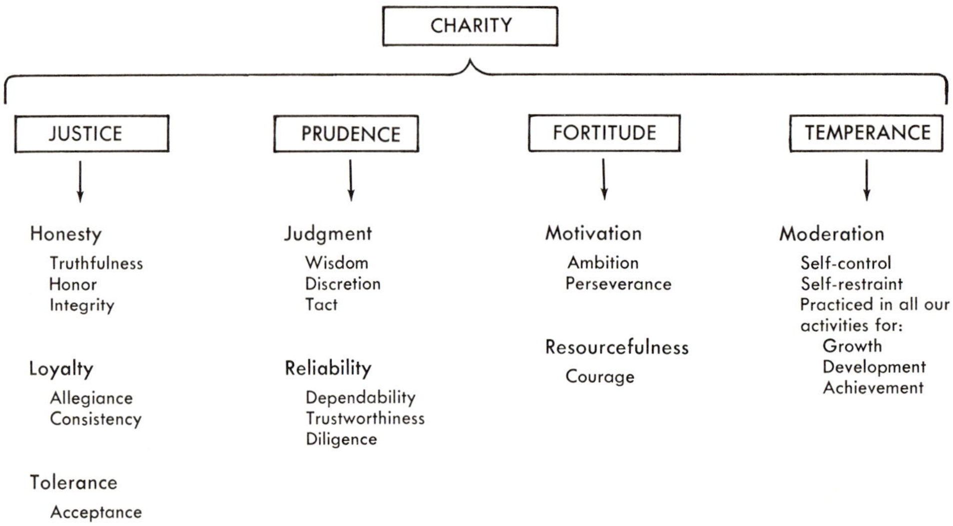

THE ATTRIBUTES OF CHARACTER BASED ON MORAL QUALITIES OR VIRTUES.

rooted in those ideals of conduct universally established and accepted by men of good will. The practice of nursing, ideally, utilizes love for one's fellow man, or the practice of the virtue of charity, as the basis of all nursing activities. Charity implies a feeling of affection or high regard. Translated into human relationships, it is the love and respect of man for his fellow man. This is the greatest virtue and serves as the foundation for a sense of values and the development of human character.

There are four virtues, or habits of moral practice, that emanate from the practice of charity. They encompass the range of human experience and are identified as justice, prudence, fortitude, and temperance. Together they provide goals for character development. The paragraphs below outline the ideal place and function of each virtue. (See figure above.)

JUSTICE governs our relations with man and the agencies within which society operates.

directs that we respect others, their rights, their welfare and their just due.

is the quality of being righteous, correct, fair, and impartial.

uses authority to uphold what is right, just, or lawful.

PRUDENCE provides for vision and a sense of balance in our lives.

integrates our life activities to achieve a harmonious and complete whole.

guides our choices of action here and now.

provides a basis for the exercise of sound judgment in practical matters.

permits us to live with good sense and perspective.

FORTITUDE provides for the control of responses made to difficulties and [illegible]

[illegible] reason in meeting [illegible] ation.

[illegible] of feelings, thoug[illegible] s in the face of di[illegible]

is an inner re[illegible] permits us to endure mi[illegible] with patience.

TEMPERANCE encourages constructive uses of the pleasures of the senses.

guides activities for growth and achievement within boundaries of self-control and moderation.

enriches human life through rational control of life's essential functions and basic emotional drives.

Attributes of character. A person who has tried to make the practice of these virtues a part of his life has such qualities as honesty, loyalty, tolerance, judgment, reliability, motivation, resourcefulness, and moderation. Your courses in the nursing program, especially psychology and ethics, will consider these attributes in detail. They will also be reviewed in your nursing classes. At this point, however, let us consider them in a general way.

HONESTY

Honesty is a most important quality in anyone who hopes to practice nursing. It means being truthful, trustworthy, and upright in one's dealings with others as well as refraining from lying, cheating, or stealing. It also implies that one's actions are free of fraud and deceit. Honesty is a quality of action centered in justice and can be discussed in terms of truthfulness, honor, and integrity.

TRUTHFULNESS is the quality of being in agreement with the facts, reality, or experience. It reflects the accuracy and honesty of a situation.

HONOR means keeping faith, making good on commitments.

INTEGRITY means that one adheres to his own set of moral values. A person with integrity can be counted on and trusted.

Honesty commands respect, for to be honest requires a high degree of self-respect and self-discipline. Honesty is so closely associated with dependability that it is difficult to imagine any truly dedicated nurse lacking either of these qualities.

The honest person is aware of his obligation to learn and know what is expected of him in the course of gaining an education or becoming skilled in practice. Ignorance of the information one is supposed to know or taking a chance in using information not clearly understood jeopardizes the safety and welfare of others. A nurse who is honest with herself, with her instructors or supervisors, with physicians, and patients avoids short-cutting and slipshod completion of assignments. She will not deliberately put off the unpleasant tasks that are part of her responsibility or "forget" to do them in the hope that someone else will perform them for her. Honesty demands that any error or possibility of error involving another's safety be reported immediately to one's teacher or superior, despite any unpleasant consequences involving the person at fault. Failure to acknowledge questionable action, neglect in recording information vital to the patient's welfare, or silence in situations that demand explanation are practices that, for obvious reasons, are unacceptable.

Honesty also involves respect for the property of others. In nursing practice this includes not only medications, equipment used in administering treatments, and prescribed tests, but also the use of linens, foods, and special equipment intended for a patient's use. It is hardly necessary to say that an honest person does not use any personal property, including food, clothing, money, or books, without express permission of the owner. The honest person also abhors any suggestion of cheating during examinations and does not represent the work of another as her own.

Evidences of honesty. Your honesty will be evident in the manner in which you deal with a variety of daily activities. Honesty has special importance when you are involved with care of material, recognition of authority, obedience, and use of time.

Care of material. Medications, hospital supplies and equipment, and all materials intended for patient care must be used properly and judiciously. It is also essential that you use care and economy in handling school and hospital equipment and in using facilities available for your daily activities. Both as a citizen and a nurse you are assuming responsibility when you accept the property or possessions of others for use or safekeeping. It is also vital that you recognize your responsibility for reporting the malfunctioning or destruction of essential supplies and equipment so that replacement may be made and adequate safeguards taken.

Recognition of authority. Honesty is closely related to justice, and we rely upon people in authority to be both honest and just in dealing with subordinates and in carrying out the responsibilities entrusted to them. People in positions of authority assume obligations as well as privileges and power; hopefully, they are aware of their obligations and are able and prepared to assume the responsibilities of the job. Often people with many responsibilities must delegate certain tasks to others who, in turn, are accountable to the person who assigned them the work. However, final responsibility rests with the person who is in charge, whether he performs all the work himself or assigns parts of the job to someone else. For example, a patient's physician may write orders for the administration of a medication. Although a nurse may be given the responsibility of actually administering the drug properly, the physician is responsible for making sure that he has ordered the correct dosage of the appropriate drug and that his orders regarding its administration were followed correctly. Similarly, your nursing program has an administrator who is responsible for conducting your educational program in accordance with policies formulated for the guidance of your total educational experience. Instructors, supervisors, and personnel assigned to various services such as student health, residence facilities, and student government have their particular roles to play. However, the director herself is responsible to the administrator of the institution for the overall functioning of the program.

Occasionally, people in positions of authority have not developed some of the qualities necessary for pleasant and productive interpersonal relations. Discourtesy and disregard for the feelings of others can create misunderstanding, unpleasantness, and sometimes active dislike between people in charge and their subordinates. However, this situation does not justify a disregard for authority in general, although certainly the manner in which authority is presented and enforced may be resented. Your own patience and courtesy can help to improve such situations.

Obedience. Relationships among people and interaction within social agencies and institutions are based upon basic rules and regulations. These rules are intended to establish a climate of mutual respect and to protect the basic rights of those persons to whom they apply. Such rules and regulations must be obeyed and applied impartially in order that each individual have some sense of order and security in his relationships with other people and with his government.

When rules and regulations are established for a good reason, rational persons can be relied upon to understand the necessity of observing them. At times you may not understand the reasons for rules and regulations, but if you trust those who are responsible for them and if they correspond to your own best judgment, you will obey. In this way you demonstrate your recognition of just and reasonable authority and your respect for it.

For nurses the acceptance of such authority is basic. Your patient's welfare, even his life, depends on the care with which you follow the principles you have been taught and on the manner in which you carry out the orders established for patients' welfare. Reasonable rules and regulations are not intended to be restrictive; they will assist you to increase your competence in providing good nursing care.

Use of time. It is important that you be honest with yourself in scheduling your time. You may plot out and develop a twenty-four hour time schedule that demonstrates your good judgment, but the way in which you actually *use* your time is what counts.

Being on time for your appointments, whether they are classes, clinical assignments, or personal engagements, is an important indication of your character. Your lack of punctuality not only seriously disrupts your own routine, but it also affects the plans of others who are depending upon you and your readiness to carry out your share of the assignments.

In hospitals, time schedules are a way of life. A patient's care, treatments, and even his life may depend on the specific schedule established for treatment and medication. You are responsible for carrying out orders by the specified time. As a member of the hospital team you are expected to be present at the time and place designated. When you fail to meet these obligations, you demonstrate not only a lack of consideration but also a serious lack of dependability.

Putting off assigned tasks will have unpleasant if not dangerous results. If your own carelessness makes you late in completing your scheduled assignments, if your medications have not been administered and checked off, or if your charting is not completed, you deprive yourself of the satisfaction that results from knowing you have completed a difficult job thoroughly and well. In addition, because you were not available, you may have lost a special opportunity for a new learning experience or a rewarding personal activity.

LOYALTY

Loyalty is the feeling of confidence, trust, and affection you have toward your family and friends and toward those who have helped, guided, and stood by you as you proceeded toward your goals. Nurses should have no difficulty in identifying the importance of this feeling. A nurse must also be loyal to herself. Such loyalty requires that you maintain allegiance to the ideals you support and maintain a constancy of belief in the sincerity of those in authority so long as your own good judgment assures that this trust is merited.

As students in nursing, and later as graduates, you must have such faith and confidence in your own judgment. This loyalty to yourself should be based on honest and sincere self-respect, which recognizes your human dignity. Respect for yourself helps you to acknowledge your rights and responsibilities in developing your talents and abilities and in deriving personal as well as professional happiness and satisfaction.

Similarly, you will develop a feeling of loyalty based on respect, trust, and confidence toward your fellow students, your school and its staff, the medical staff and hospital personnel, and your profession's standards. These standards require that you act with respect for the needs and rights of all patients, even if you do not like them personally.

TOLERANCE

Tolerance manifests itself in your recognition of the rights of others. It allows you to accept and respect others as fellow human beings entitled to enjoy the same basic rights and privileges that you claim for yourself. Of course, tolerance does not demand agreement with another's beliefs, viewpoints, practices, and habits, but it does mean that you support and protect another's *right to retain* his beliefs, points of view, practices, and habits, regardless of whether or not you agree with them.

Your practice of tolerance strengthens your awareness of justice and the effect it has on your life and on the lives of others. Tolerance is inherent in our democratic way of life. When you are tolerant and accepting of others, you recognize the dignity and respect to which all men are entitled. In denying the humanity of another you are also denying your own claim to human dignity and respect. When you accept others as fellow human beings, prejudices centered in race, color, ethnic background, creed, or political party have no place in your scheme of living. It is well to recall that the color of the human heart is identical in all men.

If you are tolerant and accepting of others, you check unwarranted, malicious, or destructive criticism of their activities. You withhold judgment of their weaknesses when you do not have all the facts for making evaluations. You give to others the chance to succeed that you would hope to receive yourself. In being tolerant, you can appreciate the meaning of the prayer attributed to the Sioux Indian Nation, "Great Spirit, grant that I may not criticize my neighbor until I have walked a mile in his moccasins."

In nursing, an accepting and tolerant attitude toward others is of primary importance if you are to establish and work within a climate based on sound interpersonal relationships. We all need to identify the place of rightful authority in our daily lives, accepting differences and exchanges of opinion and abiding by the wishes or decisions of the group.

Tolerance, as a mark of character, is demonstrated in the practice of patience, a sense of humor, sympathy, understanding, and unselfishness. These traits distinguish the truly gracious person who is able to put herself and others at ease by using them in appropriate circumstances.

PATIENCE is putting up with the thoughtless or careless words and deeds of others, bearing with unnecessary delays, interruptions, or lack of interest from others, by practicing self-control and calmness.

implies we take people as we find them and make the best of things.

A SENSE OF HUMOR is demonstrated by using one's ability to detect, appreciate, or express what is amusing or ludicrous, especially in a trying situation.

involves laughing *at* yourself and laughing *with* others at amusing instances but never *at* others to hold them up to ridicule.

SYMPATHY is putting yourself in the place of another who is experiencing grief or difficulties, and responding to them in an understanding way.

is expressed by showing compassion to a person who is in trouble.

UNDERSTANDING is perceiving or knowing the reasons underlying the words or actions of another and giving another the benefit of the doubt when interpreting the intent of words or deeds.

UNSELFISHNESS is acting in a way that shows concern and interest in the feelings and needs of others.

JUDGMENT

Judgment comes from the virtue of prudence, which itself contributes to the development of the individual's maturity. The practice of judgment, sometimes referred to as "good sense," indicates an ability to use one's intellectual capacity to form sound opinions. Making a judgment involves comparison and discrimination in order to formulate an awareness of values and relationships. Qualities involved in the use of judgment are wisdom, discretion, and tact.

WISDOM is the ability to judge soundly and to follow the soundest course of action based on your own knowledge, observation, and understanding.

DISCRETION is being careful about what you do and say.

TACT denotes one's perception of the appropriate or graceful thing to say or do without offending others or putting them in an uncomfortable position.

In nursing, the judgments you and your colleagues make with regard to your patients will be based on observation. This is the act and the developed skill of noting signs or indications that point toward an estimate or judgment of an existing situation. Over and over you will be reminded of the significance of being observant and of developing your ability to observe completely and accurately. In making observations you, as a nurse, must not only note and report the facts but also evaluate the meaning of these facts in light of your knowledge and experience, so that you may then take the appropriate course of action. The terms "signs" and "symptoms" become part of your basic vocabulary. These are the objective and subjective guideposts to a patient's reaction to illness or his responses to treatment. Every course in your curriculum and every learning experience in the clinical areas are intended to supply the basic information to which you will refer in situations that require you to make nursing judgments.

In the practice of nursing, observation demands the use of your eyes to view the world about you and to read and study all pertinent information available. It entails the use of your ears to listen to instruction in classes and laboratory sessions, to the advice of instructors and supervisors, and to the physician's orders for his patients. You must develop further skill in observation by encouraging your sensitivity to sound and to the kinds of sounds you hear, their rhythms, their intensity, or their absence. Each has significance. The observant nurse recognizes the importance of "listening with the third ear." Also, consider for a moment the contribution Laennec's stethoscope has made to medical and nursing practice.

Your sense of smell and taste provide you with additional clues as you develop your skills in observing and making judgments. Your sense of touch and the ability to use it as you administer to patients will provide still more valuable clues to help you in appraising and observing.

Your instructors understand the importance of observation from their own experience. Let their example teach you the importance of exercising discretion in learning and communicating any information related to patient care.

Skillful observation depends on your knowledge and skill which are developed and enriched through day-to-day instruction. Planned clinical experiences are yet another medium through which you may expand and increase your observation skills by applying information from your course work to an actual patient care situation.

Skilled observation requires the use of discretion and tact, because care and judgment about what you do or say regarding what you observe and the way in which you handle the resulting information are as important as making the observation in the first place.

Your tact and discretion indicate that you accept your fellow men as persons of dignity and innate worth. Tact has been identified by one author as the expression of the "educated heart." Tact is a "nice discernment of what is appropriate to do or say in dealing with others; the peculiar ability to deal with others without giving offense."* To possess the gift of tact is an asset to anyone, and it is an asset that anyone may cultivate and develop. Tact enhances the nurse's potential to serve as a competent and cooperative team member, a kind person, a valued friend, and a prospective leader.

RELIABILITY

Reliability requires prudence as well as a sense of justice, because it involves trust and integrity. Reliability means dependability and involves your use of sound judgment based upon careful observation and an understanding of any given situation in which you are required to act.

*Wolff, I. S.: The educated heart, American Journal of Nursing, 63:58-60, April 1963.

It is especially important for nurses who must be relied upon to deal with emergencies and stressful situations in a calm and competent manner.

The reliable nurse does not need constant checks on the quality of her performance in either assigned activities or those for which she volunteers. She does her best at all times and her trustworthiness is most reassuring to her patients, co-workers, and superiors.

Diligence contributes greatly to reliability. To be diligent is to be careful, persevering, and painstaking in your assignments. If you are diligent or industrious you will seek out and develop the most effective ways of using your time, rather than simply permitting time to pass.

MOTIVATION

Motivation derives from fortitude and provides incentives or moves you to plan and accomplish specific things. You were motivated to consider nursing as a career and your desire to enter this program stimulated you to comply with the school's entrance requirements. Your ability to meet this challenge by working to fulfill all the prerequisites for admission demonstrates the relationship between motivation and fortitude, because fortitude gave you the strength and *persistence* to carry through.

Properly directed, motivation is a positive force. It directs your personal reactions to the fulfillment of desires or drives that are referred to as basic human needs. Motivation can be explored in conjunction with ambition and perseverence.

Ambition. Ambition is a strong desire to succeed or achieve. It is evident in the eagerness with which people accept challenges which will bring them closer to achieving personal and professional goals. The ambitious person works to discipline himself, develops his real and potential talents, and shapes them to serve him in attaining his goals.

Motivation and ambition are the driving forces behind the development of superiority in some particular quality, skill, or ability. This desire to make increasingly better use of one's talents, to compete with others in realizing a goal, and to achieve excellence is an important characteristic that must be controlled and channeled toward the attainment of any major goal.

Perseverance. A person who is highly motivated and intent on attaining a goal must have the ability to persevere. In spite of obstacles or difficulties that could discourage someone less determined, he continues on the path he has chosen to follow, tenaciously dealing with obstacles and adhering as closely as possible to his plans and goals.

RESOURCEFULNESS

Resourcefulness involves a person's ability to recognize and deal promptly and effectively with difficulties or problems that arise. Self-control, calmness, and composure are required in making difficult decisions, and the resourceful person can call upon a reserve of inner strength to meet demands in a time of particular need. You must have the courage to face and consider alternatives which are difficult, painful, or dangerous, rather than withdrawing from action. Resourcefulness requires the utilization of information available about a given situation and using it courageously, sensibly, and constructively in dealing with the situation. The cooperation of others is vital to those who try to apply their resourcefulness. It is seen in the teamwork of those assisting a surgeon in saving a patient's life.

All of these qualities related to fortitude play a major role in your professional preparation. Learning the information and skills that are basic to the art of nursing, effectively applying nursing techniques in clinical practice, learning new skills, and finding different ways to increase your understanding of information you already have all call for a persistent attitude. Perseverance is the key to your success as a nurse practitioner. Your desire to excel and your ability to be resourceful are qualities that will stand you in good stead. If your growth and development as a nurse are based on a desire to serve others, you will be able to develop and combine these important qualities and allow them to work for you as you learn about and then practice quality patient care.

MODERATION

Moderation, which is part of temperance, allows you to maintain harmony and balance among all elements of your character and in your relationships with others by encouraging you to develop perspective and a sense of objectivity. Moderation should enable you to examine, understand, and then control your feelings so that you use them rather than become enslaved by them. Moderation is not synonymous with suppression and it does not relate exclusively to the curtailment of excesses in eating, drinking, or other such activity. Moderation involves the reasonable and appropriate exercise of ordinary emotions and feelings. The process of educating your emotions requires the practice of moderation or self-restraint and gives you much more freedom to choose and then attain your goals.

Moderation and self-restraint, important components of everyone's character, are of particular significance for the nurse. Throughout your nursing program there will be opportunities for you to identify and develop your use of moderation and self-restraint. Their practice is a life-long pursuit involving the use of your willpower or, as the situation demands, "won't"-power. By helping you to understand and control your feelings and reactions, moderation makes you better able to cope in many situations. For example, as a nurse you are expected to maintain control of your emotions in times of stress or disappointment or in the face of problems that occur with your patients. This control does not mean you are unfeeling in situations such as critical illness, impending death, or an emergency. It does mean that in such instances your self-control and the recognition of your obligations to those you serve allow you to direct your efforts toward carrying out necessary functions with assurance and calm. Your self-control allows you to restrain other factors that could have unproductive or dangerous results. Your responses to the needs of the situation serve as a golden mean between two extremes.

The nurse who practices moderation recognizes and accepts the realities of life. "Sooner or later, a man, if he is wise, discovers that life is a mixture of good days and bad, victory and defeat, give and take."* The trick is to take each day as it comes, making the most of its opportunities and learning what you can from the difficulties it presents. This may not always be easy, but it is mandatory if you are going to control and guide your actions to achieve your purpose.

The nurse who uses moderation and restraint will check her periods of moodiness and self-pity. She will work against the tendency to worry needlessly and unproductively. Persistent discouragements and anxieties are challenges that you can and must meet, and it may be helpful for you to have a conference with your counselor, an instructor, or a trusted friend with whom you can discuss and deal with these feelings.

The nurse who exercises temperance and moderation will be able to view love, faith, fear, and anger in their proper perspective as each one touches her life. She will understand her emotions and feelings as they relate to her parents and family, her patients and co-workers, and *the* man in her life. She will also understand the feeling she has for herself as a rational person. Within each of these contexts her personal conduct will be shaped by the controls and self-restraints she has developed to ensure her own well-being.

Faith is our recognition of our need to depend on others because we are human and, therefore, fallible and in need of help. Faith and confidence should develop in our relationships with teachers, counselors, supervisors, and others whom we respect and whose knowledge is greater than ours. Moderation helps us to have faith in our own ability to apply powers of reasoning in making sound decisions.

The nurse who is fearful or anxious regarding past events in her life or new experiences should take time to consider why she has these feelings. It may be advisable and worthwhile to seek help from a person qualified to help in evaluating the factors that contribute to these

*Peterson, W. In Hay, G.: This way to happiness, New York, 1968. Copyright 1967, Simon & Shuster, Inc.

feelings. Depending on the problem this could be an instructor, a doctor, a clergyman, or a psychologist. A practical look at the causes of fear and anger could reveal that you have not considered all sides of the picture. Confidence in yourself, faith in your good judgment, and the ability to view the whole picture will help to counteract fearful feelings. A more objective interpretation of the events which raised these feelings originally will contribute toward planning an effective approach to dealing with these reactions.

Moderation also has a bearing on your health. As a nurse you practice basic principles of health and hygiene for your own sake and to serve as an example for others. Details of sound, effective health and hygienic practices as well as plans for your care and treatment during periods of illness will be discussed in the appropriate classes in your nursing curriculum. Likewise, proper diet, fluid balance, elimination, and bodily cleanliness need not be discussed now. The important point here is your practice of moderation and restraint in relation to your needs for sufficient rest, adequate exercise, and time for recreation and study.

Because you are a nurse you will be expected to behave as a worthy member of the nursing profession. Members of the community will expect you to conform to the highest personal and professional standards. You have already developed some of these necessary qualities through parental and home influences and earlier educational experiences. Utilizing these as a base and developing and strengthening other essential character traits with assistance from instructors and counselors will help you to prepare the foundation for your practice of nursing.

KEEPING YOURSELF IN HAND

PERSONALITY

Generally the term "personality" is used to refer to the distinctive individual qualities that differentiate one person from another. An individual's personality is the result of integrating one's abilities, desires, impulses, habits, and physical characteristics into a harmonious whole. The effect of personality is the impression you make on others, a result of the projection of your ego or whole self. It has been noted that a person's character indicates the type of person he really is, while his personality denotes the traits he reveals to others. Ideally, character and personality complement each other. Hopefully, those qualities that identify one's personality are strengthened and highlighted in the mind of the observer by the quality of one's character.

Your personality, or other people's feelings about you, is based upon such traits as appearance, attitudes, disposition, and abilities. As we review these traits in a general way, you might make a mental inventory of qualities that contribute toward the individuality of *your* personality. Since self-respect is a strong motivating factor in human nature, it is useful to look at yourself in a spirit of constructive criticism. Self-respect demands the maintenance of a healthy body which reflects poise and dignity in action and repose. The smallest details of your appearance contribute to the impressions you give to others about yourself.

Posture. Posture refers to the habitual or assumed positions of your body in standing, sitting, or moving about. The manner in which you stand, sit, move, and generally maintain control of your body presents some clues to your personality. Posture is affected by improperly fitted clothing and footwear. In turn, the appearance you present when wearing various types of apparel is influenced by the posture you assume.

Because most nursing students have taken physical education classes in high school or college or may have enrolled in extracurricular physical education classes, techniques and recommendations for good body mechanics and posture are not included here. You are responsible for practicing a physical regimen that helps to develop and maintain good posture and physical fitness. Good posture contributes to your personal appearance as well as to your good health.

FOUNDATIONS IN NURSING—LEARNING EXPERIENCES

LIBRARY ASSIGNMENTS ARE AN IMPORTANT PART OF STUDENTS' LEARNING

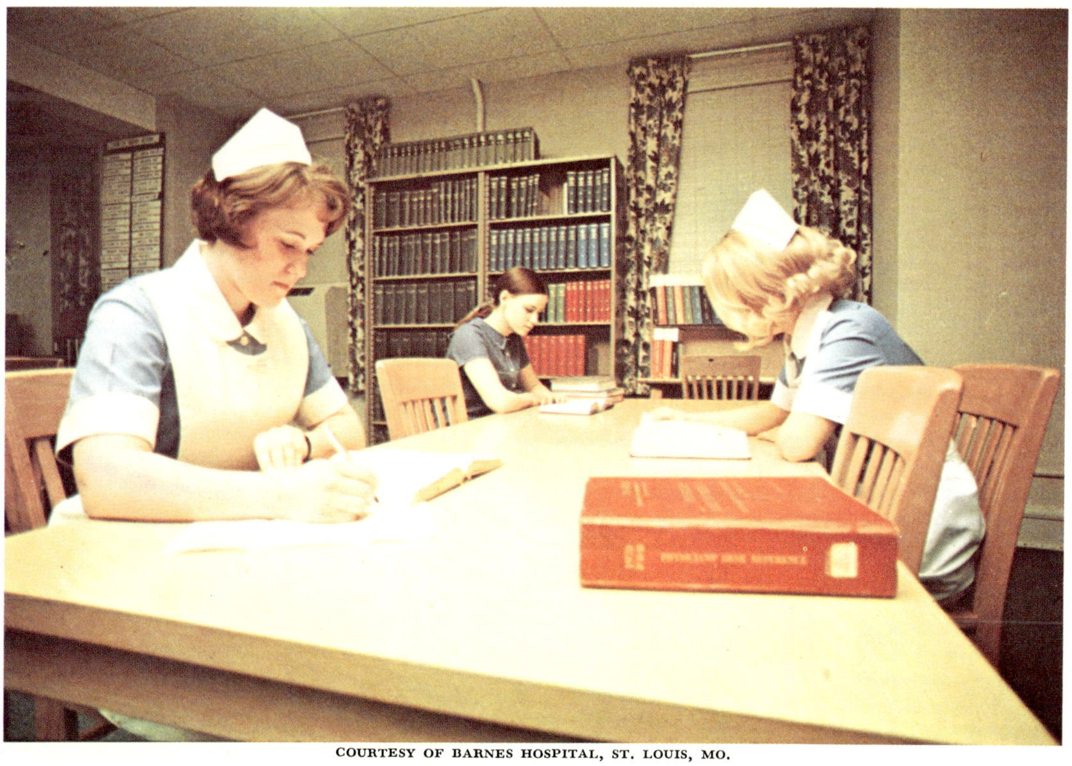

COURTESY OF BARNES HOSPITAL, ST. LOUIS, MO.

COURTESY OF BARNES HOSPITAL, ST. LOUIS, MO.

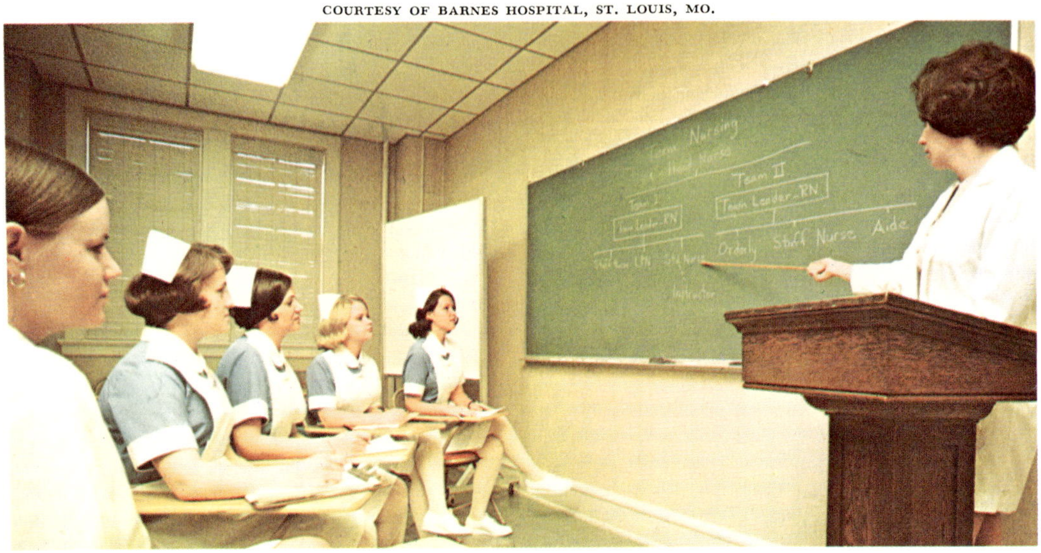

THE NURSING CARE TEAM'S STRUCTURE IS DISCUSSED
BY STUDENTS AND THEIR INSTRUCTOR

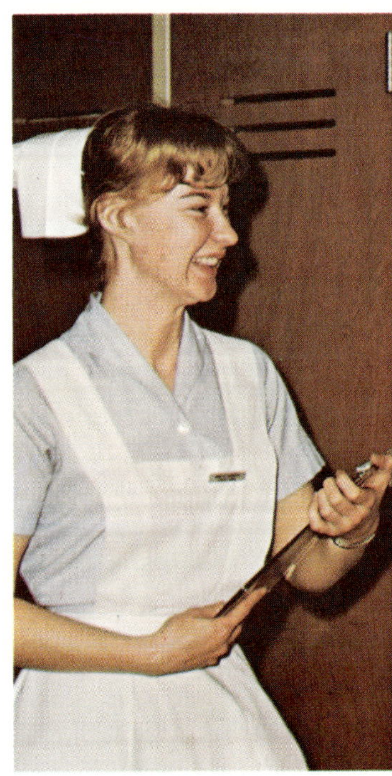

COURTESY OF BARNES HOSPITAL, ST. LOUIS, MO.

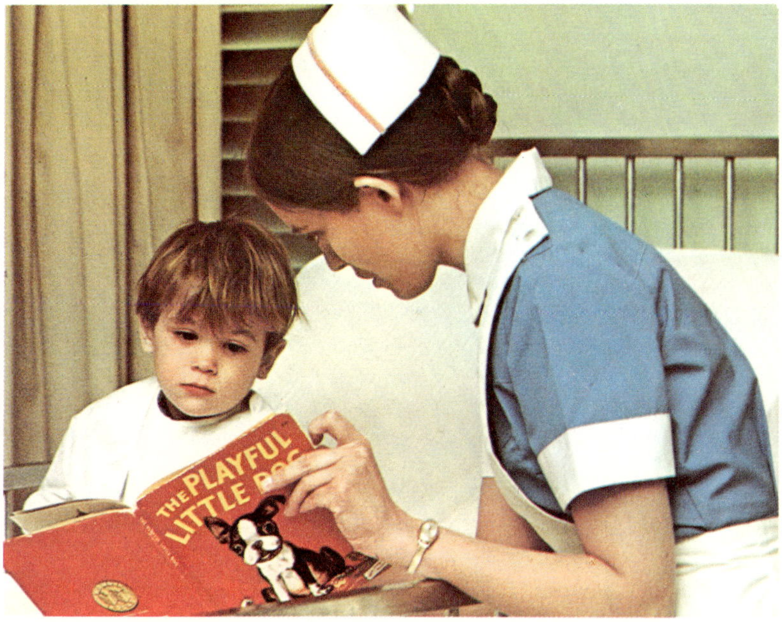

STORYBOOK READING CAN PLAY AN IMPORTANT ROLE IN NURSING CARE

RELATING TO OTHER MEMBERS OF THE NURSING TEAM

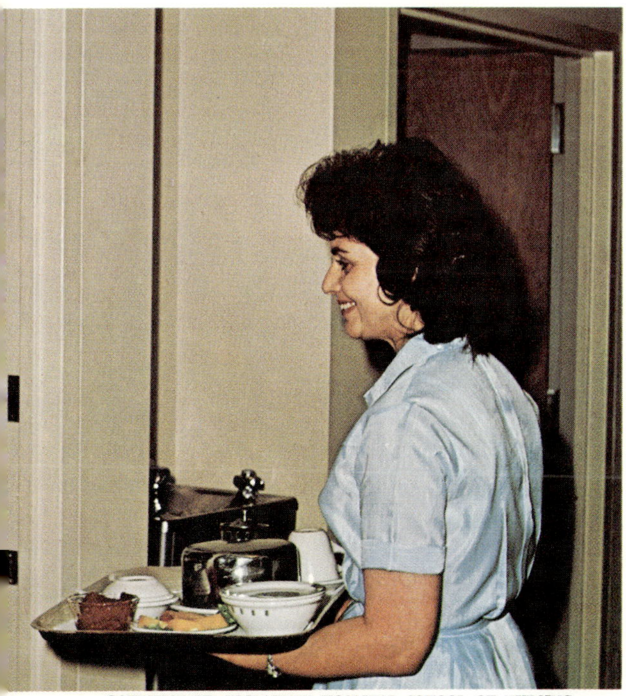

COURTESY ST. ELIZABETH HOSPITAL SCHOOL OF NURSING, DAYTON, OHIO; PHOTOGRAPH BY WALTER F. KOCH, COLUMBUS, OHIO

COURTESY ST. ELIZABETH HOSPITAL SCHOOL OF NURSING, DAYTON, OHIO; PHOTOGRAPH BY WALTER F. KOCH, COLUMBUS, OHIO

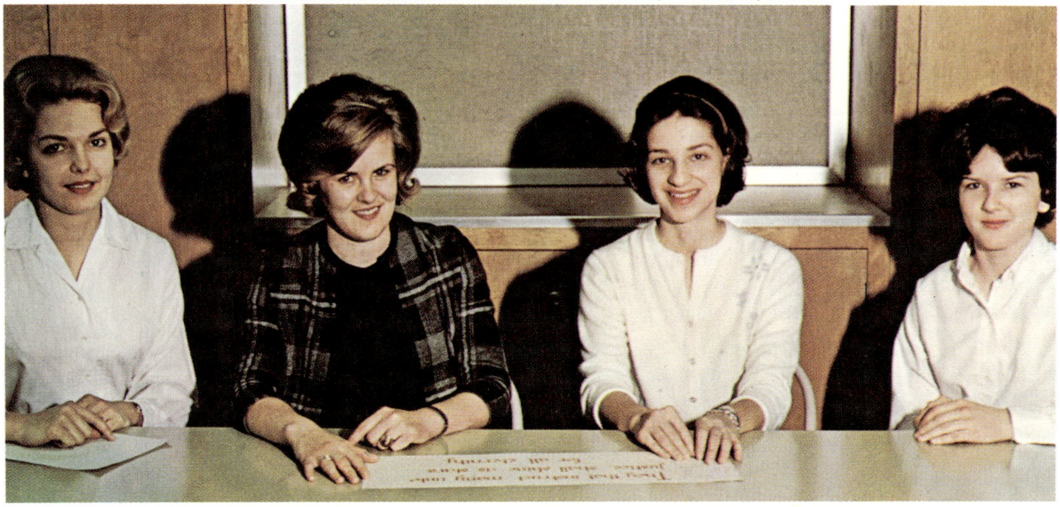

A COMMITTEE MEETING OF THE STUDENT COUNCIL

COMPARING NOTES IN PREPARATION FOR A CLASS DISCUSSION

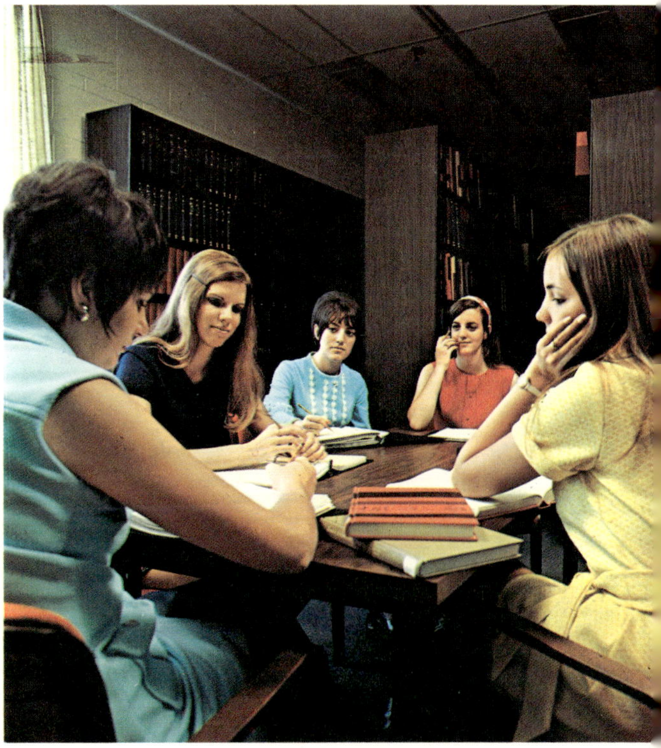

COURTESY OF BARNES HOSPITAL, ST. LOUIS, MO.

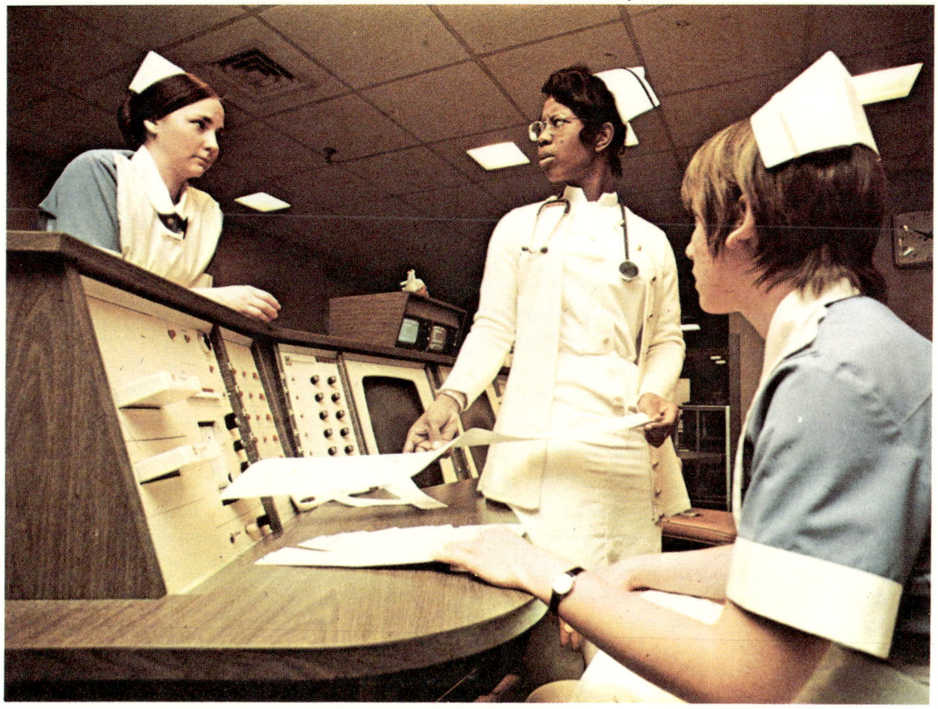

STUDENTS OBSERVE AND LEARN ABOUT THE USE OF ELECTRONIC EQUIPMENT IN A CORONARY CARE UNIT

ACCURACY IN PREPARING MEDICATIONS IS A PRIMARY RESPONSIBILITY OF EVERY NURSE

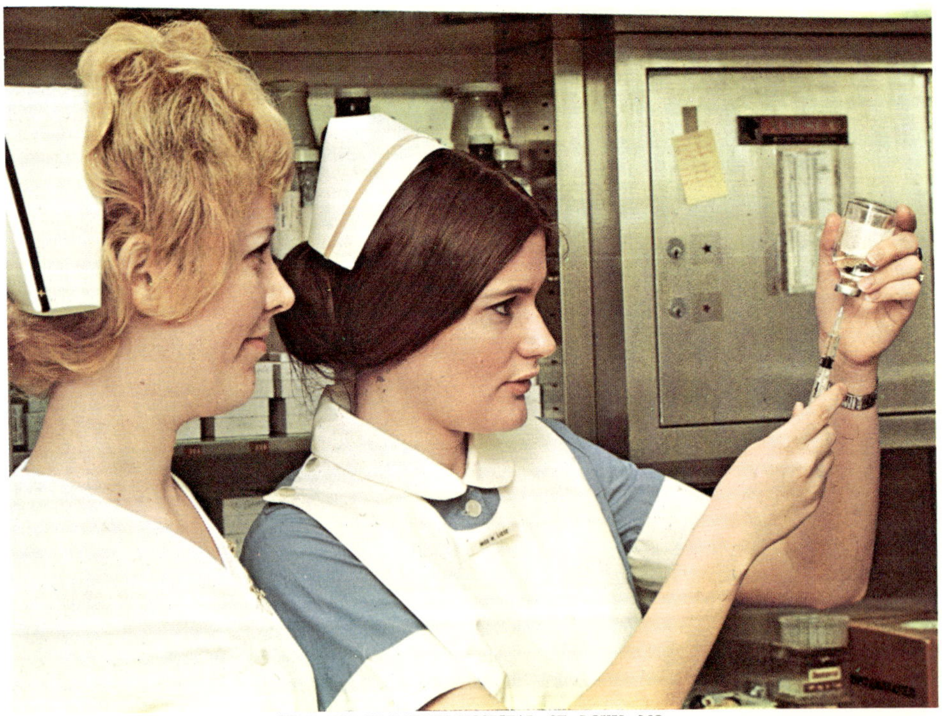

COURTESY OF BARNES HOSPITAL, ST. LOUIS, MO.

THE AGE OF "WONDER DRUGS"—
MODERN MEDICAL WARRIORS

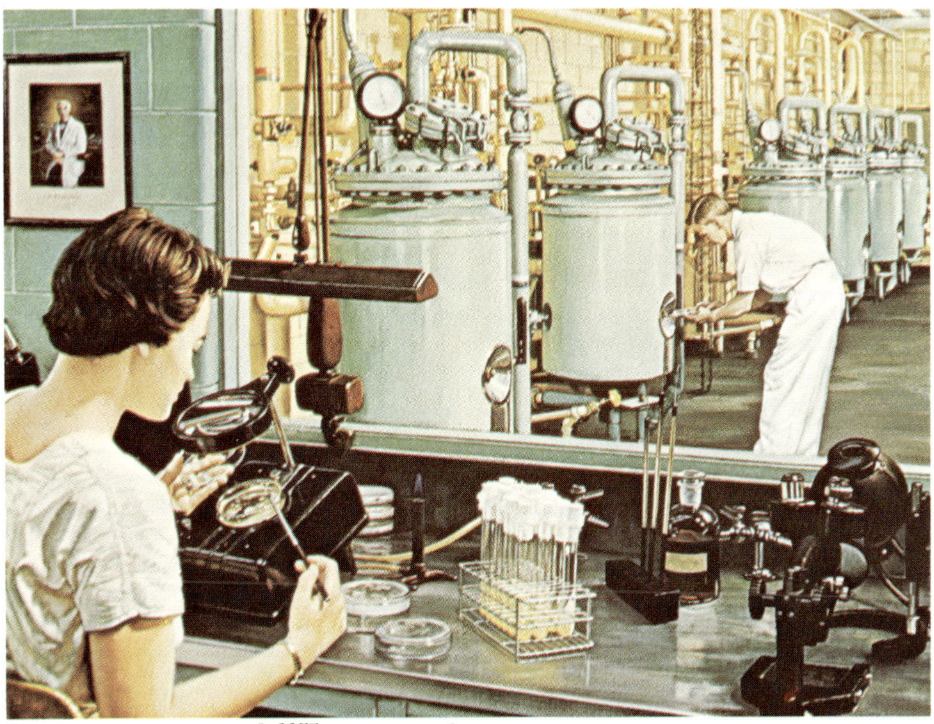

THE AGE OF "AUTOMATION"—
MODERN INTENSIVE AND CONTINUING CARE UNITS

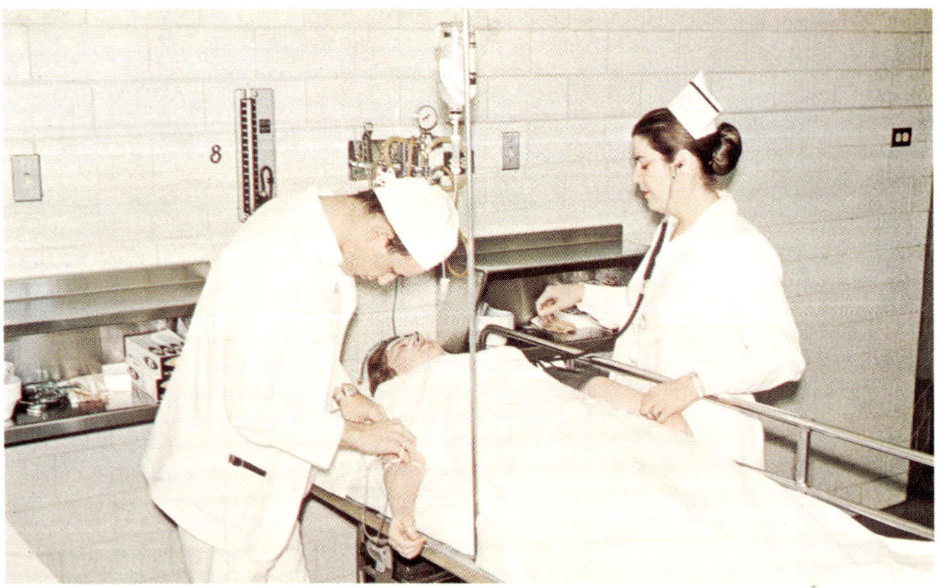

COURTESY MOUNT CARMEL MERCY HOSPITAL, DETROIT, MICH.

Cleanliness. Consideration of this topic in a text for nurses may be thought of as superfluous, yet cleanliness is one of the essential qualities we consider in evaluating personal appearance. Personal cleanliness and hygiene will be covered in detail in other classes in the nursing curriculum; emphasis here is upon the effect your personal hygiene and health has upon others you meet.

Dress. Just as self-respect is evident in good posture and personal hygiene, so is it reflected in the care you exercise with regard to dress. The following are some basic guides for personal dress:

1. Undergarments should be scrupulously clean and properly fitted for body support.
2. All articles of clothing should be neat, trim, and in good repair with special attention given to such "give away" items as shoulder straps, the slip, the heels of shoes, shoe ties or laces, and stockings.
3. The type of clothing worn should be appropriate for the specific occasion. (Proper attire serves to augment the self-assurance of the wearer.)
4. Your wardrobe need not be extensive to be attractive. Choose basic colors for your wardrobe. By adding accessories of contrasting or complementary colors you can add to the versatility of your clothing, and these items can express your mood and personality.
5. Current fads and styles need to be evaluated in light of their appropriateness and their practicality for your budget and body structure. A less-than-perfect figure can be disguised through the artful use of line, color, and texture.

The nurse's uniform. Nurses serving at a patient's bedside usually wear specified uniforms. In our society we are socially oriented to uniforms of the military services, law enforcement officers, and firemen. These all evoke a particular response in us.

For nurses and those engaged in nursing activities, the uniform has a particular symbolism. Through the centuries people who have cared for the sick have worn a distinctive type of dress. Present-day uniforms have evolved from the habits worn by the early religious orders; the nun's coif has become our cap; her scapular, our bib and apron.

As mentioned in a previous chapter, the first nurse's uniform worn in this country was designed for the first class of students at Bellevue Training School in 1873. Since that time many schools of nursing have developed distinctive school caps and pins, which reflect the school's history and tradition and which graduates cherish and wear with great pride.

White traditionally has been the color of the nurse's uniform. However, some schools have adopted washable colors for student's uniforms and some hospitals require uniforms of particular colors for wear in certain clinical areas, such as the psychiatric or pediatric units. Irrespective of color, the nurse's distinctive uniform identifies her to the patient and his family as well as to her co-workers while she is on duty.

Because the uniform is a part of the nurse's public image, nurses should respect the uniform and the traditions it represents. Both the students' and graduate nurses' uniforms should be worn only during working hours. Uniforms should not be worn with jewelry, except a school pin or name plate. A school pin or insignia of a professional organization should be honored and worn in the prescribed manner and for prescribed occasions.

The nurse's uniform cap. The cap has both sentimental and traditional significance for its wearers. While the uniforms of graduate nurses reflect the prevailing styles, the cap of a particular school usually remains the same. A nurse's cap, like the old school tie or academic robes, identifies the school at which she received her preparatory nursing education. The cap is the identifying link between the graduate and the student currently enrolled in the nursing program.

Formerly, when students entered a school of nursing they were not given a cap as part of their original uniform. The cap was to be earned after a period of "probation." Using the cap as a special award is being questioned, and there is a growing trend toward regarding the cap as part of the student's complete uniform and including it as such from the outset. This has a positive psychologic value for both students and the patients to whom they are assigned.

Some leaders in nursing have expressed the opinion that too much importance is attached to the cap, and at least one collegiate program in the country does not require caps for its students or its graduates. Male nurses do not wear caps. If your school of nursing uniform includes a distinctive cap, it should, of course, be worn in accordance with established regulations.

Because the nurse's personality is reflected in her personal appearance, the following items pertaining to the wearing of a uniform may be useful to review:

1. Every item comprising the complete uniform of the nurse should always be spotlessly clean, well fitting, and in good repair.
2. Shoes and hosiery worn with a uniform should provide for maximum comfort. The color of each is generally in accord with acceptable style or specified by regulations.
3. A uniform designated for wear in a given hospital area such as the operating room is worn in line of duty and according to established policy. It is not to be worn outside the specified department.
4. Modification of any authorized uniform to suit your individual preference is not permitted by the dictates of both good taste and integrity. Changing the appearance of an established uniform through the use of fancy handkerchiefs, jewelry, or excessive use of cosmetics negates the uniform's basic purpose and reflects the nurse's poor understanding of professional conduct.

ATTITUDES

An individual's personality is shaped by her attitudes. An attitude is defined as a manner of acting, feeling, or thinking that is indicated by your response toward another person, situation, or experience. An attitude is part of a pattern of personal behavior. It is based on opinions, viewpoints, or feelings. You develop attitudes toward life in general, toward other persons, and toward yourself in relation to your own growth and development.

Attitudes are your responses to specific experiences. They are not dormant and inactive. Every person changes his opinions and points of view from time to time as additional knowledge is gained and his understanding is broadened. Attitudes are developed by using skills, by your interest in living, and your knowledge of life. Your behavior communicates your attitudes to others, and a change in any attitude is evident by a corresponding change in your behavior.

Have you ever tried to evaluate your attitudes? As a student nurse, how do you feel about study, profitable use of your available time, or daily activities designed to ensure your well-rounded development? How do you react to your classmates, co-workers, employees serving in areas where you are assigned, and to the instructors who teach your various classes? What are your reactions to established rules and regulations, organized direction of your activities, to the demands for functioning within a structured time schedule, and reporting or "signing in"? The manner in which you respond in each of the above situations will reveal to others a part of your personality.

Attitudes are developed from awareness of yourself in relation to individuals and to situations. Attitudes are the result of an integration of the knowledge, skills, experiences, and interests acquired during your lifetime. To determine what your attitudes are at any given period, think about your own feelings about yourself and your evaluation of self as you relate to other people in both direct and indirect relationships.

As a maturing young adult, you are expected to use constructive criticisms made by others. You are also expected to analyze your learning experiences with objectivity as you work with instructors and co-workers. Your way of doing things may change. You will gain self-assurance as you learn to identify and accept your strengths and weaknesses.

The ability to understand and deal with your own attitudes should keep you near the median on the scale that balances comfortable and uncomfortable feelings. As a student nurse, and later as a graduate, the development of your attitudes will affect the rapport so essential in relationships with others. Your attitude toward a patient should reveal a warmth that communicates acceptance, sincerity, and helpfulness. Your attitudes should also allow you to be flexible in exercising judgment in your nurse-patient relationships.

New attitudes are acquired and old attitudes are changed as you mature. The proper attitude will help you to deal effectively with patients and their needs as well as with the requirements and expectations of instructors, supervisors, and physicians.

DISPOSITION AND ABILITY

You demonstrate friendliness toward others in the manner in which you meet and greet them and in the way you convey your acceptance of them. Your facial expression, tone of voice, the attention you pay to what another person is saying, and your ability to transmit sincerity and warmth are all positive factors in your personality. Willingness to help others, patience in responding to inquiries, and your ability to be sympathetic will mark you as a considerate, thoughtful person. How you participate in group activities, become involved in group efforts, share responsibility for work assignments, accept criticism, and give credit to others distinguish you as a valued team member. Your ability to establish and maintain a neat and orderly environment and your plan for work organization characterize you as an efficient worker. These positive facets of personality are pleasant to possess and to share, and their importance as elements of a nurse's personality should be evident.

Certain unhelpful or negative personality traits also deserve consideration. For example, a sullen, moody nurse who is uncooperative in her associations with classmates and co-workers or who meets requests for assistance with rudeness or defensiveness is in for a sorry time (and so are those with whom she works and for whom she cares). If a nurse responds to a patient's comments or requests in a careless manner, if displeasure or temper are shown because things do not seem to go her way, or if unjust or unwarranted criticism is voiced about personnel or the learning situation, steps must be taken for her own sake and for the sake of those around her to investigate the underlying causes and determine the best ways to help everyone concerned to deal with them.

Personality types will be studied in detail in psychology and psychiatric nursing courses. You will learn that individual personality traits may be altered through a conscientious effort to understand their causes and develop other traits to replace them. Success in such instances depends on willingness to admit that a problem exists, acceptance of help in working at the problem, and the degree to which the person truly desires to change.

These ideas about what constitutes a person's character and personality traits should become more meaningful as you correlate information obtained in classes that provide for detailed study of these subjects. At the same time your relationships with other people whose character attributes and personality traits are different from your own gives you the opportunity to note traits which you possess and which, hopefully, are positive influences for your personal happiness and welfare. You have a share of positive traits. Use them and strengthen them by applying them in your daily life.

Also, identify those traits that need to be adjusted or eliminated from your personality. Determine to do something positive about them. If you are willing to learn, willing to seek and accept the help you need, and ready to initiate the changes indicated, you can accomplish wonders. Should you possess the qualities of character and personality that will assure successful attainment of your goals in nursing, acknowledge your gift with gratitude and humility. Help someone less fortunate to develop her potential by your assistance and encouragement.

BIBLIOGRAPHY

Burton, G.: Personal, impersonal and interpersonal relations, ed. 2, New York, 1958, Springer Publishing Co.

Hay, G.: This way to happiness, New York, 1967, Simon & Shuster, Inc.

Jourard, S. M.: Personal adjustments, New York, 1958, The Macmillan Co.

Kelly, C. W.: Dimensions of professional nursing, ed. 2, New York, 1968, The Macmillan Co.

Moore, Dom Thomas Verner and Stevens, Dom Gregory: Principles of ethics, ed. 5, Philadelphia, 1959, J. B. Lippincott Co.

Ohara, F. J.: Psychology and the nurse, ed. 5, Philadelphia, W. B. Saunders Co.

Ross, C. F.: Personal and vocational relationships in practical nursing, ed. 3, Philadelphia, 1969, J. B. Lippincott Co.

Wolff, I. S.: The educated heart, American Journal of Nursing 63:58-60, Apr. 1963.

COMPLETE WORK SHEET ON PP. 313 AND 314

CHAPTER 7

Learning and working as a student in the nursing program

As a student in nursing you will frequently find that you are a member of a group, whether at home, in the nurses' residence, in a college dormitory, in various hospital clinical areas, or in other health agencies. As a member of these groups you will need to learn to accept others and to respect their rights. You also need to learn to develop the kinds of relationships that will assure opportunities for continuing personal growth as potential members of a profession. It is taken for granted each of you has had some experience in assuming responsibility, in caring for your personal possessions, in sharing, and in being accountable for materials and resources used jointly with others. However, since the nursing program will make specific demands on you, it is important to consider some of those areas that contribute to your learning and working as a student nurse.

RESPECTING THE RIGHTS OF OTHERS

Respect for the rights of others is a fundamental and necessary element in group interaction. This respect includes recognizing the property of others and the need to preserve the integrity of the environment shared by all. You must also respect another person's right to privacy and his right to courtesy. Basic to the respect for the rights of others is recognition of the inherent uniqueness of each human being.

A sense of justice and fundamental respect for other people demands that you have a similar attitude toward their possessions and your use of them. A person's property is his to use or dispose of as he wishes. It is not your privilege to avail yourself of someone else's property without permission. In turn, you have the right to expect the same respect and fairness from others in regard to your property. Borrowing, expropriation, or taking someone else's posssession without permission is not only inappropriate but is an affront to the rightful owner.

Your classes in ethics and professional relationships will consider in detail the moral and legal consequences of taking and using the property of others in an unfair or improper way. Such conduct not only indicates a disrespect for the rights of others, but also disrupts the harmonious relationships within groups. Unless controlled, it can lead to extremely serious consequences.

Successful group living depends to a large degree on the respect with which each member treats the common living areas of the group. While personal neatness and grooming present one image, the neatness and order of your living areas provide another image. The way you use and care for equipment and material available for group use and the way in which clean-up procedures are carried out after using group facilities reflect your awareness of the shared right to a pleasant, orderly environment.

People who are careless of the feelings and

rights of others with regard to shared living areas will not be welcomed by the group. It is hoped that you have developed the habit of order and have learned to care for your personal belongings and equipment.

Everyone has a right to privacy. Your instructors will repeatedly stress the importance of a patient's right to privacy and your responsibilities as a nurse to preserve and guard this right. You should also respect the right of your fellow students' privacy.

There are times when every normal person feels the need for being alone. This right to privacy, especially within the framework of group living, is most essential and should be respected. It would be expected that you observe the rules of common courtesy when the person indicates by a closed door, for example, that intrusion is not welcomed. Knocking first and requesting permission to enter is a courtesy that should be extended at any time when entering another's room. Your instructors will point out that, in general, this same courtesy is indicated when seeking admission to a patient's room when the door is closed, unless he has requested your presence by signal light or intercom system or unless circumstances dictate otherwise.

Living and working in groups is a challenge in learning how to get along with people, in developing your skills in understanding individuals, and in accepting others. Although persons differ as individuals, they all have the same basic needs. Each one desires a unique identity, acceptance, approval of his actions, and the feeling that he is important to other people. Preconceived ideas of another's worth based on personal prejudices or stereotyped thinking are unacceptable. The rights of others demand honest and fair interpersonal relationships. Certainly students in nursing will recognize that respect for a person and his rights is basic to getting along and working together for a common goal.

HOW SPEECH AND CONVERSATION CHARACTERIZE YOU

A person's voice, speech habits, and conversational abilities reveal an individual's personality and characteristics. A student is expected to be aware of the impression her voice makes on others and to develop effective speaking techniques for use in conversational exchanges.

Interest in other people can be reflected in the tone of voice, the careful pronunciation of names, and the ways in which others are encouraged to participate in verbal exchanges. Modulation of the volume and the carrying qualities of one's voice within living quarters is a *must* for people living together. It is important, also, to consider the carrying qualities of one's voice when conversing with friends, co-workers, and patients. A low, whispering, or sibilant-like type of voice can be as annoying and distracting as one that is loud and brassy. A speaking voice that is pleasant to hear conveys a warmth and sincerity to listeners and creates a positive image of the speaker.

Conversational habits also affect those with whom you live and work. Your instructors will probably discuss problems that can result when conversation is not controlled. Careless chattering and indulgence in "shop talk" can dim other qualities in a nurse's personality and may even affect her acceptance by patients and co-workers. It is taken for granted that you will avoid careless habits of speech, excessive use of slang, and the use of profane, obscene, or offensive terms. People reveal their awareness and sensitivity to others as well as their feelings about themselves in their conversation. It is also well to remember that silence, in certain situations, can be as expressive as speech.

Living and working with others require the development of a sense of responsibility for social interaction with your associates. Within a family there is a loyalty and respect toward each member that makes possible the performance of various services and acts of kindness without expectation of payment. The same loyalty and respect should be extended to your fellow students in the course of daily living.

Living with others in the nurses' residence or dormitory should generate a feeling of loyalty to the group as a whole. There are loyalties to classmates that are basic to a spirit of cooperation and identity as a class. There is a sense of loyalty and social responsiveness toward roommates or particular friends in times of stress and in times of pleasure, and these feelings are the foundations of firm and lasting friendships. This sense of social responsibility involves awareness of human and interpersonal relationships and the need for their continuing development as you move through your educational program and the experiences of daily living.

Instructors, counselors, and supervisors will continually discuss and stress the importance of recognizing and accepting other people as worthy of your best efforts in service. It is on this basic principle that the structure of personal relationships is built and developed and upon which nursing care is based.

One of the significant factors that affect both the pattern of group living and learning to work as a member within a group is obedience or the ability to be obedient. The relationship between obedience and justice was discussed in Chapter 6. The practice of being obedient is reviewed here briefly because it is important in interpersonal relationships, and it has a major effect on the working and living activities of both individuals and groups.

Obedience requires the use of willpower rather than feelings. It requires thinking and evaluation. Obedience focuses on the performance of assignments in accordance with the order or regulations of an authority, who in turn is responsible for maintaining harmonious relationships within the social order. The practice of obedience implies a willingness on the part of the one obeying, as well as a trust in the judgment and goodwill of the authority. It also implies a belief that instructions have been formulated for the general welfare. It is unfortunate when obedience is enforced upon others in a spirit of tyranny or when it is obtained because of fear or expediency. In such instances respect for the individual and his rights is absent, and those affronted are likely to respond in kind.

Certain degrees of obedience are essential in one's life. Your welfare is often involved with, and dependent upon, the manner in which you respond to authority and how you carry out the rules and regulations intended to assist you in organizing and shaping the many life situations you will experience.

BUILDING A SYMMETRICAL LIFE

Have you defined your philosophy of life? Do you understand what a philosophy of life is and how it is developed? Do you see any relationship between one's philosophy of life and one's philosophy of service? These are questions which you, as a student in nursing, should ask yourself. Philosophy is defined both as the pursuit of wisdom and the ideals and beliefs by which a person lives. Philosophy considers basic truths relating to behavior, moral values, order, and balance. The various philosophies can aid you in establishing basic values and standards of conduct, in arriving at decisions concerning behavior, and in suggesting those activities that help you to achieve your goals. Philosophy is related to the study of ethics and logic and to man's recognition of a Supreme Being or source of order in his world.

In a more personal sense, one's philosophy of life is concerned with those basic truths that contribute to personal growth in a systematic fashion and with those principles that relate to the moral values that shape the facets of character. Some consideration of how character is developed has been presented in Chapter 6.

Your personal philosophy will have a direct bearing on your philosophy of nursing and on the kind of nurse you will be. Think about the factors that motivated you to become a student nurse. What ideals prompted you to consider this career? Do you think of your commitment to nursing as being, according to one author, a combination of ego-identification and self-realization in a career having "deeper implications than just giving [you] a means of earning a living, or attaining social status"?* Is your motivation a "fractional commitment,"† to be served in pro-

*Vaillot, Sister Madeleine Clemance: Commitment to nursing, Philadelphia, 1962, J. B. Lippincott Co., p. 16-17.

†Mayes, N., Schultz, M. N., and Pierce, C. M.: Commitment to nursing—how is it achieved? Nursing Outlook 16:29-31, July 1968.

portion to other demands such as the need for a home and family? Or did you enter nursing to use your education as a basic foundation for ultimate transfer to another career choice? Answers to these questions will reveal the degree of commitment the nurse feels toward nursing.

While one can learn the theory of nursing and become proficient in the performance of nursing techniques, commitment to either a personal philosophy or a philosophy of service cannot be taught or transmitted. Commitment is inherent in one's being. It can only be developed by intense personal effort. If you are committed to nursing you will *be* a nurse rather than *act in the role* of a nurse. The decision must be yours, and it must be made fairly. The results of your decision will be evident to those with whom you live and work as well as to those whose needs you try to meet through the services you perform.

Closely allied with your development of a personal philosophy of life is the plan for expanding your spiritual life. Man is a finite being. He posseses an exquisite physical structure, an intellect, and a free will, which places him above all other creatures. His origin, his existence, and his purpose for living centers on a Higher Being who regulates the activities of the universe.

It is in the nature of man to seek answers to his questions. He strives for the betterment of his environment and aspires toward qualitative changes in his life. But in doing these things man is dependent on a source outside himself for guidance and sustenance. This source of help and support is referred to broadly as his spiritual life.

The following discourse was delivered in 1831 by John Henry Newman, who, as a newly ordained Anglican minister, served as Select Preacher at Oxford University, England. It illustrates Newman's view of the significance of the bond which exists between God and man.

> We are not sent into this world for nothing;
> we are not born at random;
> we are not here that we may go to bed at night,
> and get up in the morning, toil for our bread, eat and drink, laugh and joke, sin when we have a mind,
> and reform when we are tired of sinning, rear a family and die.
> God sees every one of us; He creates every soul,
> He lodges it in the body, one by one, for a purpose.
> He needs, He deigns to need every one of us.
> He has an end for each of us;
> we are all equal in His sight,
> and we are placed in our different ranks and stations,
> not to get what we can out of them for ourselves,
> but to labour in them for Him.

It is difficult to conceive of nurses as failing to recognize the significance of the spiritual component in their lives and the values of relating this aspect to the development of their philosophy of life. More specific consideration will be given elsewhere to provision for spiritual health in the life of the nurse as well as consideration of nurses' abilities and obligations to provide for spiritual health in the lives of the patients whom they serve.

RECREATION: A VITAL PART OF LIVING

There are many ways in which students can relax from the daily routine of work and study. Participation in group and individual sports offers an outlet for energies and enthusiasms. The active sports such as tennis, golf, swimming, surfing, skiing, hiking, or horseback riding are popular sources of exercise and fun. Dancing and teaching others the sets for square dances or folk dances are also sources of relaxation.

An interest in the arts may be stimulated or developed through visits to art museums and exhibits, plays, the opera, and concerts. Those students who have had a musical education should certainly feel justified in continuing to participate in musical groups and choirs. Lectures, demonstrations, and travelogues may have special interest for some, while others enjoy reading, movies, television, or simply talking with others.

Hobbies are another source of pleasure and relaxation. Working in arts and crafts, making decorative embroidery, sewing, knitting, or collecting stamps and coins are not only enjoyable but may also be a source of pin money if items are offered for sale. These kinds of activities and special interests can add to your enjoyment and give you the chance to share your interests with others.

An anonymous author in this "Old English Prayer" sums up the essence of a rich and full life in this way:

Take time to work—
It is the price of success.
Take time to think—
It is the source of power.
Take time to play—
It is the secret of perpetual youth.
Take time to read—
It is the fountain of wisdom.
Take time to be friendly—
It is the road to happiness.
Take time to dream—
It is hitching your wagon to a star.
Take time to love and to be loved—
It is the privilege of the gods.
Take time to look around—
It is too short a day to be selfish.
Take time to laugh—
It is the music of the soul.

DEVELOPING AN ATTITUDE FOR STUDY

To study means that a deliberate effort is made to use your mind in order to acquire knowledge and understanding. It requires that you direct your attention to the careful investigation of many aspects of a subject, not only to find out about the subject matter, but also to understand and find out more about yourself. The act of using your intellectual powers for study requires that you learn and practice definite habits of self-discipline in your work as a student.

You are preparing yourself to become an efficient and competent participant in nursing service. This identification places on each of you an obligation to apply yourself to the tasks associated with learning. To become an effective and competent practitioner you must be well acquainted and at ease with the basic elements of nursing. There are no exceptions to this principle.

It might be assumed that students in nursing programs who have completed their school's scholastic requirements and qualified for admission would have developed sound, workable study habits. Unfortunately, this is not always true. In many instances the students have not learned these habits of study during high school and, as a result, are not equipped to accept and to carry out the study requirements of the planned academic schedule in the school of nursing.

The inability of many students to take on the job of study is reflected in the attrition or drop-out rates in nursing programs. The reasons given most frequently for students withdrawing from nursing programs are "scholastic problems," "academic difficulties," or "failure to meet program's requirements."

The hypothetical cases of two students and their grade point averages described in Chapter 10 illustrate the results of effective and ineffective approaches to the demands of study. One thing is certain. Each individual must assume the responsibility of developing a technique of study that is effective and workable for *him.* The proper study techniques, when used consistently, become an integral part of a person's pattern for learning.

It is essential that each student enrolled in a nursing program work out an effective study plan as part of the daily schedule, and to make this a "top priority" matter to be dealt with immediately. Of course, students may have problems that can affect their study habits, such as poor reading skills, poor language interpretation, inadequate foundations in basic mathematics, or poor spelling. If this is the case, it may be necessary to ask for additional help from teachers or counselors, but *it is the student's responsibility to learn the techniques he needs for effective study and then apply them in the process of learning.*

Let us suppose, for a moment, that you are a student wrestling with the increasing demands your studies make upon you. You find that really learning and *knowing* course content and being prepared for class take more time and effort than you bargained for. More is expected of you now than had been in any previous educational experience. In high school you may have "gotten by" using techniques and tricks that every student tries with varying degrees of success. Now you discover that the situation is different. The greater competition within the group, and the increasing difficulty of sequential courses, and the necessity of meeting schedules for classes and clinical practice place difficult demands on you. The *reality* of your situation is that procrastination or cramming the night before an examination is simply not going to work. Such excuses as "I didn't need to study in high school so I haven't learned how," "I've been away from school for so long I'm out of the habit of studying," or "I didn't know nursing would be so hard" may cover your anxiety, but they do not help you to accomplish your work.

Why *are* you in the nursing program? In the first place you were selected because your ability to learn was shown by your high school record of achievement and by the results of the pre-entrance tests to measure your aptitude for nursing. Since you have the potential and the aptitude to be a nurse, the question you must ask yourself is "Do I *want to learn* to be a nurse?" If your present study habits are not likely to help you meet the demands of your educational program, do you want to make the effort needed to change your study habits? If you do not face up to this question squarely, and soon, the initiative will pass out of your hands. You are the one responsible for doing something positive about your study habits.

Start out by drawing up a schedule for your daily activities, dividing and allotting enough time to cover all study requirements. If you need advice or suggestions from instructors and counselors, *ask for it.* They will encourage and assist you, but you must understand that *they cannot do the job for you.*

Several publications dealing with methods of study are available in libraries and book stores. Classes in psychology and study orientation offer considerable discussion of the learning process, the use of textbooks and bibliographic resources, and ways of developing effective study habits. There is no *one* guaranteed method for successful study. This is an individual matter that you must work out for yourself. The logical approach is to identify what your study problems are, understand why they are problems, and then devise a plan to try to solve them.

The following may serve as a guide to approaching the problems of study. It may also have value for students who wish to check themselves on their established study techniques.

Why study?

The purpose of study is to learn new knowledge, to learn new ways of applying previously learned information, to use what you know to meet your immediate needs, and to build a foundation from which you may progress toward a future goal.

Study, or the acquisition of new knowledge, serves as an incentive for continued learning and personal development.

One aspect of study that is especially important in nursing is the coordination of mental ability and manual dexterity. Practice will help you to achieve the competence that identifies the qualified, skilled practitioner.

The effective use of study stimulates and encourages intellectual curiosity and the ability to use knowledge for the enrichment of one's personal life and resources.

How to develop an attitude for study

Look at your study habits squarely and honestly. Identify those factors that prevent or inhibit your intentions to study.

Take a positive position in relation to study. Accept the fact that study is work (concentration), that it involves a desire to learn (motivation and curiosity), and that it requires direction (purpose) toward a goal.

Look for ideas and try to understand the content. Do not study only for the purpose of passing a test or making a grade.

Work out a pattern for daily study that meets your specific needs.

Discipline yourself to adhere to your study plan.

Rounding out your study techniques

In class:

Pay attention in classes and participate in class discussion and activities. Prepare for class by previewing materials to be presented in class. Familiarity with content is your responsibility.

Listen to the instructor's presentation.

Take note of the way material is organized.

Pay attention to diagrams, demonstrations, use of equipment, and audio-visual aids.

Ask for clarification of subject matter presented or for additional relevant information.

Make effective use of texts and assigned references. Use your own text; underline and add marginal notes; identify key points for future review.

Take notes. Use ideas rather than verbatim statements. Stress important points. Emphasize principles.

Out of class:

Adhere to a daily schedule for study.

Choose a place for study that is comfortable and satisfactory.

Keep in mind the surroundings *you* need in order to concentrate and the availability of the equipment needed to prepare your work.

Use the particular techniques of study best suited for the requirements of each class.

Avoid wasting time.

Apply yourself to the task to be done.

Review notes taken in previous classes.

Think about the class discussion; look up errors made on quizzes or tests.

Revise and enlarge on notes, as indicated, for future use.

Preparation for the next class involves thought about the assignment and its relationship to other classes and to previous learning.

Read the text and references carefully.

Use a dictionary whenever necessary.

Apply information gained in one class to other classes.

Seek outside help from instructors if you need it.

Try to think of tests as a challenge to your ability to read, to think, and to use knowledge with discrimination and judgment.

Utilize all resources available to broaden your understanding of a subject and to serve as a basis for extending your knowledge to other areas in which you are involved both personally and professionally.

USING PERSONAL RESOURCES IN A POSITIVE WAY

Health, intelligence, peace of mind, a sense of security, and a sense of humor are all personal resources inherent to some degree in every person. It rests with each person to cultivate and strengthen his own resources and to draw upon them as he works and learns.

The use of time. The moral responsibility you have for the use of time has been presented in Chapter 6. Let us consider the use of time as a personal resource. You, as a nurse, are expected to be conscious of time in a special way because, to you, time has a different significance than it has for people in many other fields of work. You must be conscientious in administering medications or treatments on time. You must carry out procedures and nursing assignments at the times for which they are scheduled. As a student, you will be reporting for duty on time, completing your patient care assignments on time, and handing in term papers on time. Your use of time should be such that you are able to include others in your life as well as arrange time for your own needs and pleasures.

> You wake up in the morning,
> and lo!
> your purse is magically filled
> with twenty-four hours
> of the unmanufactured tissue
> of the universe of your life.
> It is yours.
> It is the most precious of possessions.
> No one can take it from you.
> It is unstealable.
> And no one receives
> either more or less
> than you receive.
>
> ARNOLD BENNETT*

Health. Good health is surely everyone's most valuable personal resource. This is especially true of nurses and other allied health personnel. Anything that interferes with health or contributes to the loss of health will lessen your ability to perform your nursing duties. Students enter

*Bennett, A.: How to live 24 hours a day, 1910. Reprinted by permission of Mrs. Dorothy Cheston Bennett.

the nursing program in good physical condition. Common sense requires that they observe the rules of physical health to maintain this prime condition.

Rest and sleep sufficient to maintain your physical reserve is your personal responsibility. Lack of rest (both mental and physical) plays a greater part in sapping vitality than any other cause. Efficiency and the ability to concentrate are adversely affected after any sustained period of work or study. This is the reason why the coffee break has become such a popular practice.

A brisk walk after prolonged study, a trip to the swimming pool, a visit to a shopping center for an interval of "window wishing" after coming off duty, a few hours on the golf course or tennis court, or puttering in the garden are all forms of relaxation to provide a change of pace in one's daily activities.

A vacation is an important means of conserving personal health. The term "vacation" means a period of rest and freedom from the usual work assignments. It is an intermission—a time for recreation through a change in environment, work activities or concentration. Hopefully, a vacation period is preceded by plans to do something different, meet new people, and broaden interests. A vacation can refresh your general outlook and should help you to return to your job with renewed vigor and interest in performing the usual tasks. When properly used, vacation periods can be sound personal investments in health and happiness.

Intelligence. Intelligence is the ability to learn or understand from experience. It is the ability to retain knowledge. Intelligence is what enables you to use your past experience to respond quickly and successfully in new situations. It involves the ability to reason things out or to think through a problem to solve it. The depth and extent of knowledge are dependent upon how well intelligence is applied. You never stop learning, but the capacity to learn depends upon the degree to which you exercise your intellectual powers.

In order to learn and work effectively you should recognize and develop your natural sense of curiosity about the things occurring in today's world and seek answers to the questions you have. The surest way of stimulating your intelligence is to look for different answers to problems and to challenge existing answers and conditions.

Peace of mind. An anonymous author has said, "We cannot control the things that happen to us, but we can control the way we face up to them." Peace of mind is as necessary as security in our lives. The two are often interrelated. Peace of mind does not come from things outside you; you must create it for yourself. Peace of mind means that the mind is free of any disproportionate degree of mental conflict, such as restlessness, uneasiness, or anxiety. Peace of mind is not compatible with strong feelings of fear, anger, jealousy, guilt, or worry.

Peace of mind is achieved by doing the best you can and *recognizing that it is the best you can do.* This requires an awareness and honest acceptance of your limitations and abilities. The three most common causes of mental upset are anxiety over past events, fear of new adjustments, and worry over anticipated occurrences. None of these negative attitudes need dominate your life if you *learn to be at peace with yourself.*

A sense of security. A sense of security also depends upon knowledge and acceptance of yourself. It is an awareness of yourself in relation to those with whom you live and work. Security has its source in self-respect and self-confidence, as well. These qualities enable you to confront and adjust to the varying conditions of life. Security means also that you have an idea of what you want your life to mean so that you may live from day to day in an organized manner.

Security shapes your ability to accept correction, rules, and new ideas. It helps you to appreciate, rather than fear, the necessity of change. The secure individual avoids complaining, sarcasm, self-pity, rationalization, and similar mechanisms that serve only to evade life situations and perhaps hurt others.

A sense of humor. Many definitions of this personal resource may be offered, and you may have one of your own. While it may be difficult to define, a sense of humor is easy to recognize. Briefly, it is the faculty for recognizing and appreciating the humorous or fanciful side of the things that make up life and daily living. As opposed to wit, which is used consciously to entertain, a sense of humor connotes kindliness and geniality and is more an expression of sympathetic amusement.

Persons with a sense of humor are in the habit of looking at life from the bright side and of seeing the pleasures and joys of living. They can enjoy the amusing aspects of everyday happenings and share their thoughts and feelings with others. They have a tolerant, accepting attitude toward themselves and others. They can laugh at themselves when the situation warrants it.

A sense of humor is invaluable in the life of a nurse. It can be a redeeming factor at the times when the going is hard. To be able to laugh at yourself and to see the humor in situations will ease many tense moments and contribute greatly to the serenity and tranquility of your life.

PROBLEM-SOLVING

The ability to face up to problems and resolve them in a satisfactory manner is one sign of a well-integrated, mature person. Problems, or challenges, are a part of daily life, and may influence your future life and activities, depending on your capacity for dealing with them. One method for dealing with problems is an arrangement of logical steps identified by the general title of "problem-solving technique." The problem-solving technique is a means of considering each aspect of the existing problem in relation to the whole. Three things are necessary for the operation of this technique. There must be an awareness that a problem exists; an ability on the part of those involved with the problem to think about it, make sensible judgments, and draw conclusions; and finally there must be an accurate determination of the cause.

Problem-solving is concerned with *what* the problem is and *why* it is a problem; *how* the problem might be solved; *testing* the proposed solution, and *evaluating* the results. The word "problem" is used in the sense of a question, subject area, or situation that requires a solution. It is also used in the sense of a question, subject area, or situation that is perplexing or difficult and about which more information or understanding is sought.

As a technique, problem-solving is universal in its application. It can be used either by an individual or by a group of persons working together to solve a problem of common concern. The problem-solving technique can be applied to almost any situation or problem whether the problem is personal or concerns aspects of professional life such as patient care and clinical practice, human relations, the use of supplies and equipment, accident control, improving nursing techniques and procedures, better ways to hold a nursing team conference, how to disseminate information to hospital employees, the reasons for patients' gripes, or how to arrange coffee breaks.

The problem-solving technique involves a careful study of all aspects of a problem and the factors contributing to it, and action, in accordance with the findings, to bring about a desired change or final outcome. The steps in the problem-solving technique are summarized in the figure on p. 94.

HOW THE PROBLEM-SOLVING TECHNIQUE IS USED

Suppose that there is a problem in your school because students fail to read the bulletin board daily in spite of a regulation requiring them to do so. As a result of this failure, students miss important notices. For example, seven students failed to report for their uniform measurements on the appointed day when the representative of the uniform company was at the school. On the surface it would appear that this "problem" is a simple one—students did not comply with a school regulation. The situation *could* be handled in a routine manner through appropriate disciplinary action. But will discipline prevent the same problem from occurring again? Past experience indicates that it will not. Let us

PROBLEM-SOLVING TECHNIQUE

1. Identify and define problem

Get the facts.

Determine what the problem is and why it is a problem.

Identify the basic problem or issue and prepare a statement of same.

2. Study the facts

Fit the facts together.

Analyze and interpret the information.

Draw conclusions based on resulting evidence.

Get additional facts, if needed.

State final conclusion.

Consider possible courses of action.

3. Take action—test your solution

Decide on a workable plan to test your solution.

Implement the plan.

Study effects of the plan.

Check results closely.

4. Evaluate results

Consider results of test.

Did it solve the problem?

Ask yourself whether your decision (solution) was effective or wise.

then try to find a solution using the problem-solving technique.

Identify and define problem. Sometimes there is more difficulty with a situation connected with the main problem than with the problem itself. The first order of business in studying a problem is to determine what the problem actually is and why it is a problem. To answer these two questions we must gather all the information we can find that has any bearing on the subject, taking care to utilize every available source. The nature of the problem will determine what information is needed as well as the sources of it. In our example, the logical sources of information are:

1. The student handbook
2. The school's administrative manual
3. Location and number of bulletin boards
4. Persons who have responsibility for the bulletin boards
5. Interviews with students for their opinions
6. Interviews with instructors for their version of the problem

The purpose of the investigation is to gather as much information and understanding as possible about the problem and its real cause. Let us assume that the following facts have been uncovered in the course of the investigation.

1. The student handbook states that all students should read the bulletin board daily. There is no explanation or interpretation of this responsibility in the statement.
2. The administrative manual for the school of nursing office contains a statement of policy that a bulletin board shall be maintained. However, no provision was found for an administrative procedure to maintain the bulletin board—the types of in-

formation that will be posted, how long items are to remain on the bulletin board, or the responsibility of adding new items and to remove items are not defined. In practice, anyone may post a notice on the bulletin board. It is not unusual to find notices posted by instructors, class officers, and alumni members next to a "want-ad," a poster for the community's Little Theatre group, or announcements of upcoming social and cultural events.

3. The nursing office secretary posts all official directives and announcements as instructed by the director. When queried on when posting is done, the secretary stated, "When I get them typed, and sometimes I have to wait until they are signed." Class schedules for the upcoming week must be posted by noon on Wednesdays. The instructors and class counselors had been in the habit of preparing and posting their own notices.
4. There are two bulletin boards. A large one, located in the main hall (class room section of the residence) opposite the director's office, is the official bulletin board. This is referred to as the "central" bulletin board. A smaller one, located in the residence near the elevator, is used only for posting the weekly class schedules.
5. Students' opinions revealed the following:
   a. The bulletin board is so cluttered that it is not easy to spot new items when they appear.
   b. Several students mentioned they "did not like to stand around reading the bulletin board when the director's door was open."
   c. A student, one of the seven "guilty" ones in the latest incident, mentioned that the notice about the uniforms was not posted when she made her daily visit to check the bulletin board.
   d. Another student volunteered that she missed an important notice because it was posted "an hour after I read the bulletin board."
   e. The location of the bulletin board meant that the students had to make several trips to the main hall each day in order to see if there was anything new posted.
6. Instructors' versions of the problem contributed the following facts:
   a. The problem is a recurring one. "Students just will not read the bulletin board."
   b. The latest incident required the representative of the uniform company, which is located in another city, to rearrange his schedule for a second trip to the school. This caused the administration considerable embarrassment.

From the above facts it would appear that the real problem is not so much the students' failure in complying with a regulation, but rather to make the bulletin board a more effective communication device.

Study the facts. When the facts are all in and studied in relation to each other, the evidence points to the bulletin board as being the basic issue in this problem. Students' lackadaisical attitude toward the regulation on checking the bulletin board stems from the disorganized, cluttered state of the bulletin board itself. The conscientious students do make an effort to consult the board each day as they have been instructed, but they react to it as a tedious responsibility. Others don't bother, and rely on getting their information from their classmates. The bulletin board is a catch-all for all sorts of information and no one is responsible for its order and organization.

The following conclusions seem to be reasonable ones in this case:

1. The bulletin board needs to be made a more effective communication device. Students need to feel that what they find on the bulletin board will be of interest and importance to them.
2. An administrative procedure should be adopted for the use and control of the bulletin board.

3. The students' responsibility for information posted on the bulletin board should be clearly spelled out in the handbook, and students should be held accountable for this responsibility.

Take action—test your solution. In this step we are concerned with solving the problem. Again it must be pointed out that the nature of the problem will determine the methods used in solving it. If the problem under study were a personal one, or one that came within the scope of your responsibility, then you would be at liberty to set up your own plan and test your solution of the problem. This, however, is an administrative problem so any solution you might propose will require administrative approval. This being the case, the plan for solving the problem will necessarily be presented in the form of a recommendation to the nursing school administration.

The plan of action for smoothing out some of the problems associated with bulletin boards is summarized below.

1. One person should be assigned the job of posting items and removing items from the bulletin board and maintaining it.
2. The central bulletin board should be divided into three sections marked NEW, SPECIAL, and PERMANENT. All items are then to be posted under one of these headings. This will result in better organization and help to emphasize new items.
3. Every item of a temporary nature should be coded with the date. The bulletin board "life" of these items should not exceed three days, after which items will be removed and filed or discarded. Directives, regulations, and other material of a more permanent nature, as well as the weekly class schedules, are to remain as long as the information is pertinent.
4. To avoid indiscriminate use of the bulletin board, all notices, announcements, and the like (except the instructors' notices) should be cleared either by the Director or someone appointed to this responsibility.
5. All new notices and announcements including changes in class schedules (when possible), should be posted on the bulletin board before 12:00 noon. This will allow students to consult the board just once a day and they will be assured of not missing any items.
6. The small bulletin board should be retained for its present use.
7. The Student Handbook should be updated to include a reference to the responsibility for students reading the bulletin board each day after 12:00 p.m.

Evaluate results. The final step in problem-solving requires that the solution be evaluated following a trial period to determine whether the solution of the problem is a workable one and whether it has achieved the desired result. If the sample we are using here had been an actual problem, and if the nursing school administration had approved and adopted the plan, it would be possible to see whether the job of problem-solving was well done.

The problem-solving technique may be used in almost any problematic situation. Tackling a problem with this technique is challenging and stimulating because it requires systematic thinking. You will be amazed at how radically different some problems will seem to you after you have pushed your thinking to develop a valid series of generalizations about the problem. As a word of comfort to the student using the problem-solving technique for the first time, it will become easier each time you use it because you are strengthening and developing your power of reasoning.

PARTICIPATING IN STUDENT GOVERNMENT ACTIVITIES

Your school has some type of student government organization. It is in your best interest to become familiar with the specifics of how your government functions and of your role in it. Students who participate in organizational activities are able to develop skills in leadership as an officer or committee chairman or member, as well as the skills inherent in cooperating as a member of a group working toward a common goal.

Student government organizations are identified under a variety of names, such as the student government association, student council, or faculty-student cooperative organization. The form of student government adopted by a specific program is expected to meet the needs of the students it serves and to provide opportunities for students to learn and work together, gaining experience in the operation of the democratic process.

In general, the purposes of student government organizations are to:

1. Serve as a channel of communication between the students and school administration
2. Provide opportunities for learning about and participating in the organization and functioning of student government
3. Aid the individual student in practicing the rules and regulations associated with good citizenship
4. Carry out the assignments of government permitted under the organization's constitution and bylaws
5. Prepare students for responsibilities of membership in their national organization

Students in nursing are potential members, upon graduation, of their national nursing organization. A student government serves as a vehicle for interpersonal communication and group action and also provides an opportunity for students to learn to work together in building and dealing with a governing structure.

The constitution and bylaws of any organization are the framework upon which its function is based. A constitution identifies the organization, defines its purposes, and establishes the rights and responsibilities of the membership. The bylaws include information and guides pertinent to the details of running the organization. The bylaws complement the constitution. When an organization's constitution and bylaws are rescinded, the organization ceases to exist.

A constitution, and particularly the bylaws, may require changing from time to time to up date them for maximum effectiveness. Changes are usually proposed by a committee authorized for this purpose and named within the constitution itself.

A constitution and bylaws define membership, the types of membership available, and the qualifications for membership in an organization. They also list by title the officers of the organization, their term of office, and the number of officers required. Duties of the officers are listed, generally, but it does not list personal characteristics needed by officer personnel for successful performance of their duties. Information about the way the organization's business is conducted, the number and types of meetings, and the manner in which they are conducted are specified in the bylaws. (A brief reference on the use of parliamentary procedures for conducting a meeting may be found in Appendix B.)

The backbone and driving power of any organization rest with its officers. Each organization will be only as successful as its officers make it, since they plan and direct the activities for the group. With a strong president to coordinate and supervise the various phases of the organization's activities, and with competent people serving as vice-president and secretary and treasurer, any organization will succeed. Without such officers to guide and urge the organization, there will be no accomplishments. On these officers rests the responsibility for a successful and enjoyable year of work. The work of officers is not glamorous or publicized, but it is of utmost importance. The true value of strong competent leaders is seldom appreciated at the time. Only when incompetent officers attempt to direct the organization do the members become aware of the importance of these people.

LEADERSHIP

Leadership requires three major qualifications:

1. A genuine interest in people and a liking for them
2. A willingness to work for and with people without benefit of publicity
3. A thorough interest in the job

Other qualifications will include:

1. Ability to make each person feel important as a participant in the group
2. Ability to contribute to the enjoyment and satisfaction of the individual members as well as the organization as a whole
3. Ability to distribute responsibility and appoint interested members to serve on committees
4. Ability to offer suggestions and assistance in an advisory capacity without "running the show"

FOLLOWERSHIP

No team can win the game with only leaders. Those members who have the aggressiveness and the interest to lead the way must have cooperative and willing members to follow them. It takes capacities which are worthwhile to make a good follower. These include:

1. Ability to understand the aims of the organization and plans of the leaders
2. Ability to cooperate in endeavors which are for group welfare
3. Ability to contribute without recognition of efforts
4. Ability to "play the game" with hope of success or winning
5. Ability to work efficiently even though the odds are on the losing side at times
6. Ability to maintain personal and organizational spirit with loyalty and interest

You cannot sit on the side lines with a feeling of self-satisfaction that "I am a member." A feeling of satisfaction as a member requires thought, action, and responsibilities which each one must share for the welfare of all.

BIBLIOGRAPHY

Berggren, H. J., and Zagornik, A. D.: Teaching nursing process to beginning students, Nursing Outlook **16**: 32-35, July 1968.

Burrill, M.: Helping students identify and solve patients' problems, Nursing Outlook **14**:648, Feb. 1966.

Collins, R. D.: Problem solving; a tool for patients, too, American Journal of Nursing **68**:1483-1485, July 1968.

Francis, G. M.: This thing called problem solving, The Journal of Nursing Education **VI**:27-30, Nov. 1967.

Hay, G.: This way to happiness, New York, 1967, Simon & Shuster, Inc.

Hayes, W. J., and Gazaway, R.: Human relations in nursing, Philadelphia, 1956, W. B. Saunders Co.

Hodnet, E.: The art of working with people, New York, 1959, Harper & Bros.

Kron, T.: Nursing team leadership, Philadelphia, 1961, W. B. Saunders Co.

Mayes, N., Schultz, M. N., and Pierce, C. M.: Commitment to nursing—how is it achieved? Nursing Outlook **16**:29-31, July 1968.

McGuire, M. J.: Mr. Roberts, please, Nursing Outlook **11**:58-60, Apr. 1963.

Moore, Dom Thomas V., and Stevens, Dom Gregory: Principles of ethics, ed. 5, Philadelphia, 1959, J. B. Lippincott Co.

Nishio, K.: Creative problem solving: a teaching innovation, Nursing Forum **VI**:432-441, Fall 1967.

Robert, S. C.: Rules of right and reason, American Journal of Nursing **60**:526-529, Apr. 1960.

Ross, C. F.: Personal and vocational relationships in practical nursing, ed. 3, Philadelphia, 1969, J. B. Lippincott Co.

Scrimshaw, F.: The parliamentarian—what she is and what she does, American Journal of Nursing **59**:373-374, Mar. 1959.

Spalding, E. K., and Notter, L. E.: Professional nursing, ed. 8, Philadelphia, 1970, J. B. Lippincott Co.

Staton, T. F.: How to study, revised edition, Nashville, Tennessee, 1962, McQuiddy Printing Co.

Thomas, Mrs. Harry Harvy: Simplified parliamentary procedure, New York, 1959, Carrie Chapman Catt Memorial Fund.

Vaillot, Sister Madeleine Clemance: Commitment to nursing, Philadelphia, 1962, J. B. Lippincott Co.

Wolff, I. S.: The educated heart, American Journal of Nursing **63**:58-60, Apr. 1963.

COMPLETE WORK SHEET ON PP. 315 AND 316

CHAPTER 8

Ethics for nursing

NATURE OF ETHICS

Ethics has been defined as "the science which guides human action and which tends to make a man's action and man himself good."* Ethics is concerned with all human action but is specifically involved with the morality of human behavior. Ethics is defined as the study of standards of conduct and the moral judgments and values upon which these standards are based. Knowledge and understanding of ethics help you to determine whether an action is good or bad. Ethical principles have their origin in customs, traditions, religion, obligations, and social and personal philosophies. Ultimately, ethical behavior helps you to order your life by indicating action commonly appropriate in given situations. The principles of ethics are most effectively applied through the use of sound judgment, the practice of honesty, and moderation (see Chapter 6).

As a nursing student you will have many opportunities to practice the principles of ethics in your personal, social, and professional life. Ethics enter into your personal life in the way you develop and strengthen your character. The qualities of character and right conduct learned and practiced earlier in your life can be strengthened and enhanced through a deeper understanding of their significance in your daily practice of nursing.

What you identify as your personal standards of moral conduct are reflected in the way you apply ethical principles in achieving your personal goals. The elements that contribute to your development as a good nurse, generally interpreted, are the same elements that constitute your character as a person. The good *nurse* is primarily a good *person*. When the qualities of moral conduct are used in conjunction with knowledge and nursing skills, you are recognized as a person worthy of identity within the nursing profession. Ability alone is not sufficient; it must be bolstered by qualities rooted in sound moral habits. Your personal ability and ethics mark your worth as a nurse.

Developing an understanding of the ethics of your chosen profession is a vital part of the nursing program. Your instructors and supervisors know that nursing education is concerned not only with specific skills and knowledge, but also with their application and use in a manner that is consistent with the highest moral standards. "To attempt to teach nursing without reference to the general conduct of the individuals concerned is like building a costly structure on a basis of sand. Lacking a solid foundation, the structure falls when a critical moment arrives."*

Living as a member of society requires the use of ethics. In this context you need to consider your moral conduct in light of your associations with others. Because ethics is concerned with what is morally acceptable, your actions

*Moore T. V., and Stevens, G.: Principles of ethics, ed. 5, Philadelphia, 1959, J. B. Lippincott Co., p. 4.

*Aikens, C.: Studies in ethics for nurses, ed. 5, Philadelphia, 1943, W. B. Saunders Co., p. 35.

as an ethical member of society in a variety of social situations are based on fundamental principles. No man is a law unto himself. What each individual *does* or *does not do* has some effect upon the lives of others. The power of example stemming from your own conduct has a definite effect on those around you. When your conduct freely and positively recognizes another's basic dignity and rights as a human being, your conduct is morally right and acceptable. Such conduct not only honors your fellow man, but it also honors you because you extend to another the recognition of those basic rights and dignities that you claim for yourself. In a social setting the practice of ethics is based on living the precept of the Golden Rule.

ETHICS VERSUS ETIQUETTE

Sometimes the practice of social ethics is confused with the practice of social etiquette. Although the two are interrelated, one is not a substitute for the other.

Ethics practiced in a social milieu is concerned with actions that are morally right and are formed on basic principles. Etiquette is a set of formal rules for social conduct based on consideration for others and designed to establish pleasant social relationships. The rules of etiquette are set by society to guide and regulate conduct and social practices. They may vary depending on the mores or customs acceptable in a particular locality or social group.

Since the rules of etiquette are based on custom and usage, both of which are subject to change, rules and standards of social behavior may be changed to meet new needs. This is evident when you compare the contents of early publications with contemporary books on etiquette.* Rules governing ethical behavior, however, tend to remain more constant because they are derived from deep beliefs and values with greater institutional support.

Conduct that is morally right and practices of social customs that enhance this conduct provide opportunities for the attainment of relationships that are acceptable from the point of view of both ethics and etiquette. On the other hand, unethical conduct can be coupled with impeccable etiquette. When considering practices involving ethics and etiquette in our society, you might reflect on the following: A lady or a gentleman, in the true sense of the term, demonstrates by his actions the proper usage of both ethics and etiquette in his relationships with others. Courteous treatment of others, coupled with genuine respect for them as human beings, is the key to honest and effective relationships.

PROFESSIONAL ETHICS

Ethics also serves as a guideline for the conduct of members of a profession. Established standards, referred to as codes of conduct or codes of ethics, set forth the rules and ordinances used for guidance of the member's professional activity. The first professional organization in the United States to adopt a code of ethics was the American Medical Association. Since adoption of the code in 1847, revisions have been incorporated to adapt to changing needs and circumstances. The current revision dates from 1957. Other professional groups with established codes of ethics include architects, attorneys, pharmacists, veterinary surgeons, teachers, hospital administrators, and nurses.

A code of ethics for the American Nurses' Association was originally formulated and adopted by the membership in 1950. The original code has undergone revisions in the intervening years, the latest being adopted in 1968. In 1959 members of the National Student Nurses' Association (NSNA) voted at their convention to endorse the code of ethics of the American Nurses' Association as applicable also to students enrolled in nursing programs. An official representative for NSNA participated in the discussions held by the ANA's Committee on Eth-

*Students in nursing programs have many opportunities to learn and practice etiquette established for correct social behavior. These opportunities include specific classes, when indicated, and experiences or assignments planned to help you apply your social skills in various situations, under the guidance and supervision of teachers knowledgeable in this subject.

ical Standards for revisions of the code in 1960 and 1968.

In an article discussing the significance of codes of ethics for the nursing and medical professions, Dr. Edmund Pellegrino points out that in each code there are elements that relate specifically to the ethical conduct and to the etiquette of the practitioner. Using the AMA code as an example, he states, "Ethics deals with the rightness or wrongness of the physician's actions in the light of principles which rise out of the nature of man as a person. It establishes nominative guides which govern specific situations in such a way that the rights of patients are always preserved."* He goes on to say that professional (medical) etiquette "deals with duties arising out of physicians' relations with each other and out of the dignity of the calling."* Dr. Pellegrino identifies some points in the code of ethics for nurses which are actually elements of etiquette, and he notes also that in nursing and medicine the "truly ethical core of the codes of both professions derives from the dignity and rights of the patient as a person."*

Nurses and physicians must cooperate in their working relationships in order to provide quality care for their patients and develop mutual respect and trust in their respective roles as part of the health team. The codes of the medical and nursing professions demand quality in practice and individual conduct. Both codes demand a high degree of personal dedication from doctors and nurses to ensure the welfare and competent care of those they are committed to serve. A copy of these codes is presented below for your information and study.

CODE FOR NURSES†

The development of a code of ethics is an essential characteristic of a profession and provides one means whereby professional standards may be established, maintained and improved. A code indicates a profession's acceptance of the responsibility and trust with which it has been invested. Each practitioner, upon entering a profession, inherits a measure of that responsibility and trust and the corresponding obligation to adhere to standards of ethical practice and conduct set by the profession.

Each nurse has an obligation to uphold and adhere to the Code in her individual practice and to ensure that her colleagues do likewise.

1. The nurse provides services with respect for the dignity of man, unrestricted by considerations of nationality, race, creed, color or status.
2. The nurse safeguards the individual's right to privacy by judiciously protecting information of a confidential nature, sharing only that information relevant to his care.
3. The nurse maintains individual competence in nursing practice, recognizing and accepting responsibility for individual actions and judgments.
4. The nurse acts to safeguard the patient when his care and safety are affected by incompetent, unethical, or illegal conduct of any person.
5. The nurse uses individual competence as a criterion in accepting delegated responsibilities and assigning nursing activities to others.
6. The nurse participates in research activities when assured that the rights of individual subjects are protected.
7. The nurse participates in the efforts of the profession to define and upgrade standards of nursing practice and education.
8. The nurse, acting through the professional organization, participates in establishing and maintaining conditions of employment conducive to high-quality nursing care.
9. The nurse works with members of health professions and other citizens in promoting efforts to meet health needs of the public.
10. The nurse refuses to give or imply endorsement to advertising, promotion, or sales for commercial products, services or enterprises.

*Pellegrino, E. D.: Nursing and medicine: ethical implications in changing practice, American Journal of Nursing **64**:110-112, Sept. 1964.

†Adopted by the American Nurses' Association, 1950; revised 1960 and 1968. From American Journal of Nursing **68**:2582-2585, Dec. 1968. Reprinted with permission.

PRINCIPLES OF MEDICAL ETHICS*

PREAMBLE. These principles are intended to aid physicians individually and collectively in maintaining a high level of ethical conduct. They are not laws but standards by which a physician may determine the propriety of his conduct in his relationship with patients, with colleagues, with members of allied professions, and with the public.

*Reprinted with permission of American Medical Association.

SECTION 1. The principal objective of the medical profession is to render service to humanity with full respect for the dignity of man. Physicians should merit the confidence of patients entrusted to their care, rendering to each a full measure of service and devotion.

SECTION 2. Physicians should strive continually to improve medical knowledge and skill, and should make available to their patients and colleagues the benefits of their professional attainments.

SECTION 3. A physician should practice a method of healing founded on a scientific basis; and he should not voluntarily associate professionally with anyone who violates this principle.

SECTION 4. The medical profession should safeguard the public and itself against physicians deficient in moral character or professional competence. Physicians should observe all laws, uphold the dignity and honor of the profession and accept its self-imposed disciplines. They should expose, without hesitation, illegal or unethical conduct of fellow members of the profession.

SECTION 5. A physician may choose whom he will serve. In an emergency, however, he should render service to the best of his ability. Having undertaken the care of a patient, he may not neglect him; and unless he has been discharged he may discontinue his services only after giving adequate notice. He should not solicit patients.

SECTION 6. A physician should not dispose of his services under terms or conditions which tend to interfere with or impair the free and complete exercise of his medical judgment and skill or tend to cause a deterioration of the quality of medical care.

SECTION 7. In the practice of medicine a physician should limit the source of his professional income to medical services actually rendered by him, or under his supervision, to his patients. His fee should be commensurate with the services rendered and the patient's ability to pay. He should neither pay nor receive a commission for referral of patients. Drugs, remedies or appliances may be dispensed or supplied by the physician provided it is in the best interests of the patient.

SECTION 8. A physician should seek consultation upon request; in doubtful or difficult cases; or whenever it appears that the quality of medical service may be enhanced thereby.

SECTION 9. A physician may not reveal the confidences entrusted to him in the course of medical attendance, or the deficiencies he may observe in the character of patients, unless he is required to do so by law or unless it becomes necessary in order to protect the welfare of the individual or of the community.

SECTION 10. The honored ideals of the medical profession imply that the responsibilities of the physician extend not only to the individual, but also to society where these responsibilities deserve his interest and participation in activities which have the purpose of improving both the health and the well-being of the individual and the community.

The International Council of Nurses adopted a code of ethics in 1953. This organization currently represents the professional nurses of seventy-four countries. At its congressional meeting in Frankfurt, Germany, 1965, some editorial clarifications were inserted in the document but no substantive changes have been incorporated. The ICN's code is drafted in general statements to facilitate its universal application as a guide for nurses to function throughout the world. Study the International Code along with the Code of the American Nurses' Association to identify commonalities and points of agreement.

INTERNATIONAL COUNCIL OF NURSES CODE OF ETHICS*

Nurses minister to the sick, assume responsibility for creating a physical, social and spiritual environment which will be conducive to recovery and stress the prevention of illness and promotion of health by teaching and example. They render health-service to the individual, the family and the community and co-ordinate their services with members of other health professions.

Service to mankind is the primary function of nurses and the reason for the existence of the nursing profession. Need for nursing service is universal. Professional nursing service is based on human need and is therefore unrestricted by considerations of nationality, race, creed, colour, politics or social status.

Inherent in the code is the fundamental concept that the nurse believes in the essential freedoms of mankind and in the preservation of human life. It is important that all nurses be aware of the Red Cross Principles and of their rights and obligations under the terms of the Geneva Conventions of 1949.

The profession recognises that an international code cannot cover in detail all the activities and relationships of nurses, some of which are conditioned by personal philosophies and beliefs.

1. The fundamental responsibility of the nurse is threefold: to conserve life, to alleviate suffering and to promote health.
2. The nurse shall maintain at all times the highest standards of nursing care and of professional conduct.
3. The nurse must not only be well prepared to practise but shall maintain knowledge and skill at a consistently high level.

*Adopted by the ICN Grand Council in Saõ Paulo, Brazil, July 1953 and revised by the ICN Grand Council, Frankfurt, Germany, June 1965. Reprinted with permission of International Council of Nurses.

4. The religious beliefs of a patient shall be respected.
5. Nurses hold in confidence all personal information entrusted to them.
6. Nurses recognise not only the responsibilities but the limitations of their professional functions; do not recommend or give medical treatment without medical orders except in emergencies, and report such action to a physician as soon as possible.
7. The nurse is under an obligation to carry out the physician's orders intelligently and loyally and to refuse to participate in unethical procedures.
8. The nurse sustains confidence in the physician and other members of the health team; incompetence or unethical conduct of associates should be exposed but only to the proper authority.
9. The nurse is entitled to just remuneration and accepts only such compensation as the contract, actual or implied, provides.
10. Nurses do not permit their names to be used in connection with the advertisement of products or with any other forms of self advertisement.
11. The nurse co-operates with and maintains harmonious relationships with members of other professions and with nursing colleagues.
12. The nurse adheres to standards of personal ethics which reflect credit upon the profession.
13. In personal conduct nurses should not knowingly disregard the accepted pattern of behaviour of the community in which they live and work.
14. The nurse participates and shares responsibility with other citizens and other health professions in promoting efforts to meet the health needs of the public—local, state, national and international.

FUNCTIONS OF PROFESSIONAL ETHICS

Codes of ethics are designed to encourage ethical professional conduct and to establish standards of acceptable behavior so that both the professionals and the public they serve know what is expected and what is not permissible. In order to do this, codes:

1. Set forth basic principles and regulations to serve as guidelines
2. Serve as resources for the orientation of new practitioners to their duties, rights, and privileges
3. Serve as guides to identify and evaluate qualities synonymous with professional conduct
4. Provide guidelines for the establishment and operation of educational programs to prepare future members for service in the profession
5. Identify common practices to be followed and those to be shunned
6. Provide a guide for considering the relationships of individuals to their employers, co-workers, society in general, and to their own profession
7. Serve as a basis for identifying standards of quality practice consistent with actions of the qualified, competent practitioner
8. Provide, by implication, for legal actions against incompetents and violators of the code and for liability of the consequences of their actions
9. Provide for due process under the law for practitioners unjustly accused of misconduct in the performance of their duties

PLEDGES OF DEDICATION

Pledges are written statements related to the more formal codes of ethics but are usually more succinct and are worded simply so that they can be readily memorized as a summary of basic beliefs and guidelines. Pledges are recited on specific occasions by members of the group to which the pledge refers, thereby providing an opportunity to think about the basic principles incorporated in the pledge and also to publicly state support of these principles.

The profession of nursing has two pledges of dedication, the Nightingale Pledge and the International Pledge. The Nightingale Pledge is frequently recited as part of graduation exercises or the capping ceremony. The Nightingale Pledge is recognized by the public as affirming the standards of conduct expected in members of the nursing profession. Memorize this pledge and think about the significance of the words whenever you have occasion to read or repeat them throughout your nursing career.

Mrs. Lystra E. Gretter, superintendent of nurses at Farrand Training School (now known as Harper Hospital School of Nursing, Detroit, Michigan) is credited with writing the Nightingale Pledge in 1893. It is patterned on the Hippocratic Oath, which is taken by physicians. The original Nightingale Pledge has, in turn, served as a source for other nursing and health care groups in their preparation of statements. Mrs. Gretter revised the final paragraph of the original pledge in 1935. This revised version is now copyrighted by the Alumnae Association of the Harper Hospital School of Nursing.

The original version of the Nightingale Pledge is included here. Study it in conjunction with a review of the code of ethics of the nursing profession and the Pledge of the International Council of Nurses.

I solemnly pledge myself before God and in the presence of this assembly to pass my life in purity and to practice my profession faithfully.

I will abstain from whatever is deleterious and mischievous and will not take or knowingly administer any harmful drug.

I will do all in my power to maintain and elevate the standard of my profession, and will hold in confidence all personal matters committed to my keeping and all family affairs coming to my knowledge in the practice of my calling.

With loyalty will I endeavor to aid the physician in his work and devote myself to the welfare of those committed to my care.

The International Pledge was proposed and written by the Ethics of Nursing Committee of the International Council of Nurses. The Council approved this version in 1965 and it has been suggested that this pledge be used at nursing graduation ceremonies.*

In full knowledge of the obligations I am undertaking I promise to care for the sick with all the skill and understanding I possess without regard to race, creed, color, politics or social status, sparing no effort to conserve life, to alleviate suffering and to promote health.

I will respect at all times the dignity and religious beliefs of the patients under my care, holding in confidence all personal information entrusted to me and refraining from any action which might endanger life or health.

I will endeavor to keep my professional knowledge and skill at the highest level and to give loyal support and cooperation to all members of the health team.

I will do my utmost to honor the international code of nursing ethics and to uphold the integrity of the professional nurse.

*Reprinted by permission of International Council of Nurses.

BIBLIOGRAPHY

Aikens, C.: Studies in ethics for nurses, ed. 5, Philadelphia, 1943, W. B. Saunders Co.

American Nurses' Association Committee on Ethical, Legal and Professional Standards: Code For Nurses, American Journal of Nursing **68**:2581-2585, Dec. 1968.

Frankfurt Congress I.C.N.: American Journal of Nursing **65**:90, Aug. 1965.

Haupt, E. A.: The Seventeen book of etiquette and entertainment, New York, 1963, David McKay Co., Inc.

Hayes, E. J.: Hayes, P. J., and Kelly, D. E.: Moral handbook of nursing, New York, 1957, The Macmillan Co.

Kelly, C. W.: Dimensions of professional nursing, New York, 1962, The Macmillan Co.

Moore, T. V., and Stevens, G.: Principles of ethics, ed. 5, Philadelphia, 1959, J. B. Lippincott Co.

Pellegrino, E. D.: Nursing and medicine: ethical implications in changing practice, American Journal of Nursing **64**:110, Sept. 1964.

Post, E. L.: Emily Post's etiquette, ed. 12, revised, New York, Funk and Wagnalls.

Spalding, E. K., and Notter, L. E.: Professional nursing, ed. 7, Philadelphia, 1965, J. B. Lippincott Co., pp. 49-64.

Vanderbilt, A.: Complete book of etiquette, Garden City, N. Y., 1963, Doubleday and Co.

COMPLETE WORK SHEET ON PP. 317 AND 318

CHAPTER 9

Some interpretations of nursing

SOME CONCEPTS OF NURSING

Nursing is concerned with people and involves the particular relationship established between people when help is needed. To nurse means to nourish, assist, hold carefully, support, tend, or care for. Each of these meanings implies an awareness of need by some person. Each connotes the establishment of a relationship between two people, one having a need and the other working to meet it. Collectively, these concepts imply a sense of accountability by the person who renders care to those she serves.

Nursing as an occupation. Nursing is a job that requires skill and time in which to learn and then to practice. In addition to the necessary satisfaction of a paycheck, nursing offers its practitioners the deep satisfaction of serving others. It is an occupation that demands both concentration on learning and dedication in practice.

Through the years the definition of nursing has been expanded and the role of nurses has accordingly become broader. Traditionally, nursing has meant taking care of patients. Today, however, it is seen by both the public and the profession as an occupation made up of many different activities. Nursing continues to focus on patient care while the variety and quality of care are extended and improved. In addition to patient care nurses also function as teachers, managers, supervisors, administrators, and researchers. Nurses who function in these assignments are identified as nurse-teachers, nurse-administrators and nurse-researchers. Although they may not be involved in offering direct care to patients, they are nonetheless important members of the nursing team.

Nursing as a profession. Nursing is a profession as well as an occupation. One author points out that "professions evolve from occupations because the services they render are deemed significant and crucial *and* because these services cannot be provided except by those who have had extensive training in the systematic knowledge of the profession."* Formerly, the term "profession" was used only in reference to education and training obtained within the areas of law, medicine, and theology—the so-called learned professions. Today "profession" is broader in meaning and use, and its interpretation is extended to include preparation for careers in such fields as architecture, business, engineering, nursing, and teaching.

The essence of a profession according to Marie Jahoda, a social psychologist, is that it is "an organization of an occupational group based on the application of special knowledge which establishes its own rules and standards for the protection of the public and the professionals. . . . A profession implies that the quality of work done by its members is of greater importance in its own eyes and in the eyes of society than the economic rewards they earn."†

An organization formed by an occupational

*Johnson, D. E.: Today's action will determine tomorrow's nursing, Nursing Outlook **13**:40, Sept. 1965.

†Jahoda, M.: A social psychologist views nursing as a profession, American Journal of Nursing **61**:53, July 1961.

group is a voluntary association of persons with comparable preparation and other designated qualifications who have united in a group with an official title (for example, The American Nurses' Association, American Medical Association, or the American Association of University Professors). The official organization establishes and enforces criteria that relate to the quality of those services which its members perform.

Today there are four separate national nursing organizations, the American Nurses' Association for registered nurses, the National Federation of Licensed Practical Nurses, Inc. for licensed practical/vocational nurses, the National League for Nursing, and the National Association for Practical Nurse Education and Service, Inc. The latter two offer membership to both nurses and laymen interested in the profession of nursing. The specific ways in which these organizations function will be discussed in other chapters.

What is a professional? The term professional has several meanings and each nurse may have her own interpretation. Let's look briefly at a few important implications.

"Professional" in the legal sense is used to identify the graduate nurse who has met a state's qualifications for licensure to practice as a registered nurse. Professional is also used to designate the level of academic preparation of the nurse who graduates from a college or university with a B.A. or B.S. degree.

After Nurse Practice Acts became part of the law in various states, nurses who were graduates of accredited schools of nursing were required to take state board examinations to establish their eligibility to practice nursing. Those who passed a state's examination were classified as registered nurses (RN). Legally they were also identified, according to Nurse Practice Acts, as professional nurses to distinguish them from nonregistered nurses. In this context, a professional nurse is a registered nurse who has met a state's requirements to practice nursing under its jurisdiction.

When used in relation to academic preparation, the term "professional" identifies an individual whose formal education and related training qualifies him to practice on a professional level. To be professionally prepared for practice in one's chosen field means that a practitioner has received academic preparation for assignments at a level commensurate with his anticipated future needs. He is trained as well as possible to enable him to function in any unusual or complicated situation that may arise.

In recent years the term "professional," when used to describe education for nursing practice, has come to reflect the concern of nursing leaders for providing students with educational preparation equal in quality to that of others, such as physicians and lawyers, whose professional training includes a broad foundation of knowledge based on the liberal arts and the sciences.

Achievement of professional preparation for nurses to function as professional practitioners in nursing is a goal toward which the American Nurses' Association is striving. It remains to be seen when this change will take place and when nurses, prepared to function in accordance with professional standards, can enjoy status and recognition based on their preservice preparation.

However, graduates of all types of collegiate or hospital-based schools of nursing who are admitted to and pass the state board examination for registration are recognized as professional nurses. Therefore, the term "professional" as applied to nurse graduates can be interpreted two ways: (1) based on academic preparation, and (2) legal recognition of qualifications to practice.

The graduate with a baccalaureate degree is entitled to be recognized as having professional status by virtue of academic achievement, but she, together with the graduates of hospital school and community college nursing programs, must qualify for legal recognition as a professional nurse by passing a state board examination for license as a registered nurse.

The various ways in which the term professional is presently used makes interpretation difficult. Nursing students should understand the meanings of the word "professional" and recognize its use in particular contexts.

The term professional in relation to performance. The word "professional" also relates to the quality of a person's performance, the completeness of an assignment, and the manner in which tasks are performed. This interpretation of the term is universal in its application. It can apply equally to a bus driver, a gardener, a service station attendant, or an astronaut. This interpretation carries the implications of deep personal pride in one's work and satisfaction in doing that work well. All nurses should identify and incorporate this interpretation of "professional" into their concept of nursing.

In this context, being professional involves the giving of yourself as part of the service you perform. It involves an awareness of the meaning of excellence. The way in which you welcome the newly admitted patient to the unit, give morning care, provide for body eliminations, attend to patients' surgical dressings, or carry out any of the tasks and services associated with the art of nursing is judged both by patients and co-workers according to their concepts of the highest standards of professional competence.

You are expected, both as a student and later as a graduate, to practice with the highest degree of quality at your command. It has been stated that "today's student will carry out tomorrow's practice about as much in the way of attitudes, commitments, knowledges and skills as she was able to secure in the process of becoming educated."* Hopefully, your application of the meaning of "professional" will be reflected in the exceptional quality of the patient care you administer throughout your career.

THE SCOPE OF NURSING

Leaders and educators in the nursing profession have attempted to define and identify not only nursing as an occupation and a service, but also the roles of nurses who function in a variety of professional capacities. Perhaps in the future it will be possible to formulate a universal definition to describe the orientation and scope of the profession and the involvement of those who serve in it.

*Maloney, E.: Interpersonal relations, Dubuque, Iowa, 1968, William C. Brown Co., p. vii.

The following definitions of nursing may serve as catalysts for your own thoughts about nursing and your place in this profession which you have selected for your career.

> Nursing is an art requiring as hard a preparation, as exclusive a devotion as any painter's or sculptor's work. For what is having to deal with dead canvas or cold marble compared to the living body, the temple of God's spirit? It is one of the fine arts . . . I had almost said the finest of the arts.

This interpretation, attributed to Florence Nightingale, considers nursing as an occupation that requires hard work, devotion to duty, and a spirit of perseverence. The patient's human needs deserve a nurse's best efforts. Generally, this interpretation is as valid today as it was when stated over 100 years ago.

The following is another interpretation of nursing as an art and a pattern of practice.

> Nursing is a helping art—a deliberate blending of thoughts, feelings and overt actions. It is practiced in relation to an individual who is in need of help, is triggered by a behavioral stimulus from that individual, is rooted in an explicit philosophy, and is directed toward fulfillment of a specific purpose.*

This next statement defines nursing as being involved with the patient as a total person as well as with the health of his family and the community as a whole.

> Nursing in its broadest sense may be defined as an art and a science which involves the *whole* patient, body, mind and spirit; promotes his spiritual, mental and physical health by teaching and by example; stresses health education and health preservation as well as ministration to the sick; involves the care of the patient's environment—social and spiritual as well as physical; and gives health service to the family and the community as well as to the individual.†

This definition enlarges on earlier concepts of nursing care and includes both health teaching and the use of preventive measures against

*Weidenbach, E.: The helping art of nursing, American Journal of Nursing 63:54, Nov. 1963.

†Gowan, Sister M. Olivia: Proceedings of the Workshop on Administration of College Programs in Nursing, June, 1944, Washington D. C., 1946, The Catholic University of America Press, p. 10.

future illness. Concern is expressed for the health environment of the patient as well as the family's needs for health services. This definition points up the importance of a broad preservice educational program to prepare nurses for practice within the context of this generous definition.

The next two statements consider nursing as a direct and compassionate service intended to supply personalized care for those who require it in time of suffering.

> . . . the purpose of nursing is to assist an individual, or family, to prevent or cope with the experience of illness and suffering . . .*

> Nursing developed in response to the need of the sick for care. It was, and still is, a reflection of man's compassion for man. This care of the sick, the injured, and the dependent has gone on even in the absence of corresponding attention to the need for measures leading to recovery or cure.†

The author of the next statement sees the nurse in the role of initiator and supporter as the patient is helped to make decisions and carry on activities affecting his life.

> The unique function of the nurse is to assist the individual, sick or well, in the performance of those activities contributing to health or its recovery (or to peaceful death) that he would perform unaided if he had the necessary strength, will or knowledge, and to do this in such a way as to help him gain independence as rapidly as possible.‡

Here the nurse's role is one of encouragement of the patient's independence in spirit and in his activities, keeping in mind the importance of his own self-esteem and his personal dignity.

Another nurse-educator expresses the purpose of nursing as follows:

> Nursing is the art of helping people feel better—as simple and as complex as this.§

Apart from these ideas about nursing expressed by members of the profession, the general public also has certain expectations. Because Mr. and Mrs. John Q. Public are in recipient roles, it is natural for them to form their opinions in terms of their experience with individual nurses and the manner in which these particular nurses did their job.

The layman expects that the nurse who cares for him and his family knows her job and will accept him without reservation as a person. He expects her to help, encourage, guide, and comfort him in accordance with his needs. He is not concerned with the educational program that prepares the nurse. His sole concern is the quality of the care he and his family receive from the nurse, and he bases his opinions about the profession as a whole chiefly on this element alone. Sometimes the layman's expectations with regard to nursing services differ from the nursing care dictated by the patient's condition or diagnosis. In this case the nurse can demonstrate her skill in handling the situation by explaining the nursing care plan to the patient, thus easing his tension and concern and gaining his cooperation.

One author may well be speaking for the layman and his interpretation of nursing when she says, "Good nursing is the product of a good person . . . A good nurse is a person who loves her neighbor as herself—who has grown from respect for herself to respect for all people. She is a person who sees helping people not as a moral imperative or as a selfish opportunity, but as a privilege and a responsibility."*

Before entering your nursing program you no doubt had your own ideas about nursing. Presumably your ideas were similar to those of the average layman. It is natural to expect that some of your ideas about nursing will change as you continue in your program and prepare for future practice as a member of the profession.

Unconsciously your feelings about nursing and your personal ideals will help you to view nursing as a career and consider its demands, its opportunities, and challenges in relation to

*Travelbee, J.: Interpersonal aspects of nursing, Philadelphia, 1966, F. A. Davis Co. p v.

†Johnson, D. E.: Today's action will determine tomorrow's nursing, Nursing Outlook **13**:38, Sept. 1965.

‡Henderson, V.: The nature of nursing, American Journal of Nursing **64**:63, Aug. 1964.

§Ingles, T.: What is good nursing? American Journal of Nursing **59**:1246, Sept. 1959.

*Ingles, T.: What is good nursing? American Journal of Nursing **59**:1246, Sept. 1959.

yourself. Nursing cannot meet all the needs of human beings in all the circumstances under which assistance may be required, but nursing does meet those needs associated with combating illness and maintaining health.

The four types of preservice educational programs that prepare students for future nursing responsibilities have been discussed in Chapter 5. One of these programs will be of primary interest to you because you are enrolled in it. On the other hand, it will be helpful to have information about the other types of programs as well. Your instructors will add relevant information to assist you in recognizing those points of interest which you may have in comparing the different programs.

Be proud of your school and your program. You chose it, you met the qualifications for admission, and were accepted. Develop a working definition of what nursing means to you and the kind of nurse you want to be. Review it from time to time and revise it if necessary; but remember that you, as a nursing student today, shape the nursing profession of tomorrow.

WORKING TOGETHER

Earlier in this chapter it was noted that the concept of nursing requires the establishment of a relationship between people to achieve its basic purpose. It was also noted that nursing involves different activities performed in a vari-

CHARACTERISTICS OF A LEADER

L	Listens with attention—is open to suggestions
E	Enthusiasm inspires co-workers
A	Analyzes situations before acting on them—able to give help and advice
D	Dependability is consistent
E	Encourages participation from co-workers
R	Responsible for coordination of group effort—respects rights of co-workers
S	Sense of fitness—utilizes good judgment
H	Hopeful for accomplishment of goal—helpful to others in reaching it
I	Impartial in dealings with co-workers
P	Patient and persevering with others

ety of work situations, which combine to make possible a high quality of patient care. People must work together to achieve this goal through the integration of their separate activities as well as through their cooperation on a person-to-person level.

Leadership—followership. If people are going to work together harmoniously and effectively, it is essential that one person be identified as the leader of the group. It is also necessary to identify those who will be followers. The relationships between the group members and the leader must be clearly defined and understood by everyone. No group can function without responsible guidance and direction, which the leaders must provide. The leader, on the other hand, must have the cooperation and trust of the group members.

In order for the group members to cooperate with each other and their leader, they must have a clear understanding of what is expected of them. A real leader plans *with* the

	CHARACTERISTICS OF A FOLLOWER
F	Follows instructions
O	Organized and ready to function
L	Listens
L	Learns
O	Observes
W	Works
E	Endeavors to do his best
R	Responsible
S	Supports the leader and carries out his assignments
H	Helps others
I	Interested
P	Participates in team's effort

group so that together they arrive at a shared idea of the best way in which to proceed. When the members of the group know what they are expected to do, each can turn to the leader for help and direction. Surely you can see that a leader who is inconsiderate, bossy, or preoccupied with power will be neither liked nor trusted. It is equally apparent that a group member who does not follow through is disliked and loses the trust and cooperation of the leader as well as fellow members of the group.

The knowledge and skills associated with leadership can be learned, but only by practicing these skills in working situations can you become relaxed and proficient in a leadership role. Your nursing program will provide opportunities for you to develop your potential for leadership. Such things as participation in student government, development of group projects, planning a party or outing, directing a musical group, or functioning as a team member in the clinical practice areas of the hospital will involve you in functioning with others in a constructive association.

Your instructors will doubtless point out opportunities for identifying and developing assignments involving the skills required for leadership. A later chapter will consider the particular relationships that should exist between those who function as effective members of the nursing team, but you are asked to study, think about, and utilize the characteristics of the person who serves in the capacity of follower or leader as these characteristics are listed on pp. 109-110.

BIBLIOGRAPHY

Clemance, Sister Madeleine: Existentialism: a philosophy of commitment, American Journal of Nursing **66**:500-505, Mar. 1966.

Coladarci, A. P.: What about that word profession? American Journal of Nursing **63**:116-118, Oct. 1963.

Darley, W.: The professions and professional people, Nursing Forum **1**:83-89, Winter 1961-1962.

Dreves, K. D.: This I believe about nursing in a changing world, Nursing Outlook **12**:50-51, Feb. 1964.

Ferlic, A.: Existential approach in nursing, Nursing Outlook **16**:30-33, Oct. 1964.

Henderson, V.: The nature of nursing, American Journal of Nursing **64**:62-68, Aug. 1964.

Ingles, T.: What is good nursing? American Journal of Nursing **59**:1246-1249, Sept. 1959.

Jahoda, M.: A social psychologist views nursing as a profession, American Journal of Nursing **61**:52-56, July 1961.

Johnson, D. E.: Today's actions will determine tomorrow's nursing, Nursing Outlook **13**:38-41, Sept. 1965.

Kron, T.: Nursing team leadership, ed. 2, Philadelphia, W. B. Saunders Co.

Lambertson, E. C.: Education for nursing leadership, Philadelphia, 1958, J. B. Lippincott Co.

MacDonald, B. D.: Nursing's many meanings, Nursing Outlook **14**:56-67, July 1966.

Major, D. M.: A profession—its growth and development, Nursing Outlook **11**:33-35, Jan. 1963.

Merton, R. K.: The search for professional status, American Journal of Nursing **60**:662-664, May 1960.

New, P. K.-M.: Another approach to professionalism, American Journal of Nursing **65**:124-126, Feb. 1965.

Perkins, E. W.: The registered nurse—a professional person? American Journal of Nursing **63**:90-92, Feb. 1963.

Saunders, L.: The changing role of nurses, American Journal of Nursing **54**:1094-1098, Sept. 1954.

Weidenbach, E.: The helping art of nursing, American Journal of Nursing **63**:54-57, Nov. 1963.

Whitaker, J. C.: The nurse as a professional person, Nursing Outlook **9**:217-219, April 1961.

COMPLETE WORK SHEET ON P. 319

CHAPTER 10

Interpreting essential academic policies and requirements

Chapter 5 dealt with various types of preservice nursing education programs. Now, let us look at those things that you should know about academic policies and scholarship requirements. Because you have been accepted and enrolled in a nursing program, you are a partner in the educational enterprise, and, as a partner, you should understand the conditions under which you were accepted in the program. You should know the academic policies and regulations that govern your education and the principles that guide the administration and affect your preparation for a nursing career. The topics included in this chapter focus on admission requirements and records, policies on attendance, grades, grading systems, and grade point averages.

THE REASONS FOR ENTRANCE REQUIREMENTS

The regulations pertaining to student selection vary among educational institutions and are based upon the demands of the nursing programs they offer. Each school determines the requirements that must be met for admission to its nursing program. Admission requirements serve as a standard for measuring the suitability of the applicant. These requirements are a means of selecting students for the nursing program who have the potential to successfully complete the curriculum.

All nursing schools require that applicants for admission furnish credentials as evidence of their qualifications. These include an official high school transcript, a college transcript, if any, a medical report, character references, and letters of recommendation. In many schools the applicant must take a battery of aptitude and achievement tests and a personality inventory.

Other entrance requirements may involve successful completion of specified courses, evidence of citizenship status, and the ability to comprehend and use the English language. In some instances a state's board of nursing may authorize the school to accept an official report of test results if the applicant cannot present an official high school transcript. The General Education Development Examination (GED) indicates an educational level equivalent to that of a high school graduate.

Many of the traditional requirements that once discouraged some people from seeking a career in nursing have been changed. Preservice nursing programs, generally, are now open to both men and women. Although a few schools may reserve the right to restrict student selection for justifiable reasons, race, creed, or national origin are generally not taken into account. There is greater flexibility regarding the age limits for admission so that an age range of 17 to 48 among students is not uncommon. Married applicants are now accepted, and students who marry while they are enrolled in the program are seldom required to withdraw. These changes have benefited the nursing profession as well as those who wish to become part of it. Many people who might once have been denied the opportunity may now study for a career in nursing. Because of the variety of programs available, the potential sources of nursing manpower are used to much greater advantage.

Most schools publish their admission requirements in catalogues or bulletins with deadlines for the submission of all materials that will be evaluated by the admissions committee. This policy provides adequate time for applicants to schedule pre-entrance tests and personal interviews, for the admissions committee to review and evaluate applicants' records and test results, and to inform candidates of the committee's recommendations.

HOW STUDENTS ARE SELECTED

You are now a student in a nursing program because your school has made a painstaking study of your qualifications and credentials and has decided that you are *right* for the program and that the program is right for you.

Each institution has an established procedure for the selection of students. Simply defined, the admission (selection) procedure is the plan followed by the school in screening prospective students and evaluating and selecting candidates for the nursing program. The sequence of the steps and the procedures used in implementing the steps will vary with the individual school, the type of nursing program, local conditions, and requirements of the state's board of nursing, but the general pattern is the same. The steps in student selection are shown below.

1. Formal application by the prospective student
2. Preliminary interview with the director of the nursing program or other designated person
3. Pre-entrance health examination
4. Pre-entrance aptitude tests
5. Review of school transcripts, records, reports, and test results by the admissions committee*
6. Check on recommendations and character references
7. Decision of the admissions committee to accept or reject the applicant
8. Notification of candidate
9. Interview with nursing department personnel, instructions incidental to dates, entrance procedures, housing, and so forth

All of these data presented yielded a composite "picture" of you on which the admissions committee could base judgments on your qualifications and potential to succeed in the nursing program.

Even though you are enrolled in a nursing program and have met your school's admission requirements, let us review in a general way the rationale behind the major pre-entrance requirements and records. So that the discussion will be as meaningful as possible, refer to the entrance or admission requirements listed in your school's catalogue. At this point you might also think about the obligations you have as a student nurse in measuring up to the standards your school has set.

The application form. The application form is one of the most valuable selection devices for determining the qualifications of applicants. It is a very personal record because in it the applicant outlines important information about herself from birth until the time she submits her application to the school. The application form furnishes the following information on the prospective student:

1. Complete identification—name, address, date and place of birth, sex, citizenship, marital status
2. Family status—name of parents and/or spouse, address, occupation, number and ages of dependents
3. Education and training—name and location of schools attended, dates of attendance and graduation, academic or major courses
4. Financial resources—sources of financial assistance during the period of the nursing program
5. Work experience—jobs held, time spent in each

*Admissions committee, as used here, is a general term for any group appointed by academic authority to select and recommend the acceptance of students for the educational program.

6. Social interests—hobbies, memberships or offices in organizations
7. References—names of responsible persons who can vouch for the character and ability of the applicant
8. Other information, as requested, relevant for the school's purposes

When completed, signed, and dated, this record becomes the formal application to the nursing program. The application form is the source of information for various office records, academic records, and reports during the student's period of enrollment. It becomes part of the student's file and is retained for reference after the student has graduated and/or leaves the program.

In completing the application form the individual often supplies information about herself that is not specifically asked for but which the admissions committee will readily recognize. Information or clues regarding the person's characteristics and ability will be noted in her care in following directions, ability to spell, her vocabulary, and her habit of neatness. A soiled, incomplete or messy application form serves as a poor introduction for a prospective student.

Official transcripts of educational records. An official transcript of high school courses, grades, and verification of graduation is required for admission to preservice nursing education programs preparing students for licensure as nurses. The high school record tells much about the applicant's intellectual ability. It holds the key to a student's potential for continuing education on the post–high school level. In evaluating your educational background the admissions committee is interested in such aspects of your academic preparation as:

1. The titles of courses taken in high school including the length and sequence of courses, the grades earned in each course, and the grade point value assigned
2. Your general academic average and level of placement in your graduating class
3. Test results and interpretations on any aptitude or achievement tests taken in high school and evidence of any particular strengths or shortcomings
4. Your academic major in high school, any changes in your major courses during your enrollment, and career, if you had decided on one
5. Any interruptions in your enrollment and the reasons for them
6. Your general pattern of scholastic achievement and ability to apply what you have learned
7. The extent of your participation in extracurricular activities and group organizations

Some applicants who otherwise qualify for admission to a nursing program must be turned down when they apply for the first time because of their general academic standing. Often the high school records of these individuals show that there was a lack of interest or lack of application in learning during the first years of high school. Later, when these students became motivated and settled down to the business of study, they demonstrated their ability to earn satisfactory grades. However, their late start and the poor grades made in the beginning resulted in an overall academic average that fell below the acceptable limit for admission to the nursing program. In such situations, prospective applicants may be counseled to postpone their intention to enter a nursing program and to consider enrollment in post–high school courses of a remedial nature to strengthen the academic background revealed by their low high school grades. Those who do not meet the academic requirements are advised to take remedial work in such areas as English usage, spelling, reading proficiency, or basic mathematics before attempting advanced educational requirements. When deficiencies in educational preparation are rectified, these applicants should reapply for admission to the nursing program. The way prospective students react to this information and accept its implications indicates, to a degree, their maturity of character and the sincerity of their desire to become nurses.

Recommendations—character references. Personal recommendations and character references can be worthwhile selection devices if the sources are candid in their statements about the individual. Many schools prefer to communicate directly with the persons who are suggested as references. In this way the school can obtain responses to direct questions about the applicant. The replies often provide supplemental information about the applicant's attitudes, personality, and character traits that is helpful in the selection process.

The number of references required is usually specified by the school. In general, the most useful sources for references are high school administrators, student advisors, instructors, former employers or supervisors, a clergyman, a member of one of the professions, and personal friends who have knowledge of the applicant's qualifications. Obtaining the permission of the person one intends to give as a reference is a courtesy the applicant should not overlook. References and recommendations are confidential and are treated as such by the school. They become part of the student's file.

Physical examination and health record. All schools of nursing require a pre-entrance physical examination as one of the conditions for admission to the nursing program. The purpose of the physical examination is to determine the state of an applicant's health and to eliminate those who do not meet the health standards established for the program. An applicant must have a satisfactory health record and an up-to-date immunization record. The latter requirement clears the student for clinical laboratory assignments in the hospital.

The health policies and health standards set for the nursing program must necessarily provide for (1) the welfare and protection of the students, (2) the protection of the educational institution, and (3) the protection of participating clinical facilities from liability and claims under the laws of the state. In addition, some states have health regulations for educational programs. For example, to enroll in school in some states the law requires evidence that the student has been immunized against poliomyelitis.

As a participating member in the educational program, the hospital and its administration have to keep in mind the legal implications of exposure to risks. Most hospitals that make their facilities available for students' clinical practice require evidence from the school that the students have been vaccinated against smallpox and immunized against typhoid fever, tetanus, diphtheria, and other diseases before they are permitted on the nursing units and assigned to care for the sick. Another requirement is a recent chest x-ray. The degree of liability assumed by the hospital as a participating unit for education and its liability for the students' well-being are generally specified in the written agreement (contract) in effect between the educational institution and the hospital.

The student-learner who functions in the hospital environment as a member of an educational program is not the *primary* responsibility of the hospital and its administration, as are the hospital's own employees. In fact, some hospitals require signed waivers releasing them from responsibility for students accepted within its environment for the purposes of education. Students' health and welfare are the responsibility of the educational institution and the students themselves.

Most schools require that forms supplied by them be used for the physical examination report. It is essential that the report be completed, dated, and signed by the examining physician. If the report shows the existence of dental or visual defects, conditions requiring surgical correction, or the need for a regimen for reducing or gaining weight, the individual is apprised of her personal responsibility for correcting these conditions before she can be admitted to the program. A widely used policy is to require that the physical examination report be submitted at the same time as the formal application so that applicants can be informed of their responsibilities before admission.

The completeness of the physical examination and the detail of the physician's report have value for both the student and the school. The final decision as to the applicant's present state of health rests with the examining physician. However, since the school is responsible for the welfare and health of the student after she has been admitted, the school is entitled to be informed of any item in the person's medical history that might be a potential health hazard. These might be a serious illness in the past, any condition being medically controlled such as diabetes, recovery from tuberculosis, a history of cardiac disease, a history of fainting or "blackouts," or treatment for mental illness. Schools may have provisions in their admission policy for accepting students, on an individual basis, who have physical or health disabilities, but before acting on these, the school needs to know the extent of the problem and its management in order to evaluate the prospective student's capabilities for coping with the demands of the nursing program.

The pre-entrance physical examination report is included in the student's permanent file. Health records of students are considered confidential and are accorded the same care given to any physician's records.

Pre-entrance tests. The use of aptitude tests for selecting prospective students is almost a universal practice among schools of nursing. Many schools use the testing services of such organizations as the National League for Nursing and the American Psychological Association. The service includes a battery of objective tests to determine an individual's aptitude in various areas of knowledge. The scoring of the tests and reporting of the test results to the school of nursing are part of the service.

The admissions committee uses the test results as a guide in selecting the most promising candidates for the nursing program. The content of these tests is intended to gauge an applicant's potential for achievement in nursing based on evidences of the person's knowledge and usage of verbal, reading, and mathematical skills, the ability to interpret written material, and use of quantitative data. The tests are scored and both raw scores and percentile rank are provided. Some test batteries include a personality inventory scored in accordance with its purposes.

Each applicant's score and percentile rank is evaluated in relation to the minimum standard of performance designated for the individual program. This measurement is the "cut-off point." The aptitude test points up those areas in which the applicant meets or exceeds the school's cut-off and those areas in which additional strengthening is needed. For example, an applicant's scores may show achievement in the area of mathematics and the solution of problems using quantitative data, but scores relating to vocabulary, reading skill, and the interpretation of printed matter may fall short of the school's cut-off point. If the applicant were to be admitted at this time, and if the weaknesses shown by the test results were not removed, the probability of the applicant's meeting the continuing demands of the nursing program and succeeding in them would be doubtful. If, in an interview, the applicant is told about the test results, and she decides to apply for admission to the program later, she may, with a counselor, plan a remedial program of study in a local college that will include vocabulary building, spelling improvement, the development of reading skills and good study habits, along with such other courses as are applicable to her scholastic growth.

If the pre-entrance tests include a personality inventory, the results, as interpreted by qualified personnel, may also identify areas where the individual needs assistance in handling problems of a personal nature.

The personal interview. The personal interview is important in the selection of students. The purpose of the interview is two-fold. It provides both the prospective student and the interviewer an opportunity to ask questions and discuss topics of mutual concern. The interview offers opportunity to personalize the admission process and to identify the applicant as a particular individual, distinct from the entire group. This interview is usually conducted by the director of the program, but a faculty member may be appointed to this responsibility. In the baccalaureate or associate degree programs, the interview may be the assignment of a member of the college's counseling staff. A summary report of the interview is usually prepared for inclusion with other entrance data.

It would be expected that this pre-admission interview had been scheduled for a definite time, and both parties had prepared for their respective roles so the outcome of the session would be mutually satisfying. The applicant should have all questions and other items she wishes to discuss clearly in mind, or better still, written down for ready reference. It is important for the applicant to understand this interview, or exchange of information, is intended for her benefit. She should make the most of the experience and be at ease. The interview and the personal appraisal of applicants is also beneficial to the school. The manner in which the interview is conducted is the interviewer's responsibility, but it should insure the development of a climate in which the applicant's identity as a person will emerge.

During the interview the applicant's reasons for wanting to be a nurse are considered, as are the evidences of maturity shown by the person. To a degree, the applicant's relationships with people and the facility for adjusting to demands and changes in one's living pattern are revealed. Without attempting to 'structure' the interview, *the interviewer* may find it helpful to check, with the applicant, data currently in her file. This technique could provide opportunity for both of them to be sure that items on the application form are complete, and that all the records and reports to be reviewed are accounted for prior to the meeting of the admission committee.

During the course of the interview it may be helpful to review with the applicant the purposes of the program, together with basic policies of the school. Nearly every applicant expresses interest in the results of the pre-entrance tests and how they affect a person's chance for admission. This is a reasonable concern. Consideration of test scores provides the interviewer with an opportunity to review, in general, the technique of testing and the purpose of the tests. It is important that the student understands that test scores are *one source* of information and they are used in conjunction with *all* of the other assembled data in selecting applicants for admission.

It is equally important for prospective students to realize that if their pre-entrance tests show ability to meet the scholastic standards of the program, and they are admitted, they will be expected to function at a level consistent with their potential. To expect less would be unfair to the student.

Some schools invite the applicant's parents to be present at the time of the interview. Depending on the circumstances, parents may or may not participate in the interview itself, but it is important, for purposes of communication and interpersonal relations, that the parents and the director of the program establish a cordial relationship. Parents are concerned about their children's career decisions. Their questions and comments are worthy of note and deserve thoughtful response. However, it should be clearly understood by the applicant and her (his) parents, that the school does not expect, nor does it intend to accept, parents' responsibility in relation to students' behavior. It is equally important to clarify how, through cooperating together in their respective roles, both the school and the parents can work for the best interests of the student.

The rapport initiated between the prospective student and the director at this interview is significant for both of them. Hopefully, it sets the stage for continuing conferences as the student progresses in her education and demonstrates the growth and development necessary for a potential nurse practitioner.

In closing this review on how students are selected for nursing education programs, it is fitting to address some questions to you. Have you stopped to think why your school chose you for its nursing program? What responsibilities did you accept when you became a student in nursing? How do you propose to fulfill these responsibilities? If you started out with sincerity of purpose, confidence, and determination you should arrive at the goal you have set for yourself—a graduate nurse, qualified to practice as a member of the nursing profession.

ACADEMIC POLICIES AND SCHOLARSHIP REQUIREMENTS

Earlier in the chapter we reviewed the reasons for admission requirements and their implications for the student. Now let us discuss what the school expects of the student regarding attendance and scholastic achievement.

ATTENDANCE

Students are expected to attend every meeting of each class in which they are enrolled and to be present for all clinical laboratory assignments. Failure to do so may result in a lowered grade for a course, and this, in turn, will affect the student's academic average. When absence is unavoidable, the student should notify the instructor in accordance with the school's policy on reporting absences. It is the student's responsibility to arrange with the instructor to make up the missed assignments and classes. *This is not the teacher's responsibility.*

Every effort should be made to build a good attendance record in both classes and clinical laboratory assignments. Although it is often possible to make up classes missed because of legitimate absence, this is not necessarily true of clinical assignments. These assignments are planned and scheduled to create a particular learning experience. "Make-up" clinical laboratory sessions will not have the same learning value, and the student is not likely to derive the same benefits as from the original class.

Punctuality is also very important, because habits of being on time are absolutely essential in nursing. A patient's life may depend on carefully timed care. Because you have much to learn, your teachers must effectively use every minute of the teaching schedule. Students should be aware of this and be on time for class. A story is told of the chemistry professor whose class started at 8:30 A.M. Each morning at exactly 8:30 the professor closed the classroom door, slipped the lock and started his lecture. Any tardy student missed that day's class. This technique may have been severe, but it was effective, and no student was late twice.

As nurses you must accept the part that time plays in your lives. You must learn to adjust to its demands if you expect to be comfortable in your work. You must remember that being on time and being dependable and effective are closely related. For the nurse, time means more than just meeting the deadline; it means being ready to start an assignment, with all necessary preparation completed at the required time.

SCHOLASTIC ACHIEVEMENT

Required standards of achievement are published in your school's catalogue, together with the policies on passing grades, the minimum level of achievement that must be maintained in order for students to remain in good academic standing, the conditions under which students may be placed on probation or subject to dismissal because of poor standing, and the conditions for repeating a course or making up a class. In other words, these are the conditions under which the two partners, the school and the student, will cooperate in the educational program.

As members in this partnership, students should have a clear understanding of how these policies apply to them personally. Students should understand (1) the basis on which the school evaluates the quality of achievement in the nursing program (system of grading), (2) how the grades earned affect academic standing (grade point average), and (3) how grades determine eligibility for promotion and graduation. Unfortunately, many students do not understand the significance of the scholarship requirements until they are faced with the alternative of "shaping up" or leaving the program because of low grades.

Grading system. The grading system used by an educational institution is established by school policy. Use of the unit credit/grade point system is practically universal for collegiate nursing programs in this country for two reasons: (1) the nursing curriculum in the college is one of many conducted by the collegiate institution, so its grades and grading system must be the same as for any other curriculum offered by the college and (2) the incidence of students transferring from one collegiate institution to another for continuing educational preparation has made it convenient for the unit credit/grade point system to be generally accepted as an evaluating device.

In noncollegiate nursing programs the grading system is established at the discretion of the individual school unless stipulated by an official agency. Nursing programs operating under noncollegiate auspices frequently use the percent scale system for grading students' work and reporting final grades. Students are not penalized because of the method used to record final grades. Grades reported on a percent scale system *can* be converted to the grade point system at any time. This conversion might be required, for example, if a student in a noncollegiate program seeks admission to a college or university.

In the grade point system, the letters A through D and F are used to indicate scholastic placement on a scale ranging from excellent to failure. Each of the letters has an assigned value based on the number of points each one carries *per unit of credit.* The grade of *A* (superior or excellent) has a grade point value of 4; a grade of *B* (above average or good) has 3 grade points; a grade of *C* (average, or satisfactory) has 2 grade points; and *D* (below average, or barely passing) has a grade point of 1. In some institutions a numeric grading system is used in which case a *1* is equivalent to an *A* and a *5* equivalent to an *F*. The grade of *F*, or failure, has no grade point value. A final grade of *D* or *F* in a course results in a deficiency and affects the total grade points on the student's academic record.

In collegiate programs every course in the curriculum carries a given number of units or credits. A unit of credit represents one clock hour per week of classroom work (lecture) or a prorated number of hours of laboratory (usually three) per week for one full semester (quarter or term) depending on the school's calendar. This unit is also referred to as a semester hour or quarter hour, again depending on the school's calendar. If, for example, a course includes two hours of lecture and three hours of laboratory assignment a week the credits assigned to it would be three units or three credit hours. Grade points are computed by multiplying the grade point value of the grade received by the number of units assigned to the course. In a course that carries three units of credit, the total possible grade points, based on the final course grade could be:

FINAL GRADE (POINTS)		UNITS		GRADE POINTS (TOTAL)
A–4	×	3	=	12
B–3	×	3	=	9
C–2	×	3	=	6
D–1	×	3	=	3
F–0	×	3	=	0

This unit credit/grade point system of marking is universally recognized in educational circles. In reviewing official transcripts or when transfer of credit is being considered, the grade granted by one institution is not questioned by another.

Other grading systems for evaluating the quality of work done by students are the percent rank and the total point rank. Noncollegiate programs may use either of these systems for recording students' grades. A perfect score on a percent rank would be 100%. A perfect score on the total point rank would be equal to the total number of points assigned to the course or to the individual testing situation. The school establishes the range it wishes to use (on either the percent rank or the total point rank) to be considered equivalent to the letter grade system. These systems are used for computing final course grades and for rating achievement on tests and examinations.

A final course grade obtained by either the percent rank or total point rank system can be equated to interpret scholastic achievement on the letter grade scale. A comparison of marking systems for grading levels of scholastic achievement, based on a hypothetical scale, is shown in the following arrangement:

LETTER GRADE	PERCENT RANK	TOTAL POINT RANK (BASED ON 300 POINTS)
A	93–100%	285–300
B	85–92%	267–284
C	78–84%	231–266
D	70–77%	210–230
F	69% or less	209 or less

The grade of *C* is recognized as a basic grade. It represents the quality of work done by the average student. A final grade of *C* granted for a course tells us that the student passed a satisfactory final examination, was usually accurate and prompt in completing assignments, demonstrated a fair mastery of pertinent skills, and presented sufficient evidence of ability to proceed to the next level of work. An overall rating of *C* (2.0) at the end of the semester, quarter, term, or academic year indicates the student's overall academic standing is satisfactory. A final rating of 1.9 or less indicates an academic deficiency. Some nursing programs require a minimum grade of *C* for all nursing courses.

A final course grade of *B* means the student did better than average work. The student made a high grade on the final examination, was accurate and prompt with assignments, and exhibited a good mastery of required skills. A course grade of *A* denotes outstanding scholarship and means that the student made consistently high grades during the grading period and demonstrated excellent mastery of skills. A course grade of *D* means the student is barely passing. In general, the student was inadequate in both knowledge and skills and did poorly on the final examination. A grade of *F* for the course indicates a failure to meet minimum requirements. Failure may be the result of consistently poor work or repeated absence from classes.

One of the mistakes often made by beginning students is that they do not see grades in the proper perspective. Some students view them as hazards in their educational paths. Others exert all their efforts toward getting good grades. Grades are important because they measure the student's ability to learn, retain, recall, and apply knowledge, but working only for grades is not the answer. Students who strive to become proficient in acquiring and using nursing knowledge and skills will be working for the right objective, and the by-product of their efforts will be good grades.

Sometimes, students who made *A*'s and *B*'s all through high school panic when they find *C*'s and *D*'s on their midterm or semester grade reports in the nursing program. This holds an important lesson for them. Students need to understand why they earned the low grades. One reason could be that they have not adjusted to a higher standard of achievement. An *A* or a *B* earned in high school is important to the student at that stage of her education, but it does not follow that she will earn the same grades in the nursing program without greater effort. Another thing the student should appreciate is that she is a member of a group that was especially selected for the nursing program; the competition is therefore greater. Students should accept the challenge presented by low grades and apply themselves to improve their knowledge while maintaining a good academic standing. Your instructors will be happy to explain the school's policies on grades and to review the procedures used for grading both academic and clinical progress and for recording the information on permanent educational records.

Earlier it was pointed out that you were admitted to the nursing program because you measured up to the admission standards of your school of nursing. Now that you are enrolled as a student, your school expects you to work up to your ability as predicted by your high school record and pre-entrance tests. The grades you make should be in keeping with your ability.

Grade point average. The grade a student makes in each course in the nursing curriculum is important. Every grade must be recorded in the student's educational record. However, a student who is knowledgeable about the way in which final grading is computed will also be concerned with and interpret properly her grade point average. Students are often under the illusion that a *B* grade in one subject will balance out a *D* grade made in another subject, and thus their standing of *C* is assured. This theory is applicable *only* if the two courses carry identical unit credits. The grade points gained by making a *B* in a two-unit course will not make up for a *D* grade in a four-unit course. In this case, for an average grade of *C*, twelve grade points are needed. The ten actual grade points (six points for the *B* grade and four points for the *D*) fall two points short of the required number for a *C* average. The grade point average is the average of *all* grades earned during one semester, quarter, or term of work. This average determines whether the student is in good academic standing (2.0) and ready to enter sequential courses and experiences.

In collegiate programs the number of units of credit students are expected to carry each semester is outlined in the program of study. This determination is made on the basis of the total number of units required for graduation. For example, if a minimum of 60 semester units is required for the associate degree, these units will be distributed over the four semesters (and any summer sessions) of the two-year program of study. If the baccalaureate program requires 120 semester units, these units are divided and distributed over the four-year period. In other than collegiate programs, the educational pattern may require a specific number of clock hours of instruction and laboratory practice during the term or the semester.

The grade point average is derived by dividing the total number of points earned by the total number of units attempted. For a *C* average at the end of a semester, a student must have earned twice the number of grade points as the number of units attempted. The higher the grades earned for a course, the more grade points are earned and the higher the grade point average. The reverse is also true. To illustrate: If eighteen units is the academic load for a semester, the total grade points *earned* must be 36 in order to attain a straight *C* (2.0) average.

The following is an example of a student's program of study and grades for the two semesters of the first year of the nursing program.

SEMESTER I	UNITS	GRADE	GRADE PTS.
Psychology 1a	3	B	9
English 1a	3	B	9
Orientation	1	C	2
Chemistry 23a	3	D	3
Anat. & Physiol. 6a	3	D	3
Nursing I	5	C	10
Total	18		36
G.P.A.		2.0	

SEMESTER II	UNITS	GRADE	GRADE PTS.
Nutrition 28	3	B	9
Anat. & Physiol. 6b	3	B	9
Bacteriology 23	3	C	6
Nursing II	7	B	21
Total	16		45
G.P.A.		2.81	
Cum. G.P.A.		*2.39*	

As shown in Semester I, this student's grade point average was obtained by dividing 36 (total grade points earned) by 18 (total units assigned for semester). Fortunately, the two *D* grades did not cause her general average to fall below a *C*. However, with a G.P.A. of a straight 2.0 there is no "cushioning" to fall back on in the next term should there by any more *D* grades. In the second semester her G.P.A. was improved by 0.81 point, which served to strengthen her average and resulted in a cumulative grade point average of 2.39 for the first year's work.

The following hypothetical cases illustrate how two students developed records of their achievement and the consequences that resulted.

Amy was in the first term of her nursing program. The units assigned to the courses scheduled for completion in her first school term totaled sixteen. Amy's instructors had discussed the school's grading system and the grade point values assigned to all courses of the nursing curriculum with the members of the class. She knew that 32 grade points would be required to balance the 16 units.

At the midterm grade period, her records showed she earned three *C*s in courses totaling ten units (twenty grade points), one *B* in a three-unit course (nine grade points), and one *D* in another three-unit course (three grade points). The grade points earned with the *B* grade maintained her overall standing of 2.0 at this point in the program, but her counselor pointed out her need to analyze her study habits and make better use of the time she had available for studying.

In the second half of the term, Amy applied herself to all her studies and worked especially hard on the course in which she had earned the *D* grade. At the same time she maintained her grades in the other courses. When the final grades were recorded, Amy had managed to maintain her midterm grades except that she had earned a *B* on the final examination in the course in which she had received a *D*. The midterm *D* and the final examination *B* earned her a *C* for the course. Because of the *B* earned in the three-unit course Amy accumulated thirty-five grade points for the semester and was promoted to the next term with a bonus of three grade points.

Amy continued with the nursing program. She added a few more *B*s and two *A*s to her record. Her cumulative grade point average showed she exceeded the school's minimum requirement for graduation. In addition, Amy's scholastic record would be a valued credential for future evaluation in the event she decided to apply to another institution for advanced education.

Lita was also enrolled as a freshman in a nursing program. Her program of sixteen units for the semester was scheduled over a 4½-day week from Monday to Friday noon. Lita applied for and obtained a part-time job as a cashier on Fridays and Saturdays from 4:00 P.M. to midnight. She was advised by her instructors and her counselor that the academic and physical demands of her nursing program required her full attention. However, she insisted she had plenty of time to study on school nights and on Sunday; that she had worked part-time during high school and passed all her courses; and besides, she wanted to be earning money. For a few weeks things seemed to go well.

When classes included written assignments and increased library research for the preparation of term papers, Lita had problems. She decided to study for classes on a day-to-day basis and to take time off from her job "later" to do the term papers. At midterm her grades for her courses were *C*s except for a *D* in a four-unit chemistry course. In a conference, her counselor suggested to Lita that her attempt to work and carry a full class schedule was too much for her. Lita stated she needed the money for a new coat and for Christmas vacation plans, but she *would* work harder on her classes.

Lita stayed up later each school night to study, but she was always tired the next morning. Two days she overslept, missing a clinical laboratory experience specially arranged for her on one day, and an important chemistry lab and a quiz on the other day.

The day before Christmas vacation ended she caught a cold. She returned to school but reported to the health service on the second day with a sore throat and severe headache. Lita's temperature was 102.6° F, so she was referred to her doctor who prescribed treatment and ordered bed rest.

After six days Lita was back in school. In the meantime her job as cashier had been filled. She had missed several classes, and her written assignments were not ready. When the semester ended, Lita's grades were inadequate to recommend her continuance in nursing. She was deficient sixteen grade points and was placed on academic probation. Lita withdrew from nursing and from college. The profession lost a potential member who, if she had attended to her studies and could have accepted counsel from those interested in her welfare, might have succeeded in completing her preservice program.

Students should realize that they are responsible for maintaining a satisfactory grade point average throughout the entire educational program. *An overall average of not less than 2.0 is necessary to meet the requirements for graduation.* If a student plans higher education, her academic record may be the deciding factor in her being accepted or refused admission to a college or university. In seeking employment after graduation, a good scholastic record is an asset that operates in the applicant's favor when being considered for a position.

BIBLIOGRAPHY

Board of Nursing Education and Nurse Registration: Laws and regulations relating to nursing education, licensure, practice, State of California, 1969.

Fivers, G., and Gosnell, D.: Nursing evaluation: the problem and the process, New York, 1966, The Macmillan Co.

Lyman, H. B.: Test scores and what they mean, Englewood Cliffs, N. J., 1963, Prentice-Hall Inc.

Nunnally, J. C.: Educational measurement and evaluation, New York, 1964, McGraw-Hill Book Co.

Rottkamp, B. C.: Attrition rates in basic baccalaureate nursing programs, Nursing Outlook **16**:44-47, June 1968.

School marks and promotions, ed. 4, Washington, D. C., 1958, National Education Association.

COMPLETE WORK SHEET ON PP. 321 AND 322

CHAPTER 11

The National Student Nurses' Association

The National Student Nurses' Association was officially organized at the National League for Nursing Convention held in Cleveland, Ohio in 1953. Supported by both the American Nurses' Association and the National League for Nursing, approximately 1,000 nursing students in convention assembled elected officers, adopted a Constitution and Bylaws, and began to plan for future programs and conventions. NSNA is the national preprofessional organization for student nurses.

HISTORY

As early as 1924 it was noted that nursing students were attending meetings and conventions of professional nurses. Because of the increasing interest, the American Nurses' Association appointed a subcommittee in 1946 to study the feasibility of admitting junior members. Their report, however, advocated organizing local student groups instead. It also encouraged the state nurses' associations to help organize these groups and to stimulate students' participation in the activities of the professional nursing organizations. Scheduled programs for students were included in all national meetings of the American Nurses' Association after 1948, and in 1949 two students were added to the subcommittee for study of the American Nurses' Association. The work of this subgroup proved so valuable that it was elevated to the rank of a full and recognized committee.

By 1950 students were expressing a desire to form their own organization. Recommendations were made at the American Nurses' Association convention in San Francisco that year that the professional nurses provide opportunities to meet the potential needs of each student, of the individual school of nursing, and of the local preprofessional nursing organizations. To accomplish this task, it was suggested that a national organization comprised of state student nurses' associations be formed. Enthusiasm for self-organization increased, and the nursing students who attended the 1952 national convention in Atlantic City voted to form a National Council of Student Nurses. In asserting their willingness to follow and also their enthusiasm to move toward leadership, these students asked that the Council function independently, but be guided and sponsored by the Coordinating Council of the American Nurses' Association and the National League for Nursing. The students began with temporary officers, many ambitious resolutions, and much hard work.

In 1953 in Ohio, the Constitution and Bylaws were adopted and officers were elected to form the National Student Nurses' Association. The parent professional organizations, American Nurses' Association and National League for Nursing, continued to offer assistance as the student organization grew. A newsletter offered a medium of distributing information and the *American Journal of Nursing* provided a section for information about National Student Nurses' Association affairs. Progress was rapid and both records and correspondence soon demanded considerable time from the staff of both American Nurses' Association and National League for Nursing. In the following year Miss Frances Tompkins was appointed coordinator. Miss Tompkins had the services of a staff consultant

OFFICIAL EMBLEM OF NSNA.
(Courtesy National Student Nurses' Association.)

from the two professional organizations and a NSNA board to promote organizational activities.

Membership exceeded 60,000 in 1955, and the Board recognized the need for a permanent mailing address. A request was made from American Nurses' Association and National League for Nursing for permission to have an office at the national nursing headquarters—10 Columbus Circle, New York, New York 10019; the request was granted and the office is still at that address. It was during this year, also, that the design of the official seal was approved for National Student Nurses' Association. It has been a symbol of pride and achievement since that time. Plans were made for elections of officers prior to the annual convention and to promote effective student organizations in schools of nursing throughout the United States.

At the Congress of the International Council of Nurses in Rome in 1957 and in Melbourne, Australia, in 1961, the National Student Nurses' Association presented the request for a proposed student unit. This request was withdrawn in 1962, however, because it was felt that such a unit might present problems too great for students to handle. Interest in international meetings has not waned because of the lack of an individual organization. Each International Council of Nurses meeting sees an ever increasing number of student nurses present and participating. The most recent, held in Montreal, was no exception.

By 1958 the National Student Nurses' Association was financially independent, and Frances Tompkins was made executive secretary. Mary Ann Tuft currently is the executive director of the national student organization. Board members were receiving and accepting additional invitations from American Nurses' Association and National League for Nursing to participate in national committee meetings. For example, in 1959 the president of National Student Nurses' Association attended a meeting called by the Secretary of the Department of Health, Education and Welfare; NSNA was also represented at the Thirteenth National Conference on Citizenship in Washington, D. C. During 1959 the National Student Nurses' Association also took legal steps to incorporate the organization and to copyright the *Newsletter*.

MEMBERSHIP

The National Student Nurses' Association has members in forty-nine states (an ADN program is opening in Anchorage, Alaska in September 1972), in the District of Columbia, and Puerto Rico. The members from the Virgin Islands were welcomed at the 1970 convention in Miami, Florida. Many states are further subdivided into districts, so that membership includes national, state, and local or district associations. Any undergraduate student enrolled in a preservice program is eligible for membership in National Student Nurses' Association, including the registered nurse enrolled in a baccalaureate nursing program. Members pay national dues of $5.00 and individual state and local dues. Membership is individual and voluntary, based on the belief that forced enrollment does not lead to active participation.

Membership responsibility includes disseminating information to other members through newsletters, local publications, and the *American Journal of Nursing;* becoming involved in activities of the organization, in nursing, and in the community; actively becoming involved in one of the various NSNA projects; and recruiting for NSNA and for *nursing.*

PURPOSE

The purpose of NSNA is to prepare student nurses for their responsibilities as registered nurses and as active members in the American Nurses' Association and National League for Nursing. NSNA also helps students to become better citizens and welds a bond among all nursing students.

ORGANIZATION

Executive board. The Executive Board of the National Student Nurses' Association includes the six elected officers and four advisors. The officers on this board are the president, first vice-president, second vice-president, corresponding secretary, recording secretary, treasurer. The advisors include an elected advisor, an appointed advisor from each of the sponsoring organizations (American Nurses' Association and National League for Nursing), and one advisor appointed by the president with board approval. The Executive Board conducts all organization business between conventions, implements the purposes of National Student Nurses' Association, makes provision for a national headquarters, and is responsible to the membership for the handling of funds, keeping of records, and the implementation of any other provision in the Bylaws. As specified in the Bylaws, each elected officer also acts as chairman of a standing committee.

COMMITTEES

Nominations committee. The committee on nominations is elected at convention. It consists of a chairman and four members. This committee meets and follows the stipulated procedure as described in the Bylaws for establishing a slate of candidates.

Membership committee. The membership committee and the chairman are appointed by the Executive Board. This important committee attempts to enroll new members each year to replace the ones who graduate. This committee plans, develops, and directs both local and national membership drives and involves members already enrolled in these campaigns.

Program committee. The first vice-president acts as chairman of the program committee and members of the Executive Board serve on the committee. This committee plans the program for conventions and the association.

Finance committee. The finance committee reviews any information concerning the organization's financial status. The national treasurer is chairman. Other responsibilities include advising state and local treasurers as to their official duties.

Bylaws committee. The second vice-president is chairman of the Bylaws committee. This important committee reviews all proposals for change in national Bylaws and relates state and local bylaws to the national Bylaws to ascertain that they are in conformity. The committee also helps local groups in writing bylaws through the development of a guide or model.

Public relations committee. The corresponding secretary is chairman of the committee on public relations. This group edits the National Student Nurses' Association *Newsletter.* At each national convention winners in state newsletter competition are announced. The competition is sponsored by this committee.

Policies committee. The recording secretary acts as chairman of the committee on policy. In an attempt to keep all policies current, this chairman reviews, revises, and submits to the board for approval any policy change deemed necessary.

ACTIVITIES

American Nurses' Association—National Student Nurses' Association Committee on Common Interests and Goals. This group was formed to promote a better relationship between American Nurses' Association and National Student Nurses' Association based on the common interests and goals of nursing and of those preparing to enter nursing by:

1. Encouraging understanding and examination of the aspirations of nurses and student nurses as expressed through the professional and preprofessional organizations
2. Focusing on ways in which the two organizations can work together to further the aims of nursing
3. Facilitating the transition from the student role and membership in National Student Nurses' Association to full professional achievement and membership in American Nurses' Association
4. Providing assistance to corresponding state and district committees (The specific functions of this committee at state and local levels should be stated, problems identified, possible solutions discussed, and a plan for resolving the difficulty developed—but the local functions should relate to guidelines as directed from the national organization.)

National Conference of Professional Students. The National Student Nurses' Association became a charter member of the National Conference of Professional Students in 1963. Student groups belonging include the student sections of the American Dental Association, the American Pharmaceutical Association, the American Law Association, the American Medical Association, and the National Education Association. This coalition affords its members the opportunity to interact and support each other in programs relating to their respective professions. Representatives of the nursing group participated in testifying before the Senate and House Appropriations Committees in June 1970. These students were appealing for full funding of Federal Health Student Loan and scholarship programs under the Health Manpower Act of 1968. The appearance of students at this hearing marked the first time that the health professions joined to support a common cause. The representative of the National Student Nurses' Association was concerned with recruitment and stated that without the aid of the scholarship funds many minority group members as well as the applicants from underprivileged areas would be lost to the health professions.

Recruitment for nursing. In an attempt to reach more men and women for nursing, the National Student Nurses' Association is vitally interested in seeing that all citizens have the opportunity to enter the career of their choice. To implement this aim, representatives work on the National Recruitment project, which is an attempt to aid any minority group obtain the preparation needed to enter the health professions. Firmly convinced that quality health care is a right of all persons, NSNA joined Opening Doors Wider in Nursing (ODWIN) to help the disadvantaged. Their work is to tutor, counsel, and give financial help as a means of showing the disadvantaged that nursing has a place for them.

Laura D. Smith scholarship. This scholarship fund was established in 1962 in memory of Laura Smith, senior editor of the *American Journal of Nursing* and an advisor to the National Student Nurses' Association. She died in 1961, and the $1,000 scholarship was established through voluntary funds. Application for this fund can be made to Nurses' Educational Funds, National League for Nursing, 10 Columbus Circle, New York, New York 10019. Registered nurses working toward a baccalaureate or master's degree are eligible, and applicants who are former active members of National Student Nurses' Association will probably get preference.

Taiwan project. An outstanding example of involvement on a very large scale is the Taiwan Project. Working in cooperation with the National Federation of Business and Professional Women, the National Student Nurses' Association helped to raise funds for the National Defense Medical Center (NDMC) in Taipei, Taiwan. This philanthropic project was undertaken on a nationwide basis in 1961. By May 1963 the goal of $25,000 had been surpassed. As a result of the interest, effort, and professional helpfulness of National Student Association members in the United States, the nursing students of the National Defense Medical Center (NDMC) have a new fifty-bed dormitory with some equipment and furnishings. The ribbon-cutting ceremony of dedication took place in March 1966, and the building was officially given the name of National Student Nurses' Association Dormitory.

Involvement. The National Student Nurses' Association holds its annual meeting just prior to the American Nurses' Association or National League for Nursing biennial conventions. Students are urged to attend these national conventions. Involvement 1970 can best be described by the review of the resolutions adopted at the 1970 convention held in Miami Beach, Florida. During this convention, 1,200 of the 1,700 student nurses attending gave proof of their "caring" attitude by their participation in the march and pledge to live for one day on the same allowance which welfare allowed the indigent in their home territory. The students then took their theme from Senator George McGovern, of South Dakota, convention keynote speaker, who urged them to ". . . help dedicate the 1970's not to weapons of death but to weapons of health, nutrition, and healing."

You, as a student in nursing, have opportunities which were undreamed of by those who preceded you. Become an active member in the National Student Nurses' Association on the national, state, and local levels. Only by involvement can you hope to gain from the National Student Nurses' Association. Membership enhances your personality development, your growth in interpersonal relationships, and in your preparation for social participation as a nurse and as a citizen. You will be fulfilling the purpose of your organization by acquiring a greater understanding of, and a respect for, nursing. You may not be able to acquire fame to the extent that your name will be recorded in the annals of history, but you can certainly step forward as a more confident graduate nurse. You can make more definite footprints in the sands of time if you share with those who travel life's highway with you.

BIBLIOGRAPHY

American Journal of Nursing, National Student Nurses' Association Page (each issue).

Ciriello, T., and Jacoby, P.: 1966 National Student Nurses' Association Convention—in retrospect, Nursing Outlook **14**:49, Sept. 1966.

Corcoran, J.: National Student Nurses' Association's first six years, American Journal of Nursing **59**:695, May 1959.

Forster, S. S.: National Student Nurses' Association's ten tall years, New York, 1963, National Student Nurses' Association, Inc.

Frackelton, D. L., and Faville, K.: Opportunities in nursing for disadvantaged youth, Nursing Outlook **14**: 26-28, April 1966.

International in scope, forward in approach. Report of National Student Nurses' Association 1963 Convention, American Journal of Nursing **63**:116-123, June 1963.

Juhre, E. M.: Clothes don't make a convention, American Journal of Nursing **54**:840-841, July 1954.

In San Francisco, this is the week that was, American Journal of Nursing **66**:1594-1599, July 1966.

National Student Nurses' Association Convention, Nursing Outlook **18**:50-51, June 1970.

National Student Nurses' Association, American Journal of Nursing **70**:1311-1316, June 1970.

Price, G.: The advisor to students, American Journal of Nursing **64**:130-132, April 1964.

Scott, H.: Convention management, Nursing Outlook **7**: 210-211, April 1959.

Students at the ICN Congress, American Journal of Nursing **61**:92-93, July 1961.

Film

Today's activity, tomorrow's progress (shows how Student Nurses' Association of New York State achieve goals); twenty-five minutes. Black and white; American Nurses' Association—National League for Nursing Film Library.

COMPLETE WORK SHEET ON PP. 323 AND 324

CHAPTER 12

The role of counseling in nursing programs

Because nursing is a demanding profession, schools of nursing are also demanding—emotionally, psychologically, and intellectually. In addition, many students are involved in an intensive period of questioning, probing, and reevaluating their lives. Therefore, these years of professional and personal growth may be difficult for students, especially if they have not previously experienced problems in coping with demands and stresses in their daily lives.

Counseling in nursing education programs is a means to an end—to help students with their personal adjustments and with achieving their educational goals. Broadly speaking, counseling in the educational situation is a personal experience in which the counselor and student consider problems presented by the student. Together they consider how the problems are affecting the student's personal life as well as how they are interfering with her adjustment to, and her progress in, the nursing program. The counselor participates in this experience by pointing out to the student, through skillful guidance of the discussion, ways in which the student can develop insight into her problem and find her own best solution.

Counseling may be very valuable to those students who feel that they need empathetic and skilled help in thinking through a matter of concern, whether it relates to their school activities or to their personal lives. Because so many students seek assistance of this kind, schools usually establish a counseling service. This service is commonly staffed by qualified and prepared counselors who are trained in administering and interpreting various psychologic and vocational aptitude tests. In addition, the service may keep a current file on jobs, career opportunities, material on advanced education, and financial assistance.

Ideally, a good nursing education program incorporates the philosophy underlying counseling and guidance into every part of the curriculum, so that necessary assistance, support, and guidance are available to help students with the developmental problems most of them share. Your school's orientation program should acquaint you with available counseling facilities, and you should take advantage of them and use them for your benefit.

Everyone needs counseling and guidance. As children you received counseling and guidance from your parents, older brothers and sisters, or other relatives. Later you received counseling from teachers, friends, and associates. Usually this kind of guidance stressed the *do* and *don't* type of advice and was intended to be accepted without questioning. Generally you accepted this counsel because you trusted the judgment of those more experienced than you. As a person grows older, a different kind of assistance in planning and living is needed. This assistance cannot and should not consist of explicit directions. For example, as prospective nursing students you probably sought someone's advice before you selected your nursing program. Hopefully, you weighed advice and alternatives and had a major role in choosing your school. Now that you are in the process of becoming a mature adult you may well need to sit down with an understanding counselor and spend some time understanding your feelings about yourself and your career.

PARTICIPANTS IN THE COUNSELING PROGRAM

The organization of a school's counseling program depends on the organization of the school and its philosophy of counseling. Some schools may include a full-time counselor as a member of the faculty. This is usually the pattern followed in collegiate programs. As a member of the faculty, this counselor has several important functions in addition to direct counseling with students. She will work with other faculty members and staff to help them with the areas in which they may advise students, serve as a member of the selection committee for the admission of new students, and participate in student orientation.

In other types of nursing programs an instructor frequently serves as counselor.

There are other personnel who may be involved in counseling programs: nurse-instructors, clinical psychologists, a physician, and members of the clergy. Sometimes the director of the student residence hall plays an important role in counseling situations. The nature of the student's problem and the particular type of guidance needed will determine which member of a counseling team might give the most effective help.

Every student should know about the many facets of the counseling program and the benefits that it can offer her. The counseling program exists to help students meet crisis situations in their lives but it also exists to help them deal constructively with their problems and adjustments in *normal* development.

COUNSELOR

A counselor should be qualified through preparation and temperament to provide advice and guidance to students involved in the broad range of problems or situations incidental to the normal maturation process. In certain areas, such as the administration of tests and the interpretation of their results, the counselor brings professional expertise and experience to bear on any given problem. The objectivity with which a counselor views a student's problem and suggests ways of formulating solutions strengthens the student's confidence in the value of the counseling. A counselor also serves as a liaison and as an advisor for others who may participate in the counseling program.

NURSE-INSTRUCTORS

Instructors have a vital role in the school's counseling program. Competent instructors have a highly developed knowledge of the subject matter and are skilled in means of transmitting their knowledge and its practical application to students. The instructors challenge their students to learn and to develop. Therefore, instructors *must* be concerned about their students' scholastic achievements and must be aware of problems students may have in learning and applying subject matter. As instructors they are the persons best able to advise and counsel students regarding difficulties relating to their course area, but students must recognize that they are responsible for requesting such counseling and guidance.

Some nursing programs use a pattern of counseling in which instructors serve as advisors for class groups, student committees, or school clubs. In this capacity the instructor's role as counselor is directed toward helping students in these groups to learn such things as group processes, identification of problems, problem-solving, group decision-making, and the planning, initiation, and the operation of student government activities. In this type of situation the instructor-advisor has a different relationship with the students than that of an instructor-counselor.

CLINICAL PSYCHOLOGIST, CLERGYMAN, AND PHYSICIAN

Some nursing education programs include clinical psychologists, physicians, and clergymen on their counseling staff. Others use the services of these specialists through a referral system. In either case the knowledge and skill of these specialists is available to students who need their services.

DIRECTOR OF RESIDENCE (HOUSEMOTHER)

The residence director or housemother has her own unique counseling function. In Chapter 7 the role of the housemother in helping new students was discussed. In some instances a resident director also functions as the school's social director and is responsible for planning and helping with various social and cultural activities and for maintaining a pleasant homelike atmosphere in the residence. A residence director's participation in counseling involves making certain that institutional regulations are understood and observed, that students' whereabouts are known when they are off campus, and, similarly, that procedures are carried out for contacting a student's parents or guardian in emergency situations.

WHY COUNSELING IS SOUGHT

Counseling can contribute to a student's ability to shape and meet educational goals and frequently can help the student to attain these goals. Counseling can have both therapeutic and preventive benefits. For example, effective guidance can assist the student in identifying personal habits or characteristics that may be obstacles to her desired academic and personal achievement. It is the responsibility of the student to identify and work to overcome these obstacles with the aid of counseling. Through counseling it is also possible for a student to discover latent abilities, which may then be encouraged and enhanced. In general, the role of counseling is to help the student to develop skills in planning her life, so that she is able to evaluate her circumstances, needs, and available alternatives. Counseling makes it possible for the student to make decisions that will yield the greatest personal and professional satisfactions.

ACADEMIC PROBLEMS

The significance of academic proficiency has been discussed in Chapter 7, but it may be helpful to stress the fact that students often need to evaluate their study habits and attitudes toward study. They must accept the discipline imposed by study and be aware of the need to develop a constructive approach to the work of studying, especially if academic difficulties are present. A student who had been able to get through high school without "cracking a book" and who had used cram techniques before tests to get grades may find that it is impossible to cope with daily assignments that require learning, understanding, remembering, and using large segments of information in a variety of classes. Such a student is under many urgent pressures and may require immediate counseling to learn how to handle the situation.

Although an instructor often recognizes the student's difficulties, her hands are tied until the student becomes aware of the need for counseling and comes to the instructor for assistance. Therefore, a student should spend some time in evaluating not only her performance but also her feelings, so that she may take advantage of the counseling facilities available and seek the help she needs from the instructor. The initiative *must* be taken by the student.

COUNSELING IN THE CLINICAL SITUATION

Students often have a difficult time in adjusting to the demands and pressures they encounter as inexperienced newcomers to the hospital environment. At this period their self-confidence may be at a low ebb, and their self-assurance needs to be bolstered by the type of counseling and guidance that only the clinical instructor can give. For example, students may feel anxious about their ability to care for patients with certain diseases, or they may worry about how they will react in performing certain types of nursing services. Students become frustrated when they cannot carry out a procedure as they were taught because of some unanticipated factors. They may find that they cannot cope with certain situations. Often, too, students try so hard to do their assignments perfectly that they fail to perform effectively—they expect too much of themselves too soon.

Your clinical instructors are interested in your learning to practice and provide quality patient care. They want you to be able to use the information you are acquiring by applying it correctly in the clinical situation, and they want you to gain self-confidence and satisfaction as you learn. They also are familiar with and can understand the problems you are having in making your adjustments. Students sometimes forget that their clinical instructors were once anxious and inexperienced students. The difficulties you may be experiencing are not unknown to them.

In order to be effective in teaching students how to put their knowledge into practice, the clinical instructor must also be able to help students to overcome their anxieties and frustrations. The relationship established between students and their clinical instructors as they work side by side should contribute to better understanding. A sound, constructive, and mutually beneficial working relationship should develop. The goal of each, the achievement of quality patient care, is attained as students learn to appreciate the instructor as a counselor as well as a clinical teacher.

Counseling and guidance are involved whenever an instructor meets with a student to review and evaluate the student's clinical record. Reviews such as this allow the student to discuss and understand demonstrated areas of proficiency as well as areas in which more effort is necessary. In addition, the student's general personal growth can also be determined. The counseling that occurs at such a session focuses on the student's interest in the course work and on her attitudes toward learning and her use of knowledge in the work situation. The kind of interpersonal relations developed and maintained with co-workers and patients is also discussed. All of these factors reflect the strengths the student has to build upon and the weaknesses she should overcome.

PERSONAL PROBLEMS

The nature of personal problems will vary with individual students, but when any problem becomes a block or a deterrent to a student's personal or academic progress, it is important that she seek help. Personal problems may involve finances or the inability to make effective use of time. They may relate to work, school, family, friends, health, or her adjustment to demands of the nursing program. In each of these instances a skilled counselor can provide guidance, encouragement, and support for the student who is trying to implement the most satisfactory solution to the problem.

THE COUNSELING RELATIONSHIP

Counseling can be either informal (incidental) or formal (planned). In the former instance the counselor and the student relate to each other on the spot, so to speak, where the meeting occurs. The guidance that emerges usually is focused upon help with an item of immediate concern. Counseling might also occur during a coffee break when both the instructor and student discuss some specific problem. Another example of incidental counseling is when the instructor and student in the clinical area review plans for patients' daily nursing care.

Emphasis in the discussion that follows will be on the more formal, or planned, counseling session. The formal type of counseling has a specific purpose, requires time for consideration of the problem, and may require a review of records or other information. For formal counseling the student makes an appointment with the school's counselor, or an instructor, psychol-

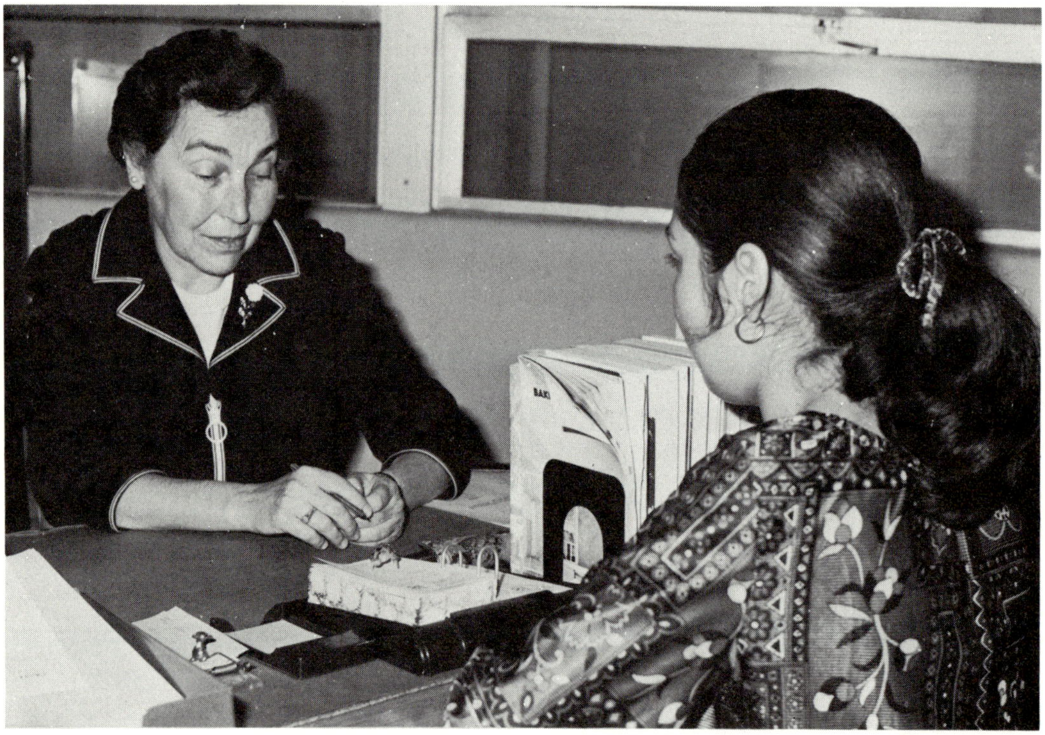

A STUDENT AND THE COUNSELOR PARTICIPATE IN A FORMAL COUNSELING SESSION.

ogist, physician, or clergyman. It is the student's responsibility to request such an appointment and, if possible, the general nature of the problem should be indicated when the appointment is made. This allows the counselor to make some plans for the meeting and to schedule adequate time for the conference.

If you make such an appointment, you should also plan for this meeting. For example, you should know why you are requesting the meeting (it may be helpful if you prepare a list of questions to assist you and your counselor to spell out problem areas). Some problems require more than one session. If this is the case, follow the prescribed procedure for making a future appointment. The *student* is responsible for making necessary appointments and keeping them. If the student does not keep appointments, she is exhibiting resistance to the counseling procedure, and this should be dealt with in the next session.

Counseling sessions are generally held where the discussion can be private and free from interruptions. Hopefully the student will soon be at ease with the counselor and will speak as freely as possible regarding all the details of the problem. Information exchanged in these sessions must be considered confidential and used in such a manner that the student's confidence is not violated. The point to remember about counseling is that the session must be "open" if positive results are to occur.

The counselor's role is to help the student develop an awareness of all aspects of the problem and an understanding of her own feelings and behavior so that she can act responsibly in developing a solution. A counselor does not tell the student what to do. A good counselor works *with* the student to develop the student's ability to deal with the specific problem at hand and to further develop problem-solving skills that will benefit the student in future areas of concern.

Counseling can only be effective if the student does her best to solve the problem. Personal growth and maturity will then result from the experience. It is a mark of personal development when a student recognizes that she needs help with a problem and then proceeds to seek it from the person best qualified to assist her. In nursing many situations appear to be problem areas simply because they are new experiences. When students take the time to analyze a problem, discuss it with another person, and see the relationship of the parts to the whole, the "problem" often becomes a challenge to be met and mastered. Whether the situation is a challenge or a serious problem, students are wise to seek appropriate help.

BIBLIOGRAPHY

Arbuckle, D. S.: Counseling, an introduction, Boston, 1968, Allyn & Bacon, Inc.

Bennett, M. E.: Guidance and counseling in groups, ed. 2, New York, 1963, McGraw-Hill Book Co.

Blocker, C. E., and Richardson, R. C., Jr.: Teaching and guidance go together, Junior College Journal **39**:14-16, Nov. 1968.

Briggs, T. H., and Justman, J.: Improving instruction through supervision, New York, 1952, The Macmillan Co.

Cristantiello, P. D.: Group process for developing a faculty advisor program, Nursing Outlook **16**:27-29, June 1968.

Daubner, E. L.: Teacher as counselor. In Lee, J. M., and Pallone, N. J., editors: Readings in guidance and counseling, New York, 1966, Sheed & Ward.

Goldstein, J.: Exploring attitudes that affect nursing care, Nursing Outlook **16**:50-51, June 1968.

Gordan, I. J.: The teacher as a guidance worker, New York, 1956, Harper & Bros.

Iafolla, M. A. C.: Guidance in nursing education, The Journal of Nursing Education **8**:15-22, Jan. 1969.

Jordan, C. H., and Kennedy, J.: Counseling that enriches, American Journal of Nursing **60**:231-233, Feb. 1960.

Kemp, C. G.: Intangibles in counseling, Boston, 1967, Houghton-Mifflin Co.

Roeher, E. C.: Orientation to the job of counseling, Chicago, 1961, Science Review Association.

Tyler, L. E.: The work of the counselor, ed. 2, New York, 1961, Appleton-Century-Crofts.

Weitz, H.: Behavior change through guidance, New York, 1964, John Wiley & Sons, Inc.

COMPLETE WORK SHEET ON PP. 325 AND 326

CHAPTER 13

Interpersonal relations

MEANING OF INTERPERSONAL RELATIONS

Interpersonal relations refers to the manner in which people respond to each other and identify with each other in situations of everyday living. The phrase also means the dynamics of *how* people interact, and *why* they react to each other as they do.

A person develops the basic patterns of relating to others long before he begins to associate with people in business or work. For example, the newborn infant has interpersonal relationships with his mother, father, and other members of his family. These relationships form the basis of such patterns in all succeeding types of interpersonal relations he will experience throughout his life. Furthermore, these early, fundamental relationships affect later development of individual characteristics associated with satisfactory interpersonal relations.

Good interpersonal relations are built on consideration and respect for other people. Respect for self and for others stems from the recognition of man's innate dignity and intrinsic worth as a member of the human race. The establishment of an interpersonal relationship includes emotional involvement between human beings because each one *is* human. Nurses, therefore, should be able to understand their obligations for relating to, or participating in, their patients' experiences without jeopardy to their own feelings and sense of identity.

The importance of sound, honest relationships between human beings cannot be sufficiently stressed. Understanding interpersonal relationships requires knowledge of theoretical content and its application in practice. To master this subject and its varied applications requires the use of a variety of learning experiences, generally directed by instructors who themselves are skilled in identifying the potential outcomes of relationships and in guiding students toward gaining benefits from them.

SOME CHARACTERISTICS OF SATISFACTORY INTERPERSONAL RELATIONSHIPS

Since interpersonal relations are the results of interaction between human beings, let us look briefly at some facets of individual personality that contribute to their establishment.

1. Self-awareness. A person can possess self-awareness only in proportion to the degree to which he is honest with himself about his basic emotions and needs. This ability depends upon personality, life experiences, intelligence, and interest in himself and others. A person who has self-awareness realizes that he needs to be accepted, respected, and appreciated by others, and he recognizes that others have the same needs. This understanding will shape his interactions with other people and will help him to develop good interpersonal relations.

2. Self-acceptance. Self-acceptance implies an awareness of both one's own strengths and shortcomings. Self-awareness also means being able to accept and live with the facts. It implies an ability to react in a way that shows he has self-respect.

As a nurse you need to accept yourself both as a person and as a professionally oriented worker. You need to believe in yourself and in your worth as a human being. At the same time you must recognize that you cannot, by yourself, supply all the answers to the world's or even one patient's problems.

All human beings have needs that must be satisfied and personal problems that require solutions. You must know and accept these needs and understand their significance before you can recognize and accept them in others. In general these needs are identified as follows:

a. A need to be recognized for one's abilities despite personal limitations
b. A need to be respected and accepted by associates and co-workers
c. A need to be accepted as a member of the group
d. A need for challenge to growth and development
e. A need for security and self-confidence

If you accept these needs in your own life, you will recognize the importance of these factors in accepting and interacting with others.

3. Acceptance of others and sensitivity to others' needs. One must be able to accept another person as having rights and privileges comparable to his own, irrespective of the other's personal philosophy, actions, or outlook. The fact that other people are different from you neither authorizes nor justifies actions and attitudes that deprive others of the same feeling of acceptance you desire for yourself.

A basic fact of social existence is the difference among people. This difference requires that those who live or work together must adapt themselves to each other. Since interaction with others is mandatory in society, it is imperative that you learn to adjust your ideas and your actions to correlate with the needs of others if satisfactory interpersonal relationships are to exist.

Elements that contribute to the acceptance of others and facilitate adjustment to human needs include evidence of respect for others and courtesy and kindness toward others. These elements in turn lead to the development of rapport and a spirit of cooperation among people. The ability to be perceptive or sensitive to the feelings of others, especially in the realm of daily work associations, is reflected in the quality of interpersonal relationships that operate among all members of a team. The qualities of loyalty, trust, and honesty are brought together in a working situation and become operational in a stable, consistent relationship. Satisfactory interpersonal relations are possible among persons whose individual differences are recognized and respected if a pattern of interdependence and fidelity to the dignity of everyone functioning within a group is achieved and maintained.

4. Respect for the job one is doing. If you are going to become a valued employee you must learn what your job entails and become familiar with its particular responsibilities and related duties. You must also be ready to accept responsibility for your actions and carry out each task to the best of your ability. In this way you show respect both for the job you are doing and for yourself as a worker. You can take pride in completing your assignments.

The manner in which you do your work and the quality of your performance tells your co-workers something about your interest in the work itself. If you are interested in the task, this interest will provide many opportunities to initiate and participate in good interpersonal relationships with many people in the course of a day's work. The display of initiative to acquire new knowledge and skills is expected if you are to grow and develop your skills in nursing, but complementing this personal development should be evidence of skills used to establish and foster interpersonal relations with your co-workers. Like other skills, this one needs to be planned for, developed, and strengthened through practice. Effective application of those elements that identify positive interpersonal relations requires an understanding of what is expected of you, an effort to achieve the right atmosphere in which to function, and a motivation to succeed. Such understanding, effort, and motivation will carry you toward the result you desire.

When these qualities are a part of your daily life, they affect the impressions you make on others. The interpersonal relations you establish as a person, as a nursing team co-worker, and eventually as a team leader will affect the role you play in the practice of nursing. Basically, the interpersonal relations you establish reflect the characteristics and attitudes you possess as a person. Hopefully these can contribute to your achieving a high quality of communication with others to ensure a high quality in the nursing services you offer your patients.

INTERPERSONAL RELATIONS IN THE CLINICAL SITUATION

In our society hospitals are recognized and accepted as institutions that provide essential health services for the public. Basically they are identified as centers organized (1) to serve the needs of those who are ill or injured, (2) to have available for immediate use all types of equipment and material required to treat all types of patients, and (3) to offer this care as an individualized service. Staff members are expected to be competent to perform necessary patient care tasks.

Hospitals also have other purposes. They serve as health education centers and as teaching areas for the professional preparation of doctors, nurses, and others engaged in caring for the public's health. They are also centers for vital research. Hospitals serve as a source of employment for many people and are major consumers of many resources and products of the community. Operating a hospital is a business venture; hospital operations currently rank among the top six industries of the United States.

Your instructors have probably discussed in detail the classification, size, services offered, licensure, accreditation, ownership, and administrative control of hospitals. You are no doubt familiar with the particular characteristics of the hospitals used for your clinical assignments and other planned learning experiences. Smooth, effective hospital or health care agency administration is dependent upon the establishment and coordination of good interpersonal relationships and communication systems among all staff personnel.

There must be a definite organizational structure upon which to base management plans for any institution, and hospitals are no exception. Organizational charts indicate the bases upon which responsibility is delegated, so that all staff members fit into the chain of supervision. Organizational charts demonstrate who is responsible for carrying out the various tasks of administrative work, direct patient care, housekeeping, dietary service, laboratory services or any one of the many services necessary to the operation of a quality patient care facility.

In the language of management operation, an organizational structure involves a concept of assignment identity known as *line and staff*. *Line* positions in an organizational pattern are illustrated by their vertical placement from the top to the bottom of the diagram. The term "line" in this context is synonymous with authority. Persons in line positions are free to give orders and to transmit those orders; they also delegate responsibility to other personnel in subordinate line positions. Relationships between persons in line positions are identified in a diagram through the use of unbroken lines. Thus the chain of command within an organization flows from the head or top position downward through administrative personnel in consecutive subordinate levels; each one in turn contributes his effort to see that the administrative order received from his superior is carried out competently and efficiently.

Staff positions within an organization pattern are associated with assignments of advising, carrying out special studies, coordinating activities that relate to the entire organization, planning, and research. The person in a staff position reports directly to an administrator. For example, the position of clinical coordinator for nursing services within a hospital is a staff position. The person in this position would report directly to the administrator of nursing services.

Any pattern of organization structure should clearly identify the official channels of communication existing within it and show how these lines of communication operate among and be-

FUNCTIONAL RELATIONSHIPS AMONG PERSONNEL IN LINE AND STAFF POSITIONS

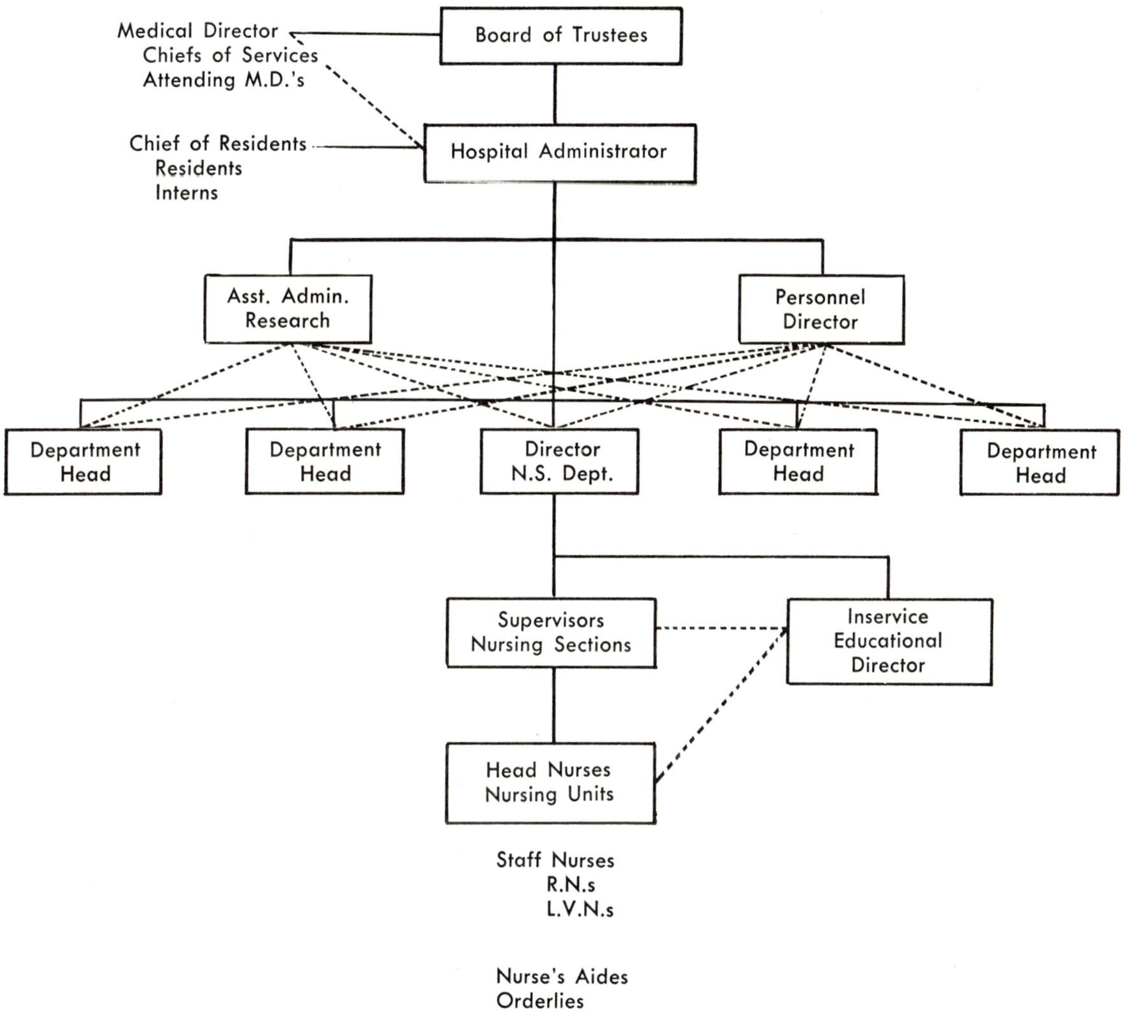

Straight lines identify positions in the line of authority and indicate who is responsible to whom, (who can give orders and who receives orders from whom). Indicate the lines of official communication in the organization.

Broken lines identify staff positions. A person in this position has advisory or general functions that cut across organizational lines.

FUNCTIONAL RELATIONSHIPS. NO ATTEMPT HAS BEEN MADE ON THIS CHART TO ILLUSTRATE A HOSPITAL ORGANIZATION OR TO SHOW GROUPINGS OF FUNCTIONS.

tween all those who are identified as members of the organization. These channels of communication are vital to the development and maintenance of good interpersonal relations among staff members of any health care facility.

No doubt all of you have been told at some time that you had to "go through channels" when you had a special request or wanted permission to do something. What does "through channels" really mean? It refers to the process of transmitting official communications from the top of the organization down through the various administrative levels to the bottom of the organization, or, upward through the organization to the top.

According to communication theory, a channel is a medium for carrying messages. The channels for official communication are determined by the formal structure of the hospital and are shown in its organization chart, in which each level of administration is delineated. The lines or directions of communication are the result of the delegation of authority and responsibility. When an individual has been given the authority and responsibility to get work done, there is an upward line of communication that he should use to transmit information to, and receive information from, his superiors. There is also a downward line that he should use to communicate information to, and receive information from, his subordinates. *The lines of authority are the channels or lines of official communication.* An official communication initiated at any level in the organization is forwarded upward or downward, as the case may be, to the next responsible person in the line of authority; the message goes through each administrative level until it reaches the person who has been *delegated the authority and responsibility to act upon it.*

It is suggested that you study the organizational pattern of the hospital with which your nursing program is affiliated. Doubtless there is a master chart showing the overall structure, including the hospital's governing board, the hospital administrator and his assistants, and the specific areas of service within the hospital for which each is accountable. Note the placement of the medical staff as a unit for service and its relationship both to the hospital administrator and to the governing board.

Additional diagrams showing details of the organization pattern such as the placement of the department of nursing services and the dietary, housekeeping, and maintenance departments can demonstrate the significance of lines of authority to and from the person in charge, the concept of line and staff relationships, and the provisions in effect for communication from high to low levels and among personnel on all levels.

Do you detect any correlation between the diagram illustrating the organizational pattern of the hospital's services and the importance of a plan of maintaining communication among all personnel who make up its working force? What is the significance of establishing and maintaining good interpersonal relations among various departments and within each department of the total organization? How can problems develop if authority throughout a department or the whole organization is not clearly defined, if lines of communication from superior to subordinate and between persons with comparable responsibilities are not clear, or if relationships between people serving within the organization break down on a person-to-person basis? Answers to these inquiries will reveal that there is a definite relationship between the quality of interpersonal relations and the degree to which good communication exists throughout the group.

INTERPERSONAL RELATIONS IN THE EDUCATIONAL SETTING

An organizational structure exists also in the nursing school to give structure to the students' educational program. In general, the organizational structure serves the same purpose in a school as in a hospital. The type of nursing education program and its relationship to an administration within a college or a hospital establish the requirements for patterns of authority and responsibility. These factors are reflected in the organizational chart. The diagram illustrating the organizational structure is likely to be found in the office of the nursing director. Study this diagram and try to identify the provisions made for the establishment and maintenance of communication and the relationships dependent on it.

Line and staff relationships and the accompanying patterns of communication are significant. They contribute not only to harmonious operation of the educational unit within the parent organization but also to the maintenance of good relationships with the hospital personnel responsible for the areas used as nursing practice laboratories.

Interpersonal relationships established by faculty working together for the benefit of the students' welfare are strengthened when faculty members understand their role as supervisors and their responsibility for carrying out their activities under the aegis of the head nurse assigned to the hospital's clinical unit. *When the clinical instructor is on a nursing unit working with students, she is in a staff relationship to the head nurse of the unit.* In this capacity the clinical instructor has nothing to do with the administration of the nursing unit, but she can suggest and advise on matters that affect students' clinical practice. With the head nurse she plans which patients will be assigned to which students and coordinates with her those aspects of an individual patient's care that will be performed by the students and for which the regular nursing staff will be responsible.

The head nurse of a patient care unit works in the line of authority that passes directly from the administrator of the hospital to the director of nursing service to the section (division) nursing service supervisor and then to her. All messages or information from a higher authority come to the head nurse first; she in turn informs the members of her nursing staff. The head nurse is responsible for keeping the division supervisor informed about the condition of patients, how work is progressing, what factors may be preventing work progress, any incidents or mistakes that may have occurred in her area of responsibility, and all other matters of an official nature pertaining to the patients, the personnel in her jurisdiction, and the operation of the unit.

Personnel assigned to the nursing unit report to the head nurse. Each one is individually responsible for keeping the head nurse informed on all matters pertaining to her work and the care administered to assigned patients. When nursing care assignments are made to nursing care teams, an intermediate line of communication, through each nursing team leader, is set up between the head nurse and the nursing team members. The leader of each nursing care team is responsible for keeping the head nurse informed about the condition of all patients under the care of her team and for reporting on the activities and problems in her assigned area. Individual team members report to the team leader; she in turn incorporates this information in the report she makes to the head nurse at the close of the duty tour.

The student's line of communication. With this background in mind we need to look at communication lines as they apply to the student who is working in the clinical area but is not an assigned member of the nursing staff. To whom does the student report when she is practicing on the nursing unit? A student's first line of communication is to the clinical instructor. Students receive their assignments from her and report directly to her concerning all matters involving the care of patients, requests for help in performing nursing procedures, and the recording of care given. However, the student also has a communication line to the head nurse when she is practicing on the nursing unit because *the head nurse is the person ultimately accountable for all patients on that unit.*

As a student, you will be expected to demonstrate your understanding of proper communication by observing certain procedures based on necessity and common courtesy. You should report to the head nurse when you arrive on the unit for your clinical practice and again at the close of your practice period. If you are unable to complete any part of your assignment, if you have some pertinent information or observations about the patients, or if there is a request made by a patient that you are unable to fulfill, you should pass this information to the head nurse (or team leader), in addition to telling your instructor about it before leaving the nursing unit. You must remember that communication and the maintenance of interpersonal relationships are important parts of the job of nursing.

RELATIONSHIPS BETWEEN INDIVIDUALS

Within the world of the hospital you will encounter some unusual interpersonal relationships, which are created by the particular circumstances that exist; these relationships are affected by the situations in which they occur and reflect the way in which you respond to them and allow them to influence your daily life.

The most obvious relationships involving nurses are those developed with patients. Throughout your nursing program instructors and clinical supervisors will discuss the significance of the nurse-patient relationship and the importance of accepting patients as individuals and of establishing rapport with them. As one nurse-educator points out, "Acceptance is not just being nice to people. It is a principle of action in which the nurse perceives and works with the patient as he really is."* The development of rapport with patients will influence your success as a professional and will contribute to the skill with which you evaluate a patient's needs and give him the necessary personalized care. Nurses, both as students and as graduates, are responsible for determining the degree of involvement they develop in this type of relationship so that the relationship is a positive experience for both patient and nurse.

The nurse-patient relationship is intended to be a helping relationship. It is a two-way experience unique to the participants. It might be compared to a situation in which each person channels something of himself into a pool and thereafter withdraws new knowledge, better understanding, and new strength from this common resource to meet the daily demands. Because of this relationship each participant can share in the privilege of bringing out the best qualities of the other. However, it is imperative that nurses use caution and good judgment in the management of this relationship. The nurse must avoid extremes of either underinvolvement or overinvolvement in a patient's life as long as a need for the relationship exists; she must also refrain from assuming the highly inappropriate possessive "my patient" attitude.

Another type of helping relationship is the one that exists between doctors and nurses in the performance of their respective professional duties. While this association affects each one personally, its primary focus is to benefit the patients whom they are trying to assist. Both the doctor and the nurse are expected to recognize and accept the supportive role each plays as part of a professional team providing health care. They must cooperate fully to meet the needs of the patient. Because of his preparation in the field of medicine the physician is liable for the patient's welfare in terms of medical diagnosis. He is responsible for evaluating the condition of the sick person, making the medical judgments, and ordering those treatments, medications, and other procedures which in his professional opinion will most benefit the patient. It is the doctor's prerogative to specify exact techniques to be used in caring for the patient, the times at which certain procedures are to be performed, and the priority for implementing medical orders. In these instances the nurse functions in a subordinate position to the doctor; her services are performed under his supervision and are adjunctive to his role in the professional relationship.

There are also instances when the nurse functions in a situation distinct from the physician's activities. The nurse is accountable for her activities as a professional employee, for evaluating her responsibilities toward co-workers and patients and for making discriminating judgments pertaining to the kinds of nursing care the sick person needs in response to his condition. She is responsible for initiating and following through with a plan of nursing care that dovetails with the medical care plan so that the coordinated efforts of all those involved in caring for the patient will produce a positive result.

*Connelly, M. G.: What acceptance means to patients, American Journal of Nursing **60**:1754, Dec. 1960.

It is easy to see that the establishment of any plan for interpersonal action intended to benefit the patient demands that both doctors and nurses practice the elements of good interpersonal relations discussed earlier in this chapter. The results may well include such benefits as a firm basis for positive patient reaction to the quality of care received, co-workers who understand the benefits accruing when everyone works for a common purpose, and a public with a favorable evaluation of the institution in which such good professional interrelationships exist and are evident.

Personnel on the nursing staff within a hospital or clinical agency are identified by job titles and are responsible for the assignments associated with each title and job description—for example, director of nursing services, head nurse, staff nurse, or floor nurse. Irrespective of title or position, however, each staff member needs to develop and foster harmonious relationships with others so that the standards of nursing care for which she is responsible will be maintained.

Earlier in this chapter we looked at the ways in which the effective functioning of an organization depends upon identification of the flow of authority and the flow of communication in direct line from top administration to those in subordinate positions. The relationships established among staff members and the morale of the group will determine the effectiveness of any authority and communication channels. This effectiveness in turn will determine the quality of care available. The pattern of relationships and communication found in a single hospital unit can affect the operation of other personnel groups in other hospital units. The effects of good staff relationships are not lost on the workers, the administration, the medical staff, the patients, or visitors. Most important for the individual, however, is the awareness that his efforts as a team member are significant and that his efforts, when combined with the efforts of others, can effect a positive result.

Throughout their educational program, nursing students are assigned to clinical experiences that involve a continuing series of interpersonal relationships. These include relationships with nursing instructors and supervisors to whom they are directly responsible, nursing service personnel and medical staff members on clinical divisions with whom they work and share a variety of learning experiences, and patients for whose care they are responsible and whose daily progress must be reported to instructors, head nurses, and/or team leaders. Understanding and accepting the need for these relationships are fundamental to the successful performance of one's nursing assignments, as well as to laying a foundation for the continuity of positive relations.

The importance of establishing a pattern of communication whereby one person responds constructively to another is emphasized in all nursing classes and clinical assignments throughout the course of a nursing program. Each participant must recognize his role and responsibility for developing a viable relationship. It is this interaction among people, together with the related communication of ideas, that serves as a foundation for the good, satisfying relationships in both professional life and personal life.

BIBLIOGRAPHY

Burton, G.: Personal, impersonal, and interpersonal relations, ed. 2, New York, Springer Publishing Co.

Connelly, M. G.: What acceptance means to patients, American Journal of Nursing **60**:1754-1757, Dec. 1960.

Crow, L., and Crow, A.: Understanding interrelations in nursing, New York, 1961, The Macmillan Co.

Davis, A. J.: The skills of communication, American Journal of Nursing **63**:66-70, Jan. 1963.

Hall, B. L.: Human relations in the hospital setting, Nursing Outlook **16**:43-45, Mar. 1968.

Hayes, W. J., and Gazaway, R.: Human relations in nursing, ed. 3, Philadelphia, 1964, W. B. Saunders Co.

Kron, T.: Nurses' aides need clearer directions, American Journal of Nursing **63**:118-119, Mar. 1963.

Maloney, E.: Interpersonal relations, Dubuque, Iowa, 1966, William C. Brown Co., Publishers.

Peterson, G.: Working with others for patient care, Dubuque, Iowa, 1968, William C. Brown Co., Publishers.

Rasmussen, E. H.: Changing organizational relations, American Journal of Nursing **62**:73-77, Oct. 1962.

Ujhely, G. B.: Determinants of the nurse-patient relationship, New York, 1968, Springer Publishing Co.

COMPLETE WORK SHEET ON PP. 327 TO 330

CHAPTER 14

Communication

THE IMPORTANCE OF COMMUNICATION IN NURSING

A nurse must be able to communicate accurately and effectively in almost every professional activity. This ability is the most essential skill a nurse can have. The frequently mentioned skill of "working with people" requires an ability to transmit information to the proper people and to put across your own ideas and understanding. Knowledge alone is not sufficient; to succeed in nursing, you must combine your knowledge with the ability to apply and share it clearly and efficiently.

In the course of a day's work, every nurse gives and takes orders, complies with requests, and makes oral and written reports. As a team leader the nurse is responsible for the activities of the other team members under her direction. In order for them to meet her expectations for quality patient care, she must make assignments, clarify misunderstandings, and discuss solutions to problems in a manner that is thorough, consistent with doctors' orders, and tactful. She must know about the care and use of an array of complicated equipment and must be able to instruct other personnel in its proper care and application.

Events that require explanations occur constantly in the nurse-patient setting. The nurse is responsible for explaining to patients the reasons and the procedures for various tests and treatments. These explanations are given in order to solicit the patient's active cooperation. Only by giving cooperation can the best results in each treatment plan be achieved.

The head nurse is a first-level manager in the hospital administration; she directs the work of the nursing unit, interprets administrative policies and procedures, helps to resolve any misunderstandings among personnel, and supervises the coordination and performance of the many activities within the unit. All of these functions require the use of one or more basic communication skills, because professional effectiveness depends greatly upon the ability to communicate with each person encountered in the course of the working day.

You will have many opportunities to develop this fundamental skill as you build your professional knowledge and clinical experience. Just as you learn to adapt your general professional skills to specialized use, you will also learn how to use your communication skills and techniques in relating to patients and co-workers on the nursing unit.

In this chapter we will discuss person-to-person communication and will briefly explain some of the important points of communication theory in order to give you an insight into the communication process. You will then be able to develop and improve your capacity to share your ideas, knowledge, and feelings with others. You may wish to supplement this material by reading some of the numerous articles and books on the many aspects of communication.

VERBAL AND NONVERBAL COMMUNICATION

The word "communication" is generally used to mean intentional, verbal messages of one kind or another. During most of your waking hours you are engaged in some form of communication behavior—speaking, listening, reading, or writing. What reaches you through the use of words, however, is only part of the picture. There is also the nonverbal communication that occurs in each interaction that adds dimensions of meaning to the verbal message. Your "Thank you" may reveal that you did not really appreciate the favor done for you; "Hello" on the telephone may be short for, "Who's this bothering me now?" You assume that the other person takes your "Thank you" and your "Hello" in their conventional meanings, but the nonverbal messages in your voice and manner may reveal far more about your meaning than the words alone.

Each encounter you have with others provides additional information about them and influences your perceptions of them. Every action, incident, or event—however minor—communicates information that you perceive, often unconsciously, through one or more of your senses. These nonverbal signs may go unnoticed or be misunderstood if you have not learned to observe them.

Nonverbal communication, as the name implies, is any communication that involves indicators other than words. Gestures and movements of the body are all expressive of an idea or an emotion. One's posture, manner of dress, manner of speaking, all communicate nonverbal messages to the observer. Gestures may accompany verbal communication and reinforce words, or they may substitute for, or even contradict, a verbal message. They can be deliberate—such as a shrug of the shoulders or raised eyebrows—or they may be mannerisms of which you are not aware.

Nonverbal communication invariably accompanies verbal communication when two persons engage in face-to-face conversation. Nonverbal meanings are conveyed by facial expressions, by inflections of the voice, and by emphasis given to what is said. You usually look at the person to whom you are speaking to see whether he understands you and to determine whether he agrees or disagrees with you. If a person were to say to you, "What did you do to your hair?" he could mean either "How pretty you look," or "Ugh, you look frightful." You can tell what he really means as a result of knowing him and of listening to the way he says it—by the tone of voice, inflection, and expression. Sometimes the nonverbal message is conveyed so strongly that it overrides the words a person might be speaking. A startled glance, a blush, a look of distaste, and a grimace all serve as meaningful messages in and of themselves.

You use nonverbal signs as clues in evaluating how other people feel toward you, toward what you do and say. You must realize that other people will interpret your gestures and expressions in the same manner.

PERSON-TO-PERSON COMMUNICATION

At times we all have trouble getting other people to understand what we say, and we have difficulty understanding them. As one author notes, "You have only to cast your mind back over your dealings with other people to realize that faulty communication has much to do with creating disorder in human affairs."* Every day we communicate with many different people in many different ways for hundreds of different reasons. For the most part we take our capacities for speaking, listening, reading, and writing so much for granted that we are seldom aware of the complexities involved in communication. We usually give thought to the *way* people communicate only when we are on the receiving end, and then only when we have trouble understanding the other person.

Basically, communication means conveying ideas and information by one person to another. One of the definitions Webster gives for communication is, "interchange of thoughts or opinions; a process by which meanings are changed through a common system of symbols (as language, signs or gestures)." In communication ideas must travel between a sender and a re-

*Hodnet, E.: The art of working with people, New York, 1959, Harper & Brothers, p. 84.

ceiver; that is, between a speaker and listener or a writer and reader. In order for true communication to take place, the receiver needs to understand the idea that the sender is trying to get across.

The mere fact that two individuals are engaged in sending and receiving messages is no assurance that communication is actually taking place. Unless there is understanding resulting from these interactions there is no communication. The other person may not agree with what you are saying, but as long as he *understands* what you are saying, communication has taken place. The test of the effectiveness of your communication depends on how the other person is able to pick up your message, although his reaction will depend upon his own feelings and ideas.

You communicate for many reasons: to get the things you want, to get or give information, to convince someone, and to express your feelings and opinions. The response you want from the other person is understanding, acceptance, and the desired action. However, the fact that you have expressed an idea does not guarantee that you will elicit the desired response or even that every message you send will be understood or acted upon at all.

To communicate effectively you must understand the complex processes involved when ideas are expressed. Factors vital to effective communication are the following:

1. How well meanings of words are understood
2. How thoughts are organized
3. How messages are constructed
4. How well one person understands another's meaning
5. How well attitudes and prejudices are understood

However, before these aspects of communication are considered, let us look at what actually occurs during the transmission and reception of messages. By knowing something of the process of communication and the steps involved, you will have a better idea of what happens when you communicate with someone.

The communication process.* Plainly stated, communication is concerned with the transfer of meanings. When two persons engage in the act of communication, the sender changes ideas into words, and the receiver changes the words back into ideas. The meaning apprehended by the receiver must be the same as that intended by the sender, or there is no communication between them.

Although every communication differs from every other one, certain elements and conditions must be present in order for communication to occur. There is always a *sender* (someone who has a reason or purpose for communicating), a *message*, and a *receiver* (the person from whom response and action are expected). The message (the sender's thoughts) has to be put into the form of a *code* so that it can be transmitted. A code may be any set of symbols that can be structured in a way that will express the message and be meaningful to someone. If, for example, the sender wants a glass of water, he may transmit his message in the form of spoken words, written words, or pantomime. Finally, the message must be put into some *channel* so that it reaches the other party. The channel serves as a carrier for the message (for example, airwaves or sound waves). The physical and mental activities performed by the sender in encoding and transmitting the message and by the recipient in receiving and decoding the message and responding to it constitute the *communication process.*

A description of what occurs in the process of communication is outlined in the following situation. Suppose you and your roommate Carol are in your room studying. Carol likes the radio playing while she studies. Ordinarily the radio does not bother you, but this evening you are having difficulty concentrating because the music is distracting you. You decide to ask her to turn off the radio. You are now ready to act as a communication sender. You have a purpose—to get Carol to turn off the radio. Your message has to

*Material for explanation of the communication process is adapted from Berlo, D. K.: The process of communication, New York, 1960, Holt, Rinehart & Winston, pp. 23-39.

be put into some physical form so that it can be transmitted. In this case the code is spoken words. Your speech mechanism is the encoder. Your central nervous system orders your speech mechanism to construct a message to express your purpose. Obediently, your vocal cords produce the message: "Carol, do you mind turning off the radio? I know it isn't loud, but I'm having trouble concentrating."

The message is transmitted via sound waves through air so that Carol's ear can receive it. This is the channel. Carol's hearing mechanism acts as the decoder. The vibrations that Carol's ear receives are forwarded in the form of electrical impulses to her brain, which she experiences as sounds. The brain translates the sounds into words and reassembles them into the whole idea of the message. Carol's nervous system responds to the message. It agrees with your observation about the radio, and she decides to comply with your request. Carol orders her speech mechanism to produce a message: "Sorry, I'll do it right away." With Carol's response the communication process is completed for a single communication. During the process of communication Carol received your message, decoded and understood it correctly, and responded in the way you intended. This is communication. The process is a complicated one, though it is over in far less time than it takes to describe it and, as you can see, much of the process requires no conscious effort.

A special point needs to be mentioned. In describing communication it is necessary to talk about the actions of the sender and of the receiver separately, as though a speaker, for example, initiated communication and a listener was the end of communication. In the dynamic sense these are not independent behaviors but are part of the *communication process*. The person who had been a sender at one moment has become a receiver the next, and the messages he produces are determined by the messages he has received. In any ordinary conversation, beyond those requiring no more than a nod or a "yes" or "no" answer, the same individual can and often does act as both sender and receiver several times during the same conversation.

SOME FACTORS TO KEEP IN MIND WHEN YOU COMMUNICATE

Now that you have some understanding of the communication process, let us explore ways in which you can apply this understanding in order to improve your own ability to communicate. Everyone has a tendency to blame the other person when there is a misunderstanding or a breakdown in communications. If a classmate does not understand what you tell her, your reaction is: "Why don't you pay attention?" When a patient fails to follow your instructions, your defense is: "But I explained it to him." If an aide has difficulty in comprehending your instructions, "There is something wrong with her." Or when you find it difficult to follow a speaker, you blame him and give up trying to listen to what he is saying.

Make your intent clear. Communication is impaired at the *sending stage* if the sender does not have his purpose clearly in mind before he attempts to communicate. Communicative purpose is simply what the sender wants to have happen as the result of his message—what it is he wants the receiver to know, to do, or to accept. The sender's purpose or reason for communicating *is* his message.

A message is what you mean to say, but it is not always what you do say. For example, a nurse has just refilled a patient's water pitcher and has noted his fluid intake. Before leaving him she says, "Remember, you are scheduled for tests in the morning, so don't drink after eight o'clock." The patient followed what he thought was the nurse's instruction—not to drink any water after 8:00 P.M. However, he accepted and drank a glass of chocolate milk when evening refreshments were passed out to patients. The nurse failed to get her message across to the patient, and he missed the point of her instruction, which was to not drink *anything* after 8:00.

The sender cannot send *meaning* to the receiver. One important aspect of communication theory is that meaning is not transmittable—only messages are transmittable, and meanings are not in the message. A message is an *expression* of the sender's thoughts or ideas. In producing his message, the sender has his own meanings for the words he uses. He chooses words and arranges them in sentences in the way he hopes will express his message. The receiver who decodes the message attaches *his own* meanings to the words he translates. There is understanding between them only if the receiver has meaning for the message and if his meanings match those intended by the sender. If the receiver's interpretation of the message is different from that of the sender's, or if he does not understand the words the sender uses, there is no communication.

When you have something important to communicate to someone, clarify in your own mind what you want to say and then plan how you will say it. When you explain something to a patient or instruct an aide in the performance of a certain task, think of what the person needs to know about the subject. In composing your message, it is important to relate the content to the receiver in terms of his knowledge level and background experience with the subject, and to consider his feelings about what you are going to tell him. Because you want the receiver to respond in a certain way, you try to anticipate how he will accept and respond to your message so that you can make your message both understandable and acceptable to him.

Since the purpose of communication is to convey something to someone, it is important to use clear, exact words that will be understood by the receiver. A person thinks and comprehends the thoughts of others in terms of the words he knows. Therefore, it is important to use words that are part of the receiver's vocabulary.

As mentioned earlier, when you communicate you cannot know whether the messages will be accepted, rejected, or even understood by the receiver. Although meaning cannot be transmitted, you can facilitate the transfer of understanding by structuring your messages in such a way that your intent will be clear to the receiver.

Choose the right time. Communication is rendered ineffectual from the start if the timing is not right. Communication is a two-way process and as such requires the cooperation of both the sender and the receiver. If a person does not want to listen or is unable to listen—for example, because of his emotional state—he will not get your message.

Many of the annoying misunderstandings and mix-ups in communication occur when the recipient's attention is occupied with another matter. For example, an aide asks the head nurse for permission to leave early in the afternoon. The head nurse, who is busy writing a report, answers, "Go ahead." Later that afternoon when she looks for the aide to find out why she had not put the clean linen away, she remembers what she said to the aide. When she told the aide to "go ahead," she did not fully realize what she was saying.

In the clinical setting the factor of time is always an important consideration, and judgment is required in deciding on an appropriate time to instruct or explain something to a patient. In orienting a new patient and in explaining hospital regulations and policies, for example, the nurse may observe that the patient appears nervous and upset. In this situation she might better wait with her explanation until the patient is calmer and can attend to what she is telling him. If a patient is to have a particular test or examination that requires detailed instructions about his responsibility in the procedure, the nurse should make certain that she explains the procedure at a time when she has the patient's full attention and when the patient has the opportunity to ask questions to clarify any confusion that may exist.

Attitudes and prejudices. Attitudes are more or less the controlling factors in the ways in which you communicate with and respond to other people. Broadly speaking, "attitude" refers to a disposition, an inclination, or a tendency to act toward something in a particular way. An attitude is a point of view. Each individual builds up attitudes that are derived from his past experience, his social and cultural background, and his knowledge level. Attitudes may be strong or weak depending on the individual's experience with the subject and the pleasant or painful reactions he has received in the course of his involvement with it. You have acquired attitudes about many things—food, dress, cats, politics, religion, war, nationalities, unions, authority, bus drivers, and so on. Some sample expressions of attitudes are: an individual feels antagonistic; an individual feels favorably disposed; an individual feels skeptical.

Prejudice is a particular kind of attitude. Prejudice means prejudging or making up one's mind in advance of the evidence with no intention of changing an opinion, regardless of any facts or pertinent information to the contrary. The prejudiced person uses labels, stereotypes, and generalities; what is seen or heard is judged in relation to these labels, stereotypes, and generalities. Prejudice is a learned behavior; it is an emotional one because it is irrational. It prevents you from knowing things as they really are, because you hear only what you want to hear, and the rest is lost or distorted.

A sender's attitudes affect both the way he produces his message and the way the receiver responds to it. For example, if the sender does not have a good opinion of the receiver, this unfavorable feeling will influence what he says and how he says it. When the listener realizes this, he will be more critical of the sender's message and less likely to accept what he says.

When a person listens he evaluates what he hears in relation to his own background and experience, and he takes the sender into account. It is difficult for the receiver to separate what he hears in the message from his feelings about the sender. How many times do we permit an individual's statement or expression to turn us away from him? In the listening situation this sort of thing happens more often than any other. Unfortunately, a person is not always aware of the strength of his own attitudes and prejudices and how they affect perceptions and efforts to relate to others. He may even think of himself as a completely objective listener.

Attitudes are often indicated unintentionally by choice of words. At a Parent-Teacher Association meeting a teacher remarked with regard to a parent's proposal, "She is only a housewife—she's never had any experience in this matter." Imagine the effect of this remark upon all of the parents in the group. The teacher had, in effect, discounted anything they might have to contribute.

You also reveal your feelings about your own importance when you overuse the words *I* or *my* in general conversations. Again, there are people who tend to aggravate and alienate others, not so much by what they say as how they say it. The message may be acceptable, but the manner and tone tend to irritate others. When this happens, the listener is prone to respond to those aspects of the message rather than to the words themselves. The more you know about your own attitudes and prejudices the more conscious you will be of the ways in which they color your thinking. Only insofar as you are sensitive to yourself will you be able to check and control the tendency to distort or misinterpret what another person is saying.

How you use feedback. When a sender transmits a message it is important that he knows whether or not he is getting through to the receiver. He discovers this by interpreting the cues or the feedback that he receives from the other person.

In communication terminology *feedback* refers to the interdependence of action and reaction in a communication situation. A simplified explanation of the concept is the following. In a two-way conversation, A produces a message. The message is perceived by B, who reacts and responds to it. Then A uses the information he receives from B to shape *his* response to B's message. The cycle is repeated as many times as is necessary until the communication is terminated. In the back and forth exchange of messages, each person's response is influenced or affected by the feedback he gets from the other person. Feedback is necessary to the communication process. Sending a message is only one part of the communication process. It is not completed until feedback is received.

Feedback may be conscious or unconscious, verbal or nonverbal. You use feedback all the time, whether you are aware of it or not. Earlier we mentioned the communicative qualities of facial expressions, gestures, manner of speaking, and body movements to transmit meanings. In presenting his lecture a teacher may note expressions of puzzlement on the faces of some of the students. This signals to him that these students do not understand what he is talking about. In this case the teacher may decide to backtrack and explain some point, or he may ask the students if they have any questions.

How feedback is used can either facilitate or impede communication. Most of the time communication is taken for granted, and important cues may be missed, especially when feedback is received. If you listen only to the literal meaning of what the person says, you may miss the meaning he is actually trying to convey. You need to develop the habit of listening for different levels of expression and meaning. People attach different meanings to commonly used words and phrases, and you need to understand clearly what the words mean to the person using them. Sometimes it is necessary to ask the other person, "Did I get this right?" or, "I'm not sure that I got that. Is this what you mean?" This is the counterpart to making your own meaning clear, which was discussed earlier.

Sometimes a response is actually two messages, and if you fail to "hear" one of them you thwart communication. For example, a head nurse asks a new aide at the close of her first day on duty, "How did it go today?" The aide answers "So-so, I guess." If the head nurse is alert and does not take the aide's words at face value, she will ask the aide what she meant by "so-so" and will learn that the aide had a perfectly miserable day and is not planning to return to work the next morning.

If you are not sure the receiver has understood your message, you can ask the other person for direct feedback. If the communication involves directions on how to perform a procedure, explanation about some detailed routine, or a complicated order, you may ask a person to repeat in his own words the information he has been given. This is more satisfactory than merely asking him whether or not he understands or if the instruction is clear. If the receiver states in his own words the content of the message the sender will know what the receiver has heard and whether or not he understands.

How you use language. Normally words serve us well and we can understand each other; but it sometimes happens that words that are unfamiliar or that suggest a different meaning to the receiver are used. In such cases the words themselves prevent the communication process or distort the meaning of the message for the receiver.

As previously stated, meaning is not transmittable. In communicating, the sender selects his words and constructs his message in a way that he hopes will elicit the correct understanding of his meaning from his receiver. Communication is successful only if the receiver takes meaning from the message and if his meaning is similar to that intended by the sender. If you are to make yourself understood and understand other people, it is necessary to know something about the use of words. You must know what gives them their special meanings in different situations, the various ways in which they are used, and how words can take on nonverbal meanings.

Language and meaning. Words get their meaning from the way they are used by people in speaking and in writing. It is important to remember that words are verbal symbols used to represent things: objects in the physical world, concepts, ideas, or feelings. A word symbolizes your *concept* of the thing, not the thing itself. The word and the thing become related only when people agree to a certain relationship between the two. For example, there is no absolute connection between the object known as a bed and the word "bed" except that that particular word has been set aside in the English language to serve as a symbol of the object.

Part of the problem in using language and in making yourself understood concerns the multiple meanings of words. People often use different words to mean the same thing. For example, one person may use the term *spigot* and another may be more accustomed to use the term *faucet.* A certain type of iron frying pan may be a *skillet* to one cook and a *spider* to another. In hospitals the familiar four-wheel cart used to transport patients may be called a *stretcher,* a *litter,* or a *guerney.* Many of the words used in ordinary conversations have extended meanings and are used in different ways with different meanings. The words that have many meanings are usually the short ones, the words everyone knows. For example, the dictionary lists 104 meanings for the word *run*. To compound the problem, two or more words that have different meanings are pronounced the same: hare and hair; mete, meet, and meat; heir and air; capital and capitol. Although these words are spelled differently they sound the same.

In order to use language effectively you must be aware of the alternate meanings of words and consider the receiver, who must decode your message and translate what it means. A word may have a specific meaning for you, but it is not safe to assume that it will have the same meaning, or any meaning at all, for the listener. Your intention in using a particular word may have to be explained. Again, if you use words that can be interpreted broadly, the listener is required to fill in his own meaning for the message. Thus the foundation is laid for misunderstanding on both sides. As a nurse you may block communication if you do not translate medical and nursing terms into meaningful language for the patients. Too often it is assumed that patients know what is meant not only by medical and anatomic terms but also by unofficial abbreviations of medical terms and hospital jargon.

Denotative meaning. Basic to understanding the meaning of words is knowledge of the difference between denotative and connotative meanings. When you think first about the meaning of a word you think of the denotation, or what it has come to mean as a result of the way in which it is used.

Denotative meaning refers to the object-word relationship. When you use the word "bed" you refer to the object in the physical world that this term stands for. It is this denotative or identifying meaning of words that the dictionary records and tries to describe. The thing that the word stands for is called its *referent.* Pointing out or identifying the referent gives a word its primary or core meaning—its denotation.

Words vary as to definiteness of meaning, depending on the exactness with which they bring to mind their specific referents. Such words as *Pennsylvania Avenue, cable car, stethoscope,* and *three-ring notebook* have specific meanings, because you can readily identify the objects spoken about. Words such as *neatness, pain, reliability,* and *humor* have less definite referents; meaning is dependent on the user's past experience with the word. Meanings for words that refer to general or abstract concepts have the least definite referents and are the most difficult to agree upon. Some examples of these so-called abstract words are: *beauty, wealth, courage, patriotism,* and *freedom.*

Connotative meaning. Besides denotative meanings, words also have secondary or implied meanings because of the association of ideas they evoke. Connotative meaning is based on the relationship among the object, the word, and the person. It is usually related to personal experience. Connotative meaning refers to your personal feelings about the object or concept or how you perceive it as a result of your personal experience. For example, a student nurse exerts special effort to make a very ill patient comfortable; when she is finished and ready to leave she remarks, "Now, rest in peace." Obviously, the student meant to convey her wishes for comfort and relief, but her words meant something entirely different to the patient, who associated the words "rest in peace" with the familiar response in a prayer for the dead. The patient thought the nurse was telling him he was going to die. A word may suggest what the person's past experience, his temperament, or his imagination has given it for him. The fact that the sender may not experience the same association of ideas is a frequent cause of misunderstanding.

Besides the special associations words have for a particular person, many words have acquired connotations from the way the word has generally been used. For example, the words "childlike" and "childish" have the same denotative meaning in that they both refer to characteristics or qualities of childhood, but "childish" suggests characteristics that are unfavorable or unpleasant.

Some words are used for the connotation they carry. Synonyms generally refer to the same idea or subject, but one cannot be used in place of the other without changing the sense of the statement, for example, angry-annoyed-indignant; cross-grumpy-sulky-sullen; languor-listlessness-boredom.

Words that conspicuously suggest connotations are sometimes referred to as "loaded" words. These words suggest an attitude or a feeling of the person using them and would stimulate a similar positive or antagonistic attitude or feeling in most listeners or readers. Advertising and propaganda of all types make use of words whose associative ideas have strong positively or negatively loaded connotations.

It was mentioned earlier that the usual meaning of a word can be inverted or changed by tone of voice or facial expression. Meaning can also be changed by the circumstances in which the word is used. Note the difference in meaning between: "Tomorrow we will *review* Chapter 5 in class," and "It is time to *review* your progress."

Both denotation and connotation must be considered. You want to express your ideas, but you must also remember the import of emotions and feelings in determining meaning. You must choose the words that will be most likely to bring about mutual understanding.

Meaning from context. From this brief review of the meanings of words you may be wondering how people can use words and make sense with them. If individual words can have many meanings and if several different words can have a common meaning, how is communication possible? Words get their meaning from the context in which they are used. As isolated entities words have little or no communicative meaning.

If someone asked you the meaning of *light*, more than likely your reply would be "How is it used?" Thoughts are expressed in groups of words—in phrases, clauses, and sentences. Words only have possible meanings until they are used with other words around them. The placement of a word in the sentence determines its meaning to a great extent. The following sentences show how the context determines the meaning of the word:

1. The *light* was dazzling when it burst upon us.
2. She wore a *light* blue ribbon in her hair.
3. Let's *light* a bonfire.

How you put your words together (grammar) and in what order (syntax) they are put together are important if your message is to convey your meaning accurately and if the receiver is to interpret the meaning intended.

Word usage. Word usage refers to the choice of language that is appropriate to the communication situation. It was pointed out earlier that a person interprets meaning according to what the words mean to him. Therefore, in order to avoid a breakdown in communications, a sender should adapt his language to the receiver and should use words the receiver is accustomed to and can understand.

The more words you have at your disposal, the better able you are to express your thoughts and ideas, provided that you use the specialized elements of your vocabulary in a proper context. In using words you must consider the effect they will have on the receiver. You must remember that there is a wide vocabulary difference among people; words that are quite familiar to one person may not be understood by someone else.

How do you go about adapting your words so other people will understand your messages? The function of language is to make yourself understood, so your first aim should be to use plain, direct, uncomplicated language whenever possible. For the rest, you must learn to depend upon your sensitivity and the clues received from the other person. If a patient complains about his "stomachache," you would use his phrase in discussing his complaint with him. However, in reporting his complaint to a doctor the situation would call for a more exact description, and the more specific description of "pain in the epigastric area" (if such were the case) would be the appropriate language for a professional communication between doctor and nurse.

To communicate meaning, words must be used accurately in context. Effective word usage demands that the words be appropriate for the purpose and for the situation in which they are used. The following statements all tell us the same thing, but the context clearly illustrates why they are not always interchangeable.

1. He had a cholecystectomy last year. (Professional speech and writing)
2. He had a gallbladder operation last year. (General conversational speech and writing)
3. He had his gallbladder out last year. (Colloquial speech)
4. He had a G.B. last year. (Operating room shop talk)

Medical jargon and slang. Jargon, or shop talk, is language used by members of a particular profession, trade, or calling. The language typically includes the names for materials, equipment, and procedures used in the work of the group. The terminology is often unintelligible to an outsider. Medical jargon plays a big role in the speech patterns of hospital personnel. At this stage in your nursing studies you are probably well indoctrinated in this language, and such expressions and abbreviations as *IPPB, Code 9, MI, BMR,* and *NPO* are no doubt part of your professional vocabulary.

Medical jargon is a distinctive vocabulary and is appropriate only when talking with other medical and nursing colleagues who understand the language. It should not be overused or allowed to spill over into ordinary conversations. Jargon is a very useful and efficient language if you use it where and when it is appropriate. It should not be used in communication with patients. A patient should not be forced to figure out what you mean when you ask him if the lab has taken his CBC yet. Terms that are commonplace to those who know the jargon can be confusing, if not downright alarming, to other people.

You should not assume that all personnel working on the nursing unit are familiar with the technical names of equipment and the various medical expressions and abbreviations. If you find it necessary to use these terms when you are giving directions or explanations or answering questions, make certain that the person understands what you are telling him.

Slang and other types of "in" talk, on the other hand, are extremely informal forms of language and have limited use in purposeful communication. In general, slang words are newly made-up words, old words with extended meanings, catchy words or phrases, or standard words used in different ways with changed meanings. The real objection to the use of slang is that the connotations of words are so short-lived that their meaning is lost in repeated use. Although very sparing use of slang can enliven casual conversations, a person who uses this type of language constantly becomes tiresome to listen to. One's judgment and sense of fitness actually dictate the language that is appropriate in any situation.

How you speak. Most people take speech for granted. They pay little, if any, attention to how they talk and how they sound to other people. However, there are some basic elements to be reckoned with in this sphere of communication. The speaking voice is generally broken down into four separate but interrelated elements. These are volume, rate, pitch, and quality. The proper use and control of these elements contribute immeasurably to the sound and the effectiveness of one's voice.

Volume refers to the loudness, the fullness, and the quantity of the voice sounds. Loudness or softness of speech results from the amount of air moving through the voice passage and from the force with which words are spoken. Speaking in too loud a voice is irritating and tiring to the listener; talking in too low a tone is equally as annoying, because it is difficult for the listener to hear what you are saying. It is naturally desirable for a speaker to be easy and pleasant to listen to. Learn to regulate the volume of your voice to the level that is best suited to the listener, the occasion, and the surroundings. Try to develop the habit of noting when a listener seems to be having difficulty in hearing you. Many people are hard of hearing and are sensitive about it, and they may not ask you to speak louder. You may need to adjust your voice to the changing conditions of noise. If you are asked to repeat yourself, it is a cue that you must talk *over* the noise around you. If your listener cannot hear you he may not ask you more than once to speak louder.

Finally, he gives up and acts as though he understands. Be sensitive to sudden, loud, and competing sounds that drown out key words. "The patients in rooms 409 and 411 went home last evening. Please clean these rooms [the food cart rumbles past] before you start your other work." If the maid does not hear the words "before you start your other work," she will miss the point you wish to make.

Each person has a rate of speaking that is natural for him. It is important that the hearer be able to keep up with what the speaker has to say, so that the rate of speech does not detract from the clarity of what is being said. The human ear is probably the best instrument for gauging the correct rate of speech. If you find that you are frequently asked to repeat something and are sure that you are speaking loudly enough, chances are you are speaking too rapidly. The rapid speaker creates tension in the listener because he has to strain to take in all the words the speaker is saying and probably has to guess at his meaning as well. Speaking too slowly also irritates most listeners and makes speech dull and uninteresting to follow.

Rate of speaking and enunciation are closely related. A common fault of many fast talkers is that they do not pronounce their words distinctly. The consonants are generally the most important sounds in distinguishing words, yet these are the easiest sounds to slur. Read the following:

1. Shadda goat th' store fort close'.
2. Sh'gonna put th' picher inner room.

The first sentence is probably understandable even though the words are slurred. In the second sentence, however, it is impossible to know if the speaker is talking about a pitcher or a picture. From these examples you can see how careless, slurred speech can lead to needless misunderstanding.

It is also important to pronounce initial consonants distinctly. This is why, when you spell out a name over the telephone, for example, you should say "T" as in Thomas, "B" as in Baker. The words serve as a check and identification of the two sounds. Rate of speaking should not interfere with clear tone, distinct enunciation, and good diction.

Pitch refers to the tone of the voice compared to the notes on the musical scale. The pitch of the voice is determined by the length and tension of the vocal cords. A woman's voice usually has a higher pitch because of the physiology of her voice mechanism; a man's voice is deeper because the vocal folds are longer and thicker. Pitch accounts for the distinctiveness of each person's voice. An optimum pitch is one that is produced in an easy, relaxed manner and is pleasant to listen to. An excessively high pitch should be corrected. Not only is it irritating to the listener, but it also projects the image of immaturity.

When speaking we are concerned not only with the basic pitch of the voice but also with the changes that occur during speech. A pitch that is too high is monotonous and does not allow for the variations and inflections that make communication effective. Pitch distinguishes between such things as questions and exclamations and can be used to give emphasis. Say the following phrases, emphasizing the italicized word. Jim's father gave him a *car;* Jim's father *gave* him a car; Jim's *father* gave him a car; or Jim's father gave *him* a car.

Different qualities of tone and pitch reveal the emotional state of the speaker. Tension affects tone; the vocal chords tighten and literally squeeze the voice. Stress also affects the pitch and the nasal quality of the voice. Note how people in arguments raise their voices and how the harsh tone, high pitch, and nasal intonation communicate irritation and anger. Most of us should try more often to speak in a level tone that shows no undue emotion. If you make an unemotional statement of fact, as you should in most situations, the listener will usually respond in kind. A quiet tone helps reduce tension not only in yourself but also in those with whom you are speaking.

Voice quality reveals or suggests to the listener the feelings and attitudes of the speaker. You respond not only to the words of the speaker, but also to what you "read" in his voice. For example, a patient can receive as much encouragement from the doctor's calm, confident tones as he does from what the doctor says.

The impressions that you form of a person are usually based on how he sounds to you. A person with a "whiny" voice is regarded as a chronic complainer. The person who habitually uses the high loud tones of conscious superiority may be tolerated, but he is not generally liked by his associates. A person expresses warmth through his voice. When he smiles something happens to the quality of his voice that evokes a friendly response from the listener. On the other hand, if the individual is insincere or unfriendly, his voice will generally communicate these qualities.

If a tape recorder is available you may wish to make a recording of your voice and listen to it with a critical ear. This will help you to hear how your voice sounds to other people. You may learn much about your voice and about your way of speaking. You may find that you mumble or slur your words, that your pitch is thin, nasal, or breathy, or that you preface your spoken sentences with "ah" and "uh." Another method you may find helpful is to occasionally inquire of people in whom you have confidence, "Do I speak clearly? Do you understand all I say? Do you have to strain your ears and guess at my meaning?" The results of a few such inquiries may greatly surprise you.

How you listen. Communication is blocked when either participant in the interaction fails to receive (hear or listen to) a transmitted message. There is an important distinction between failing to hear and failing to listen. Hearing and listening are both concerned with the perception of sound. *To hear* is to have such perception by the auditory sense. Hearing is a passive process, resulting automatically when the auditory nerves are stimulated. For example, you may hear a clock chime in the background or hear traffic on the street outside. Listening, on the other hand, is an active process. It requires a receptive attitude and encompasses all the processes by which meaning is attached to sound. *To listen* implies giving close attention to what is heard. After recognizing word sounds, the listener must search out the meaning the other person is trying to convey. It is said that we hear with our ears but listen with our entire being.

Many factors affect people's ability to hear what is going on about them. Defective hearing can be a communication barrier. Imperfect hearing can be present to a greater or lesser degree without one's being aware of it. Again, people who are hard of hearing may be sensitive about it; they often try to cover up by acting as though they can hear. A person who has impaired hearing may distinguish sounds of certain pitches but not others.

When you are conversing with someone, it is important to look at your listener. Avoid looking away or talking with your back turned. As sound waves strike the eardrum they may be distorted by the way they are uttered or by disturbances in the air through which they travel, with the result that there can be a wide discrepancy between what you say and what the listener hears.

Environmental factors such as the sounds of other people talking, the hum of an air conditioner, or music playing can be disturbing to people with normal hearing. Unfortunately, many people cannot tune sounds out. Sounds annoy or distract them into daydreaming and they often fail to listen when remarks are addressed to them.

Not listening, or half-listening, is a common fault of many people and a major cause of misunderstanding and breakdown in communication. Much of the difficulty we have in listening is caused by the fact that the speed of thought is several times faster than the speed of speech. When we are listening, it is easy to let the mind wander and think of other things instead of concentrating on the speaker. Close attention is necessary for listening. If a person is ill, tired, bored, or preoccupied with other matters he may not expend the necessary energy in listening. He may not listen because of the inadequacies of a speaker who mumbles his words, has a monotonous voice, or has some unconscious mannerism or nervous habit that serves to distract the listener's attention.

A common fault of poor listeners is the habit of interrupting the person who is speaking. In doing this, one violates the purpose of communication, blocks the sharing of ideas, and fails to consider his own responsibility as a listener. When you interrupt, you are really saying that you know what the other person means and you prevent him from explaining his meaning fully. You also indicate that you are not genuinely interested and do not have the courtesy to wait to present your own views or opinions.

Talking too much can be a serious deterrent to effective listening. Most people concentrate more on their talking skills than on their listening skills. When you are concerned with what you are going to tell others, you do not give yourself a chance to think about what the other person is saying. This can cause you to assume an understanding that you do not possess. Everyone has had his own experience with the person who is so anxious to prove his quickness of thought and understanding that he assumes what you have on your mind and says it for you.

Your attitudes and prejudices can cause you to be selective in your listening. You listen for the facts and the ideas that substantiate your preconceived beliefs. On the other hand, when a person expresses an idea or opinion that is contrary to what you believe, you may be so affronted that you do not hear anything else he says. You stop paying attention and begin to think how you can refute his statement rather than trying to understand his point of view.

We discussed earlier the importance of context in understanding the meaning of words. It is also important to learn to listen "in context." To listen only for words and facts is not enough; you should listen also for feelings and attitudes. Emotional and interpersonal meanings especially are often conveyed in the larger context and not by the literal meaning of words.

In this chapter we have noted the importance of communication in nursing, how one operates as a communicator, and some of the barriers to effective communication. You cannot expect that you will always be understood when you try to communicate. Communication is situational. You cannot expect that you will always communicate effectively after learning a few principles and rules, but you *can* learn to be more skillful in your use of the tools of communication, language, speaking, listening, and observing.

BIBLIOGRAPHY

Barbara, D. A.: The art of listening, Springfield, Ill., 1958, Charles C Thomas, Publisher.

Berlo, D. K.: The process of communication, New York, 1960, Holt, Rinehart & Winston, Inc.

Chase, S.: Power of words, New York, 1954, Harcourt, Brace & Co.

Cohen, M. S.: Easy to listen to, American Journal of Nursing **66**:1999, Sept. 1966.

Hayakawa, S. I.: Language in thought and action, New York, 1964, Harcourt, Brace & Co.

Hodnet, E.: The art of working with people, New York, 1959, Harper & Brothers.

Kron, T.: Communication in nursing, Philadelphia, 1967, W. B. Saunders Co.

Lewis, G. K.: Nurse-patient communication, Dubuque, Iowa, 1969, William C. Brown Co., Publishers.

Linehan, D. T.: What does the patient want to know? American Journal of Nursing **66**:1066-1070, May 1966.

Lockerby, F. K.: Communication for nurses, St. Louis, 1968, The C. V. Mosby Co.

Pei, M.: Language for everybody, New York, 1956, The Devin-Adair Co.

Perrin, P. G.: Writer's guide and index to English, Chicago, 1942, Scott, Foresman and Co.

Perrin, P. G., and Smith, G. H.: The Perrin-Smith handbook of current English, ed. 2, New York, 1966, Bantam Books, Inc.

Travelbee, J.: Interpersonal aspects of nursing, Philadelphia, 1966, F. A. Davis Co.

Wiskell, W.: Do they understand you? New York, 1960, The Macmillan Co.

COMPLETE WORK SHEET ON PP. 331 AND 332

CHAPTER 15

Communication skills and techniques

In the preceding chapter we discussed some elementary communication theories and looked at some key elements of the communication process. In this chapter we will concentrate on communication skills that you will need to develop and practice in working with others on the nursing unit and in communication with your patients.*

Most people are aware that they do communicate with others in the course of daily interaction. However, simply because a person does a thing does not mean he does it skillfully. Skill in communicating involves more than the ability to use the four *verbal communication skills*—speaking, listening, writing, and reading. Skill in communicating requires (1) an awareness of the underlying reasons or rationale for communicating in various situations; (2) awareness of how much, if any, communication is actually taking place; (3) ability to transmit a message in a manner that will elicit the desired response; and (4) awareness of the emotional reactions and responses conveyed by nonverbal communication.

The term "communication skills," as it is used here, refers to various methods or ways of communicating that are used selectively and deliberately by the nurse to achieve some specific purpose or goal. Skill in communicating involves the practiced and sensitive use of specific techniques designed to achieve the desired results in accordance with the demands of the situation. It is skill that differentiates the awkward attempts of the beginner from the finished performance of the practiced nurse. Techniques are the means by which the results are obtained; they are not goals in themselves. A truly skillful practitioner uses basic principles and modifies details to fit a specific situation. The skill represents a unified and integrated whole into which the separate parts fit as details of the total act. To achieve the desired results, it is necessary that you have a clear idea of what your goal truly is. You must then be able to use a variety of techniques based upon a good understanding of *how* and *where* each technique can be most effectively used. Some communication skills that serve a practical function in "how to communicate" in varied situations are discussed in the following paragraphs.

GETTING INFORMATION

Questions are an integral part of daily conversations. You need only recall several of the conversations in which you shared today in order to recognize the extent to which all of us use and depend upon questions in everyday living. Questions such as "How are you?" or "How have you been?" are a common form of greeting when friends meet. In casual conversation with a classmate you may well ask, "Are you ready for the exam?" or "What are you doing after class?" Questions play a major role

*Special communication skills and the techniques for using them are not dealt with here. It is presumed that this aspect of communication will be enlarged upon in other classes, where these skills will be discussed as they apply to the care of patients with special problems in communicating.

whenever you make plans. On making a date for lunch you might ask your companion, "Where would you like to go?" or "What time shall we meet?"

Questions are important in the give-and-take of social conversations, but they are also a vital part of the nurse's work. They are basic in fact-finding, interviewing, and counseling. You need information upon which to base your actions. Often a person fails to get the necessary information because he does not ask questions in the proper way. In the previous chapter we mentioned the importance of constructing messages in a manner that makes the purpose or intent of a communication clear to the intended receiver. We also stressed the importance of trying to anticipate the receiver's reaction by careful wording of the message so that the desired response is achieved. Questions must also be posed with the other person in mind. The choice of words and the direction of thought should be geared to the person who must answer the question.

There are several steps involved in asking questions effectively. First you must have a clear idea of exactly what you want to find out from the other person. The kind of information you want depends upon a variety of factors. Do you want facts and information? Do you need clarification? Do you need to understand another's thinking? For any given purpose you can convey your desire for information by constructing one or another of several question types. In doing this you have an infinite number of choices in selecting and arranging the words used to frame the questions. Choosing the right question form for the purpose or objective you have in mind has an important bearing on the kind of answer your question will receive. Let us look at the different question types. How do they differ from each other? How do we select a type and use it?

Question types. The key to effective questions lies in their construction. When you ask someone a question you are really requesting him to think about the subject you introduce. You can request someone to channel his thoughts in order to get the information you wish through the way in which you construct your question. The way in which you put your question determines the kind of answer that you will receive.

In general, there are two basic kinds of questions: structured and unstructured. A structured question is one that requires a fact or specific information in answer. For example, "Where were you born?" directs that the answer include the name of the city or town and the state or country. "Why did you come to the hospital?" indicates that the patient mention the symptoms, condition, or illness that caused him to be admitted to the hospital. A question such as "Are you ready for the exam?" might elicit the answer "Yes," "No," or "I think so." A structured question requires that the answer lie within a fairly circumscribed range. The person answering the question has merely to respond with the fact or information asked for.

An unstructured question, on the other hand, is one that is designed to stimulate the other person to talk about the subject rather than answer with a specific fact or with a "Yes" or "No." A question such as "Why do you think your grade is unfair?" permits the person to explain or give the reasons for his feeling that the grade was unfair. The question, "What seems to be the trouble?" encourages the person to discuss what is bothering him or causing him difficulty. In an unstructured question, the questioner indicates the area in which he is seeking information, but the other person is free to organize his thoughts and answer the question as he interprets it.

Some distinguishing characteristics of structured and unstructured questions are summarized on p. 157.

The degree to which a question is structured depends upon the kind of information being sought. A direct question—"How old are you?"—is a highly structured question because the questioner demands a specific fact. A less structured question—"How does it feel to be twenty-one?"—is one in which the questioner throws out an idea to the other person in order to encourage discussion of a topic.

The following conversation between a coun-

Structured questions:	*Unstructured questions:*
1. Ask for specific information or facts within a restricted range of possibilities;	1. Stimulate discussion within a broad area with no restrictions on the direction of the discussion;
2. Are the source for the structure of ideas because the questioner directs the thought;	2. Depend upon the answer for the structure of ideas, because the person answers the question according to how he interprets it;
3. Require that the response be directed only to the information that is asked for. The answers are short and require no explanation.	3. Require only that the person answering starts at some relevant point and develops and expands the thought.

selor and a student nurse illustrates the use of both question types.

COUNSELOR: "Can you tell me about your study habits?" (The counselor opens with an unstructured question because she wants to give the student a chance to discuss and explain.)

STUDENT: "I don't have what you would call a routine. I usually try to study from 7:30 to about 10:00 P.M. When I don't, I set the alarm for 5:00 A.M. Mom doesn't like me to go back to the library at night, so I try to do my library assignments in my free hours between classes."

COUNSELOR: "What about priorities? Do you find yourself spending more time on certain subjects than on others?"
(Counselor continues with another relatively unstructured question, but one that narrows the area of discussion because she wants to get a more definite picture of the student's study habits.)

STUDENT: "Generally I concentrate on the subjects in which I have a test coming up. Otherwise, I try to read over other assignments if I can't actually study them."

COUNSELOR: "How much time do you spend studying anatomy, would you say?"
(Counselor moves to a structured question in order to acquire specific information.)

STUDENT: "Ruth Brice and I study together and ask each other questions. I'd say we spend about an hour each time going over the assignment."

COUNSELOR: "Considering your standing at the midterm and your grades on the two quizzes since then, do you think you are spending enough time on your anatomy assignments?"
(Here the counselor asks a very structured question so that the student will give careful thought to the effectiveness of her present study habits and then make necessary revisions for the future.)

In this situation the counselor might have opened the discussion with a highly structured question, but if she had, the student might not have started thinking actively about her study habits—which was the counselor's primary purpose in this conversation. Thus unstructured questions are valuable aids in encouraging and stimulating thought, whereas structured questions generally require that the response consist of already known material. Skillful questioning requires that you understand *when* to use one or another of these techniques and know *what* it is you want to accomplish before you begin your questioning.

Techniques for asking questions. Skillful questioning more often than not is based on assessment of the particular situation rather than on any prescribed rules and formulas. Getting the proper information depends very much on whether you put the *right* question to the other person. When you try to elicit information from someone, you are actually asking him to do something for you; essentially, you are asking him to think about your ideas and prepare a response to your request. In addition to its explicit message, your question also carries an implicit message—the demand for an answer.

In asking questions you should never give the impression of probing or pumping for information. Since each question is a demand that the other person supply information, it is important to relate to the respondent tactfully and to consider his feelings. You should never use him only as a source to satisfy your needs and curiosity. Keep this in mind when you must question patients, co-workers, and subordinates, as well as friends. For example, you are guilty of pumping if you become so preoccupied with acquiring information that you ask another question immediately after receiving the answer to your previous question. Questions of an imperative nature can give the impression of probing for information and have all the characteristics of an interrogation: "Why do you say that?" "Don't you want to explain?" "What do you mean?" "Can't you tell me more?" Again, some questions that are asked for clarification may seem probing in their demand: "Are you a regular church member?" "Do you drink much?" "Have you always been as heavy as you are now?" Brusque and forceful questioning can be frightening and create needless anxiety, causing the respondent to withdraw. It is advisable to remember that courtesy in questioning is helpful as well as proper.

To draw out information. In general, the more unstructured the question the more information you are likely to get. *In formulating questions to draw out a respondent, word the questions so that the person must explain what he means rather than merely supply a specific fact or a "Yes" or "No" answer.* The following are examples of unstructured questions: "What do you plan to do?" "How do you feel about being transferred?" "What happened?" "Why did he leave so early?"

Questions involving *when* and *where* are more highly structured, because the framework of the question must be observed in the answer. For example, if a patient asks you, "When shall I take this medicine?" he would expect your answer to include the number of times and the specific hours at which he should take the medicine each day. Another kind of highly structured question is one that gives the person a choice of two or more possibilities and implies that he has merely to make a choice. If you were settling a patient for the night and you said, "It's almost nine-thirty. Don't you want to go to sleep now?" you give him the option to answer "No, thank you, I would like to remain up for a while longer." Similarly, you can see the difference between saying "May I talk with you a few minutes about your diet?" and "I would like to speak with you about your diet." The question allows for a "Yes" or "No" answer, and there might be circumstances in which a statement would be preferable.

While the interrogative words *why* and *how* are generally used in eliciting an expanded answer or explanation in certain kinds of communication situations, questioning in this manner may defeat the purpose for asking the question in the first place. It may actually block the conversation by making the respondent feel defensive. For example, asking "Why?" often stimulates partial answers or superficial reasons, or the person may invent causes to please the questioner or to avoid answering.

Nurses who really understand the meanings of *how* and *why* questions use them very judiciously. A *how* question implies that the person knows the process and the steps by which something has happened. A *why* question asks for reasons, causes, explanations, or conclusions. Both types of questions are highly structured. If the respondent has adequate information and the ability to analyze the situation, he could be expected to answer a *why* or *how* question directly. If he does not have the necessary information, asking a *why* or *how* question is inappropriate and may leave him feeling inadequate or even resentful. Asking a patient who has soiled his bed why he didn't signal for assistance is in effect asking a question that is extremely difficult, if not impossible, for the patient to answer. Besides, there is always the danger that the nurse's tone and inflection may imply censure, thus making it even more difficult and embarrassing for him to answer or explain.

To get clarification. Unstructured questions are useful for getting clarification of something the other person said. The technique for using unstructured questions in this way is to *repeat certain key words or phrases* of the person's previous answer in your next question. This indicates your interest and implies that you would like to know more about what he thinks or how he feels. For example, if a person says, "I'm in a funny mood today," you might draw out his feelings by asking, "What do you mean by 'funny mood'?" Another use of the technique is to repeat the person's statement in the form of a question. To the patient who says, "I don't feel like eating," you might respond, "You don't feel like eating?" to get him to explain further. Or, if a person says, "I'm sorry about the way things turned out," you might draw him out further by responding with "Sorry?"

Another way of getting clarification is to *summarize* your understanding of what the other person meant ("Are you saying . . . ?"). If he agrees, your question is a highly structured one to which he can merely reply with "Yes" or "No," or to which he can add further thoughts. If he disagrees he is faced with an unstructured question and must explain the basis of his disagreement, give you another explanation of what he means, and possibly add new information.

To get another's thinking. Questions are also helpful in understanding a person's thinking on some matter. One technique for using unstructured questions is to preface the topic word or words with the phrase "What about" or "How about": "What about the plans for the school dance?" "What about chaperones?" This is a way of asking the other person to start at some relevant point and explain his ideas or opinions.

Additional kinds of questions and techniques are available, but the intention has been to show that you need not and should not question randomly when you try to get information from someone. In using these or any other techniques it is always necessary to consider your purpose in asking the question, decide the best way to present it, and evaluate the results. The answer you receive depends a great deal upon your question and the manner in which it is received and understood.

GIVING INFORMATION

Thus far we have discussed some techniques of obtaining information from others. Now let us look at the processes involved when questions are asked of you—when you must give information.

The basic goal in giving information is to communicate what is asked for in such a way that it will be understandable and useful to the person receiving it. In giving information your concern is to help the other person to increase his knowledge so that he will be in a better position to act more responsibly than he would if he were less well informed.

Make sure you understand what the person wants to know. When a person comes to you for information, it is easy to come to a premature conclusion about what he means or about the problem he is presenting. Sometimes a person fails to give the desired information because he does not understand the question or because he does not take the time to really listen to what he is being asked.

Sometimes the question is unclear or can be answered in more than one way. You must be careful not to *assume* that you understand what the questioner means. Do not hesitate to ask that a question be repeated. Ask for more details if necessary. You may have to restate the person's ideas to make sure you understand them correctly. Such statements as, "Did you mean . . . ?" and "Are you asking . . . ?" are helpful in gaining clarification. You should always take time to answer every question as carefully as possible.

Cultivate the habit of listening for implicit messages when you listen to questions. The explicit message is the question. The implicit message can be communicated through the context, pacing of ideas, or pauses, as well as through the words themselves. The individual's implicit message expresses his real feelings or the things he wants to know. Suppose one of your classmates received two *F*'s as midterm grades. She is very worried about her standing and she asks you whether she should tell her parents. The explicit message is: should she inform her parents about her failing grades? Her implicit message is a plea, first for understanding, then for advice—hopefully of a particular kind.

When a person asks for advice he may want someone else to shoulder the responsibility for whatever decision he makes, or he may ask for advice in order to bolster the opinion he already has. In responding to questions involving advice, it is important to make a distinction between giving information and giving advice. To give advice is not always helpful. In a situation such as that in the preceding paragraph, you would be of more help to your classmate by giving her a chance to talk and think her problem through and let her come to a decision on her own.

The ability to give useful information requires that you develop the habit of analyzing questions. What is the person saying? Why is he saying this? What is implied? What does he *really* mean?

Present the information in a useful manner. When you understand the question and have the pertinent information that is being requested, your next task is to present it in an understandable and usable manner. Remember that you have not really answered the question if the person does not understand the information you have given him.

In giving information, always keep in mind that the other person may have different experiences, values, and outlook. He is likely to use different words to say the same thing. Try to look at the information you are presenting from his frame of reference. In order for the other person to grasp your information, he must fit it into his way of thinking. Giving information or an explanation that the person is not able to accept or is unprepared to use is a waste of time and effort. It is not just a matter of hearing what you say—the person has to be able to imagine the information in use in some situation that involves him.

In some situations it will be helpful to present your information in different ways using slightly different words and phrases. Using analogies and examples in some instances is also helpful. When giving information, avoid the temptation to impress others with your knowledge. Sometimes a person's desire to demonstrate superior knowledge of a subject involves the use of difficult words and lengthy explanations. As a result, his statements are incomprehensible and unnecessary to the person seeking specific information. The simpler you keep your language, the more likely you are to be understood.

Unfamiliar situations tend to induce anxiety in many people. In the absence of any concrete information about what to expect, they will often imagine the worst. Although specific, sound information about the situation or what will probably take place will not prevent all anxiety, such information can do much to alleviate uneasiness. In giving an explanation or information of any kind, the type and extent of explanation must be geared to the individual's need and ability to comprehend. For example, patients are frequently subjected to diagnostic or therapeutic measures with which they are partially or totally unfamiliar. Particular care must be taken in judging the type and extent of explanation given to patients. You err in answering patients' questions if you give a lot of information or give it in a highly technical form. A factual description of an impending action or procedure is not the sort of information to allay a patient's apprehension. Generally, it is sufficient to give the patient a summary of what is done, what is expected of him during the procedure, and the approximate length of time it will require. However, you should remember that, although a procedure may be simple or routine to you, the patient may see it as complex, difficult, and frightening.

In the preceding chapter we discussed the importance of words and meanings. Since abstract words have a wide variety of meanings, and since we think in specific images, it is quite likely that a nurse using an abstract word has a different image in her mind from that of the patient listening to her instructions. Some abstract words that must be clearly defined when giving information are: a *few* minutes, a *small* amount, a *large* amount, and for a *short* while. Also, in giving information do not overlook the significance of *small* details. These are relatively simple points, but to neglect them causes needless difficulty for many people. You may neglect to mention details because of your familiarity with what is being asked. You may not stop to realize that the person asking the question is unfamiliar with things that are everyday knowledge to you. For example, if you explain to a patient that a particular pill is to be taken three times a day, you should further explain by saying, "Take one after each meal." This elaboration is a way of repeating the idea of three times and gives the patient a schedule to follow.

In certain situations it will be necessary for you to know whether the person understands the information. A good procedure is to have him repeat to you the information you gave him. It is often assumed that a person understands what is said when he does not. The person may not want to expose his ignorance, or he may not want to impose on you any further. He may even be afraid to ask you to repeat the information, especially if you are in a position of authority. The person may nod or act as if he understands, even though he does not understand at all or may have a distorted impression of what you said. When you give information to another, do not assume that it is understood until you have his reaction to it.

Share the reasoning behind the information. In many communication situations you must share the reasoning behind the information you give with those you are trying to help. This is necessary in order to gain their cooperation and to counteract any negative attitudes they may hold toward the information you give them. Events that require explanation of hospital regulations and policies, for example, are constantly occurring in the nursing unit setting. In addition to other duties, the nurse is responsible for the interpretation and enforcement of hospital policies and regulations. Informing personnel, patients, and their families about pertinent rules and procedures requires more than just quoting the information verbatim from a directive or manual. Giving the exact, correct information is not enough to ensure cooperation in abiding by the regulations. It is also necessary to make sure the regulations are meaningful to those involved. You must remember that if a person understands the purpose of the regulations or policies he will be much more willing to cooperate. If the person understands how the regulations function to his benefit he will develop a justified confidence in the hospital, its administration, and its personnel.

When people are not adequately informed about regulations they tend to view them as restrictions and to fight them. Authoritarian presentation of any limits on the person's actions, with no explanation or additional information, seldom helps others to see the limits as meaningful or worthy of their cooperation.

GIVING DIRECTIONS

Giving directions is a specialized form of information giving; the receiver is expected to comply with or follow the directions or instructions as given. Directions include explanations of a nursing technique or how to perform some task. Teaching a patient to prepare, measure, and administer his own insulin is essentially a matter of giving directions. Giving directions can also be as limited as ordering a cup of coffee in the snack bar.

Skill in giving effective directions entails encouraging an attitude of acceptance in the other person, presenting the information in a way that is understandable to him, and making clear to him the significance of the information. In general, people are more inclined to follow directions or to comply with orders if they understand why compliance is important. A patient, for example, will work harder at some imposed task or exercise if he knows how it will help him to get well. Personnel will follow policies and procedures more carefully if they understand the reasons for them and have some appreciation of how they relate to their own welfare or contribute to the welfare of the patients.

Be specific when giving directions. This suggestion is important whether the activity is a simple order or a complex procedure. If you want a person to follow your instructions, he must know what he is to do, and when, where, and how he must do it. When you instruct a person in the use of equipment or in the performance of some nursing procedure, all necessary articles should be assembled and pretested before the demonstration is held. When teaching patients procedures they will perform at home, the best results are achieved when the equipment and the conditions under which it will be used are as similar as possible to the home situation.

Present the steps in logical order. The receiver may become confused if you have to go back to previous information because you forgot to include an important point. Make it a practice to emphasize what to do, rather than what not to do. If the instructions include a demonstration, make running comments on the materials used, the processes taking place, and the anticipated results. Demonstrations assist learning because the listener can see as well as hear what should be done. This active mental impression fortifies his verbal knowledge. If the directions include many steps or if they require memorization of specific values or measurements, it is a good idea to ask the person to write them down as you give them or to give him an instruction sheet that will serve as a reference if he has to refresh his memory.

Pace your instructions so that the recipient can absorb what you are telling him. In order to absorb the information he has to think about it; he cannot think about one idea and listen to the next at the same time.

Use language understandable to the recipient. Because directions or instructions seem simple and routine to you, do not assume that they will be simple to someone else. Always consider the background and knowledge of your recipient when giving any type of directions or instructions. Avoid the use of jargon, abbreviations, or technical terminology unless you are sure that the person understands the terms. It would be meaningless to instruct an aide in how to record fluid intake and output if she had no concept of what the symbols *cc.* or *oz.* mean.

Explain the meaning of all new words or words used in an unfamiliar way. A patient could be left in a very bewildered state if you did not explain your instructions to "scrub the area with pHisoHex." The patient's interpretation of "scrub" might be entirely different from your meaning of the word. Also, you owe the patient an explanation of the nature and use of pHisoHex solution and the chance to repeat the explanation if necessary so that he is able to impress it on his memory.

Wording of directions is very important. The words *must, shall, will,* and *is to* are used when some action is mandatory. *May* is used when the action is recommended, while *should* indicates that the action is recommended if circumstances permit.

Make provision for feedback. As mentioned previously, it is important to know whether your directions or orders are actually understood by the other person. The fact that the person does not ask questions does not always indicate understanding. Sometimes the lack of comprehension makes the person unable to ask questions, or he may think he understands when actually he does not. Sometimes you may have to question him to find out whether he knows exactly what you expect him to do. One tactful way of doing this is to ask him to tell you how he is going to carry out your instructions.

The axiom, "No order is complete until the person reports back," has particular application in nursing. Head nurses and team leaders who supervise the work of other personnel must know whether their orders and assignments are being followed in order to ensure continuity of patient care. No assignment or order should be considered fulfilled until a report has been filed regarding what steps were taken and what the result has been.

GIVING REPORTS

The ability to give a concise and accurate oral report is a communication skill of the utmost importance to nurses and is vital to good management and administration. Oral reporting is a method of giving personnel the information they need to carry on with their activities quickly and effectively. No group effort is possible without this form of communication; each person must be kept informed, and a constant exchange of information is essential to prevent errors. In most cases, errors can be traced to a breakdown in communication.

You will give reports on many occasions in the classroom, the hospital, and at meetings of committees, associations, and other groups. The same basic technique is applicable to all types of reports.

A report is essentially a statement or summary of pertinent facts or information. In order to be effective reports should be complete and timely and should include all vital information in sufficient detail to communicate the required information. Good organization is a primary requisite for effective reports whether they are oral or written, formal or informal, brief or lengthy.

Organizing your material. If you are to give an oral report, think through the information and organize your thoughts clearly and logically. Decide on the main points in the report. Shuffle and reshuffle these points until you have them in the right order. For the purpose of clarity you need to develop a logical sequence in which one item follows another naturally.

When you have crystallized your thinking and your plan is clear, your next problem is to select those facts that bear directly on each point you plan to develop. Your source may be experiential information, facts you obtained from written records or reports, or answers to questions you have asked. Choose only the ideas or information that will make the point clearer to the listener. Brevity is important not only in the use of words, but also in the amount of material to be conveyed. Your listeners will get more from your report if you keep it as brief as you can. Too many details will be confusing and boring. Prepare an outline or notes to glance at as you make your report. In this way you will cover all of the major points and avoid confusing your listeners by repeating or backtracking to add material or pick up points you missed.

Delivering your report. When you give a report, the full responsibility for communication rests with you. Instead of talking *to* one person you are talking *to* a group. As a reporter you will probably be doing all the talking; there may be no feedback from the listeners to indicate whether you are getting your message across. Indeed, you cannot be sure that those who appear to be listening are actually concentrating on what you are telling them. As was mentioned earlier, communication is a two-way process—you cannot force people to listen to you. As the communicator, you can attract and develop their interest and make sure that what you say is useful, easy to grasp, worth your time in telling it and worth the time your audience gives to listening.

In giving a report, concentrate on a lively sense of communication. Talk *to* your listeners, not *at* them. Watch your audience and observe their facial expressions, attitudes of attention, and signs of restlessness. Maintain the proper eye contact. Do not address your remarks to just one or two persons. Vary your tone of voice; avoid droning or talking monotonously. At best, a listener's attention is unstable and continually drifts away and back to the subject at hand. Your voice and manner of speaking can contribute to his inattention and make him even less inclined to listen.

Pacing can make the difference between a stimulating report and a dull presentation. If your conversational pace is too slow, the listener's attention will wander; if the pace is too rapid, he will not have time to absorb the ideas that are coming at him and he may become annoyed and give up trying to listen. If listeners cannot follow your line of thought they will probably tune out, preferring to give their attention to personal concerns or to events going on around them.

Unfortunately, many nurses see reporting as a routine task. Skill in giving effective reports requires practice; once learned, however, this skill will contribute immeasurably to your efficiency as a nurse and to the effectiveness of your leadership in nursing practice.

A good place to begin to practice this skill and gain facility in reporting is the patient-condition report. The purpose of the patient-condition report is to orient personnel coming on duty to the existing situation on the ward or nursing unit and to give them the information they need to carry on with the care of patients. Hospitals have different systems and different tools for recording doctors' orders and the care and treatment given to patients. In some instances the entire medical and nursing plan for each patient is recorded on individual cards and placed in a particular type of card file. It is also fairly standard practice in hospitals for the person reporting to refer directly to these cards when giving patient-condition reports.

To give a good patient-condition report you must be able to present the information so that it will answer as many questions as the situation demands without going into unnecessary detail. If you want to give a logical presentation that your listeners will understand and be able to follow, you must have a mental outline of the points you want to cover. This will help you to order your thoughts and will help your listeners to absorb what you are telling them.

The following is a logical sequence for presentation of facts and information about each patient: (1) an appraisal of the patient's condition at the present time, (2) a summary of what was done to and for him and why it was done, (3) a reminder to personnel regarding changes in doctor's orders, new orders for medicines and treatments, and the time at which these orders were initiated, (4) a reminder to personnel about events scheduled or coming up, and (5) a statement about preliminary preparations accomplished or not, and the reasons.

Barring the common obstacles to communication (language, not listening, and so on), an oral report can be considered very complete when the listener has no questions regarding major points of information. One or two questions would indicate that the report is quite satisfactory. Written reports, on the other hand, should be in sufficient detail so that no further questions need be asked or additions to the report made. In an incident report, for example, the details should answer the "five W's"—what, who, when, where, and why. All of these details are necessary to make this type of report more clear and complete.

You will need patience and practice to learn and develop communication skills. These skills will be truly useful to you when you understand *how* and *why* you are using them. Get into the habit of applying them in your daily conversation.

BIBLIOGRAPHY

Aasterud, M.: Explanation to the patient, Nursing Forum 2(4):36-43, 1963.

Bain, B.: The therapeutic role of the staff nurse, Nursing Forum 2(2):91-97, 1963.

Bursten, B., and Diers, D.: Pseudo-patient-centered orientation, Nursing Forum 3(2):38-50, 1964.

Elder, R. G.: What is the patient saying? Nursing Forum 2(1):25-37, 1963.

Ellis, G. L.: Communications and interdepartmental relationships, Nursing Forum 5(4):82-89, 1966.

Hays, J. S.: Analysis of nurse-patient communications, Nursing Outlook 14:32-35, Sept. 1966.

Hodnet, E.: The art of working with people, New York, 1959, Harper & Brothers.

Kron, T.: Nursing team leadership, Philadelphia, 1961, W. B. Saunders Co.

Kron, T.: Communication in nursing, Philadelphia, 1967, W. B. Saunders Co.

Lewis, G. K.: Nurse-patient communication, Dubuque, Iowa, 1969, William C. Brown Co., Publishers.

Lewis, G. K.: Communication: a factor in meeting emotional crises, Nursing Outlook 13:36-39, Aug. 1965.

Logan, H., and Blochman, L. C.: Are you misunderstood? New York, 1965, Wilfred Funk, Inc.

Mahoney, S. C.: The art of helping people, New York, 1967, Association Press.

Nirenberg, J. S.: Getting through to people, Englewood Cliffs, New Jersey, 1963, Prentice-Hall, Inc.

Schmahl, J. A.: Ritualism in nursing practice, Nursing Forum 3(4):74-84, 1964.

Skipper, J. K., Mauksch, H. O., and Tegliacozzo, D.: Barriers to communication between patients and hospital functionaries, Nursing Forum 2(1):15-23, 1963.

Siggins, C. M.: A professor of English looks at communication skills, Nursing Outlook 9:666-669, Nov. 1961.

Stephens, R. R.: In the middle of the muddle, Nursing Forum 3(4):29-35, 1964.

Travelbee, J.: Interpersonal aspects of nursing, Philadelphia, 1966, F. A. Davis Co.

COMPLETE WORK SHEET ON PP. 333 AND 334

CHAPTER 16

Working in a team

The team approach to nursing care is the result of an experimental study initiated in 1949 and conducted by the Division of Nursing Education of the Teachers College of Columbia University in New York City. A nursing team is a group in nursing service whose assignment involves working together under the direction of a leader to provide nursing care for designated patients.

Many duties once performed by nurses are now assigned to other personnel. Housekeepers, dietitians, nurse's aides, and licensed practical nurses are only a few of the specially trained staff members who work with registered nurses and physicians to meet the total needs of patients during their hospitalization. Many hospitals conduct active in-service training programs to recruit and train people to do these important jobs. All these people working together in a team relationship can make an effective contribution to quality patient care.

TYPES OF TEAMS

Hospitals, clinics, convalescent and rehabilitation units, health agencies, and physicians' offices are centers in which patients receive most of their health supervision and nursing care. In each of these centers the number of personnel and their responsibilities vary according to the services offered by the agency. Administrators and supervisors are responsible for the direction of the staff and for maintaining a smoothly run organization.

Hospital administration team. In a hospital the administrator functions as the head of the entire organization; he is the leader of the hospital's team. Heads of departments within the hospital are each responsible to the administrator for their department's effective functioning and for the quality of the services provided by the departmental staff. Administration involves planning, organizing, directing, coordinating, and controlling the operation of the varied departmental functions. Consideration must also be given to the interrelationships among all departments within the institution. This teamwork makes hospital patterns of organization (Chapter 13) workable.

Nursing service administration team. It is the responsibility of the personnel in charge of the various nursing units in a hospital to administer nursing services beneficial to patient welfare. Assistant directors, department supervisors, and head nurses are responsible for administering segments of the entire nursing service department. They are accountable to the director of nursing services. Throughout all of its levels the nursing service administration team is concerned with the atmosphere in which its nursing staff serves. The means by which the needs of all nursing service employees are met, including provisions for effective communications, for staffing patterns, for the morale of the group, and for solving nursing service problems, are basic concerns of this type of team. This team functions for the benefit of the institution and the persons working under its jurisdiction, as well as for the benefit of patients. The emphasis here is on the people who perform services and on the assignment of duties that ensure their competent performance. The nursing service department team is *one* of a group of teams operating within the hospital organization.

Health team. The health team, which is led by a physician, may also include registered nurses, dietitians, social service workers, physical, occupational, and other specialized therapists, psychologists, counselors, and members of the clergy. In some instances members of the patient's family are included on this team.

The health team has several goals. One goal is to assist individuals and communities to maintain a state of good health. However, when an individual is sick, the goal is to help him to return to the highest possible level of health. This includes supervision of any necessary rehabilitation. A community's health team is usually under the direction of a public health officer, who can identify community health problems and plan procedures for solving them. In hospitals, health teams under the leadership of physicians plan and implement programs and procedures that will help patients recover from illness and encourage their rehabilitation.

The working organization of the health team is relatively informal because its structure and the work of its members are tailored to meet the changing needs of individual patients. Each team member is capable of working independently, but each one's particular assignment is coordinated with the others under the leader's direction.

Each member of the health team is responsible for providing a particular type of assistance to meet patient needs. The physician coordinates all individual efforts to produce total patient care. The team leader may meet with individual members as well as with the whole group. Both the structure of the health team and the members' participation are broad in scope.

Specialized groups may be organized within the health team to function on specific phases of the total assignment. This team-within-a-team approach is a method by which the services of many people with different abilities and skills can be directed toward achievement of a central objective—high quality patient care. Using the team-within-a-team approach the physician makes one type of contribution, the dietitian and her staff make another type of contribution, and the registered nurse, who also heads the nursing care team, makes a different type of contribution. All work toward the objective of better patient care.

NURSING CARE TEAM

The nursing care team functions in the hospital on a team-within-a-team basis. The team consists of registered nurses, practical or vocational nurses, nurse's aides, and attendants who function under the direction of an assigned leader. Student nurses may also be members of the nursing care team. The leader is usually a registered nurse experienced in patient care administration or a senior student nurse in a registered nurse program who works closely with her clinical instructor. The number of team members is not as important as the understanding each has of ideal nursing team care and of her own role in making the ideal successful in practice.

A nursing care team functions *as a group* to use their nursing knowledge and skills to meet the nursing needs of those patients for whom they are assigned to care. The patients are selected by the team leader, subject to the approval of the unit's head nurse. The team leader is responsible to the head nurse for the team's performance and for her supervision of it. The use of the team concept for nursing care presupposes that the capabilities of each team member are fully utilized for each patient's benefit. The anticipated result of a team's functioning is the administration of a superior quality of *patient-centered* nursing care not attainable under other patterns of nursing service.

EVOLUTION OF THE NURSING CARE TEAM

This particular team approach has evolved because of several major changes in the nature and scope of health care. These include the increased numbers of patients admitted to hospitals and other health care facilities, the increasing variety of extended care facilities, and the need for staff members with a variety of specialized professional nursing skills who are able to administer the many new procedures being developed for diagnosis, treatment, and rehabilitation. In essence these factors mean that more skilled personnel are needed in many occupational categories to provide more and different kinds of care for increasing numbers of patients. Because there are not enough registered nurses, teams including licensed practical (vocational) nurses and other allied health personnel have been formed to meet the needs. A national report reveals that, of the total number of registered nurses in the United States in 1969, those actually employed in nursing numbered 680,000.* The Division of Nursing of the Bureau of Health Manpower predicted that 850,000 registered nurses could satisfy only the nation's *minimum* nursing service requirements in 1970,† while the minimum number of registered nurses who will be needed in 1975 is estimated at 1,000,000.* Effective and proper planning for assignment of nursing care team groups may provide one of the best solutions to this pressing problem.

THE TEAM'S PURPOSE

A nursing care team's primary objective is to provide nursing care. Although this point is obvious, some of the elements involved include the *method* by which care is provided. This method is essential because inherent in it are the relationships and respect developed among the team members. The team approach also allows better utilization of personnel. The nursing team is more effective than the traditional methods of nursing care because the team members receive more supervision.

Careful planning is necessary in order to create a successful nursing care team. Maximum use must be made of the skills each member brings to the team effort. In addition, the kinds of work done by each team member and the support and cooperation each receives from fellow team members must be clearly and sensibly organized and well understood by all participants. The team's effectiveness can only be maintained and improved if its activities are reviewed and evaluated daily. In this way team members can adjust their plans for nursing to meet constantly changing patient needs.

Because a highly effective level of interaction must exist among group members, communication plays a vital role. The leader is responsible for one aspect of this communication. She must advise the team members of significant observations they are to make as they administer care to patients. Another aspect of communication is the team conference at which time all team members discuss their observations.

ORGANIZATION FOR SERVICE

The person assigned to lead a nursing care team should be involved directly in patient care. She must possess expertise in clinical knowledge and the application of nursing skills.

The head nurse on the unit is *not* the leader of the nursing care team. She is the administrative leader of her unit and is responsible for its overall administration, the assignments and performance of all personnel who report to her, and the nursing care of all patients on her unit. If nursing care teams are used on a clinical unit, the head nurse should be able to take advantage of them as one method for the organization of nursing care administration. She assigns the leader of the nursing care team and delegates responsibility for the team's supervision to its leader who, in turn, is directly accountable to the head nurse.

Unless the head nurse and team leader understand and appropriately use the nursing care team, the plan will become just another means of staffing the unit, rather than being an important, viable program. Dr. R. Louise McManus says, "Merely assigning professional nurses, practical nurses, nurses' aides and student nurses to

*American Nurses' Association: Facts about nursing, a statistical summary, 1969, The Association.

†U. S. Department of Health, Education and Welfare, Public Health Service: Nurse Training Act of 1964 Program Review Report, Washington, D. C., 1967, The Department.

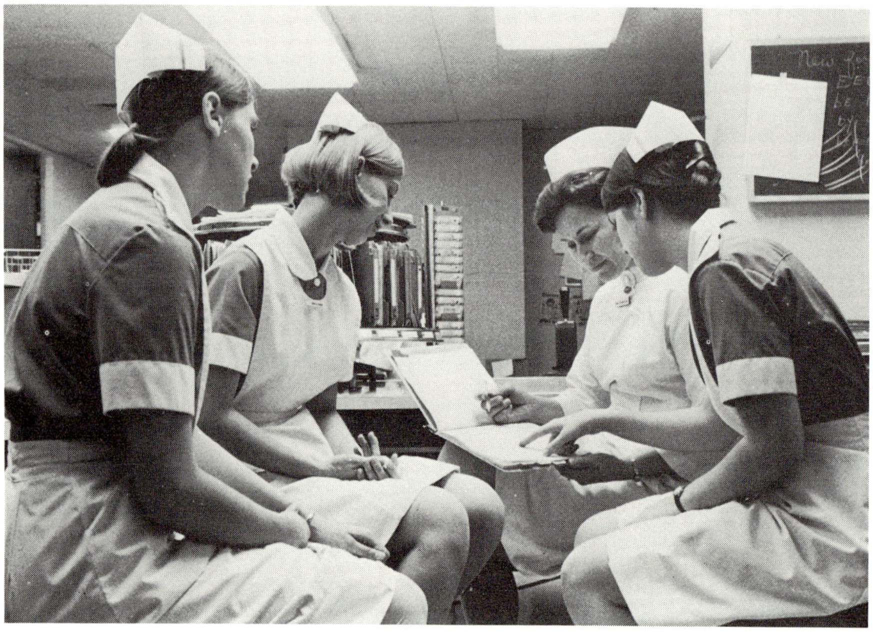

THE NURSING CARE TEAM CONFERENCE. TEAM LEADER AND MEMBERS DISCUSS PATIENTS' CARE.

work in the same ward unit does not necessarily make a team. Unless the workers or players are united in a common purpose, unless they know the roles they are expected to play and are all familiar with the roles, unless they know the signals and willingly accept and follow the leadership of the team captain, there can be no team."*

Team leader. The head nurse of the clinical area in which nursing care teams function appoints the team leaders. These leaders are authorized to organize their teams' tasks in relation to patients' needs. The leaders assign jobs to the team members best able to do them and plan for implementation of the assigned tasks. Each team leader maintains close communication with the head nurse; she reports the team's progress, plans, and problems. It is her job to see that her team functions *as a team,* rather than as a group of people operating independently of one another. For this reason, assignments are based on the skill and ability of each team member rather than upon seniority or other status elements. Team members and the leader are accountable to each other, as well as to the head nurse. There must be a sense of shared responsibility in order to maintain group morale and so that together the team members administer quality nursing care to all their patients. In short, a team leader's plan for nursing care involves a positive relationship and a responsibility to the administration, to the members of the team, and to the patients who are the recipients of the team's ministrations.

The team leader serves in a dual capacity, directing the team's total activities and main-

*Lambertson, E. C., Nursing team organization and functioning, New York, 1953, Bureau of Publications, Teachers College, Columbia University, p. iv.

taining positive relationships with those in her own group and with the head nurse. She must also maintain staff relationships with other teams. Her capacity for making judgments, her awareness of the significance of "little things" as keys to possible problem areas, and her nursing knowledge and potential for leadership have all been factors in her appointment as leader.

A nursing care · team leader's functions, broadly interpreted, include the following:

1. Selecting, with administrative consent, the patients who will receive her nursing team's care
2. Studying and evaluating the patients' needs for nursing care in relation to the abilities of the team members
3. Developing a nursing care plan based upon her evaluation
4. Reviewing with team members the methods they will use as a team and allocating individual assignments in accordance with the abilities of each team member
5. Directing, coordinating, and participating in carrying out the overall nursing plan
6. Accepting responsibility for the quality of each member's work
7. Serving as liaison between the team and administrative personnel and other team groups
8. Providing time for daily conferences after the team's assignments are completed, and maintaining records of progress and plans for the group's effort

WORKING IN A NURSING CARE TEAM

Your assignment as a nursing team member, and in some instances as a team leader, can provide a valuable learning experience. Through its pattern of clinical assignments and rotations, your nursing program will provide specific opportunities for you to be a member of nursing care teams under the guidance of your clinical instructors. Teachers in today's nursing programs know that they are responsible for providing learning experiences that will prepare you to function as a nurse practitioner in realistic nursing service assignments after graduation. If your nursing program is based upon a philosophy of nursing service centered around patient care, you may be assured that your instructors will cooperate with head nurses and team leaders in clinical divisions to plan and provide for your participation in nursing care teams.

You will learn to identify your role as a student when you become a member of a nursing care team. You are legally and ethically responsible for fulfilling your tasks.

You will be given many kinds of assignments that are designed to help you to obtain essential learning experiences. Included are functional and case assignments, as well as assignments to a nursing care team. Each experience demands that you apply the full range of your knowledge and technical skills in order to derive the greatest advantage, because each experience is planned with a definite goal for you in mind.

Making beds, serving meals, recording T.P.R.'s according to schedule, and administering medications are all parts of a nursing unit routine. These are functional assignments in which you will learn to complete certain tasks within a specific time schedule with concern for the patient you serve as well as for getting the job done well. Functional assignments are essentially work centered. In performing them it is important that you do not lose sight of the patient and his needs.

When a nurse is assigned to a particular case she becomes responsible for giving all necessary care to that patient during her duty hours in that clinical area. Because nursing responsibility on case assignments extends beyond purely technical duties and involves the exercise of judgment, cases should be given to those with more preparation and experience. The registered staff nurse, the private practice nurse, or the senior student under the guidance and advice of a clinical instructor function well and profit immeasurably in this kind of learning experience. Senior student nurses can use nursing case assignments as a means of broadening their understanding of the details of a patient's illness and his reactions to being ill and to the care he receives. In addition, the student has an opportunity to prepare a detailed written report on the nursing care administered and on the value of the assignment as a learning tool.

Participation in a nursing care team makes unique demands upon each member. In order for the team to function, personal interaction among the members and between each member and the team leader must be smooth and constructive. Consequently, each participant in a nursing care team must acquire, develop, and use good communication skills and must demonstrate professional competence.

The team leader is expected to exercise good judgment in evaluating changes in a patient's condition, in choosing a method of nursing intervention, in determining priorities, and in deciding when a physician should be called. Team membership gives each person in the group the opportunity to develop an understanding of his identity within the group both as a contributor and as a cooperating member. It is a challenge to work as part of a team and to see how each individual effort can be blended to achieve good patient care. In order for this process to work with a minimum of friction and difficulty, each member of the team must understand and accept the basic ground rules and her own role as either member or leader.

A strong rapport develops among team members through their combined efforts. In addition, every team member can share in the enormous satisfaction that results from such a successful cooperative effort, so that work on a nursing team is rewarding personally as well as professionally.

OPPORTUNITIES FOR PERSONAL GROWTH AND DEVELOPMENT

There are many opportunities for nurses to grow and develop personally as well as professionally. This increasing maturity is evident in a willingness to learn and apply new skills. As future nurses you should develop such character traits as honesty, loyalty, tact, and the ability to cooperate in your daily interactions with co-workers and patients.

As a team member you will be able to combine your knowledge and skill with your ability to make judgments and decisions and to relate well to others. As a team member you will learn to accept and successfully discharge the following responsibilities:

1. Accepting and performing assigned duties
2. Understanding the significance of each member's contribution to the team effort
3. Developing effective communication and positive relationships between yourself and your associates
4. Maintaining the patients' welfare as your chief concern
5. Reporting and reviewing activities in planned group conferences
6. Assessing and evaluating your own and the team's work in providing total nursing care and in order to meet patients' changing needs

Functioning in a nursing care team either as a member or the leader offers many challenges. Several resources in the chapter bibliography provide excellent information on the many elements that make participation in a nursing care team a rewarding personal experience. It is taken for granted that your instructors are planning to schedule some experiences in team technique for nursing care.

As students you are learning to synthesize and use your knowledge. Your instructors, supervisors, many of your classmates, and co-workers help you, both directly and indirectly, to profit from your experiences of learning and working in groups. The manner in which you use successive learning experiences to advantage and the methods you use for developing successful social relationships are actually preparing you for team action. How you utilize the results of your education for service will be up to you.

BIBLIOGRAPHY

American Nurses' Association: Facts about nursing—a statistical summary, 1969 edition, The Association.

Brooks, E. A.: Team nursing, 1961, American Journal of Nursing **61**:87-89, Apr. 1961.

Byers, V. B.: Nursing observation, Dubuque, Iowa, 1968, William C. Brown Co., Publishers.

Cook, B. J. M., and Festog, E. J.: Two head nurses talk about team nursing, American Journal of Nursing **63**:93, Nov. 1963.

Corona, D. F., and Black, E. E.: One hospital's approach to team nursing, Nursing Outlook **11**:506-507, July 1963.

Davis, A. J.: The skills of communication, American Journal of Nursing **63**:66, Jan. 1963.

Douglass, L. Mae, and Bevis, E. O.: Team leadership in action; principles and applications to staff nursing situations, St. Louis, 1970, The C. V. Mosby Co.

Ehrlich, I. F.: Supervision, process not position, American Journal of Nursing **68**:115-119, Jan. 1968.

Komorita, N.: Nursing diagnosis, American Journal of Nursing **63**:83-86, Dec. 1963.

Kron, T.: Nurses' aides need clearer directions, American Journal of Nursing **63**:118-119, Mar. 1963.

Kron, T.: Nursing team leadership, Philadelphia, 1966, W. B. Saunders Co.

Lambertson, E. C.: Nursing team organization and functioning, New York, 1953, Bureau of Publications, Teachers College, Columbia University.

Levine, M. E.: This I believe . . . about patient centered care, Nursing Outlook **15**:53-55, July 1967.

McAnulty, E.: Can a team leader become involved? American Journal of Nursing **65**:128, July 1965.

Melody, M., and Clark, G.: Walking-planning rounds, American Journal of Nursing **67**:53-55, Apr. 1967.

Moxley, J. H.: The predicament in health manpower, American Journal of Nursing **68**:1486-1490, July 1968.

Newcomb, D. P.: The team plan, New York, 1953, G. P. Putnam's Sons.

Peterson, G.: Working with others for patient care, Dubuque, Iowa, 1968, William C. Brown Co., Publishers.

Swansburg, R. C.: An experiment in team nursing, Nursing Outlook **16**:45-47, Aug. 1968; **16**:42-43, Sept. 1968.

Swansburg, R. C.: Team nursing: a programmed learning experience, Units 1-4, New York, 1968, G. P. Putnam's Sons.

U. S. Department of Health, Education and Welfare, Public Health Service: Nurse Training Act of 1964 Program Review Report, December, 1967.

Williams, M. A.: The myth and assumptions about team nursing, Nursing Forum **11**(4):61-73, 1964.

Wood, M. M.: From general duty nurse to team leader, American Journal of Nursing **63**:104-105, Jan. 1963.

Yanick, M., and Podobrinker, N. S.: Don't you miss patient care? American Journal of Nursing **67**:1260-1262, June 1967.

COMPLETE WORK SHEET ON PP. 335 AND 336

CHAPTER 17

Legal aspects of nursing practice

PURPOSE OF LAW

In a democratic and constitutional society basic tenets of the law serve the twofold purpose of protecting individuals from society and of protecting an individual from the aggressive acts of others. Laws establish the framework within which the various community groups interact, they provide the rights and privileges for each citizen, and they contain provision for equal justice. When the due process of the law is disregarded or ignored, chaos results.

Systems of law are categorized according to the way in which the law originated. *Common law* brought from England by the early settlers, is based upon custom and the records of previous court decisions. Its basic principle is *stare decisis,* "the previous decision stands." *Statutory law* is a body of law enacted by federal, state, and local governments. As a nurse you practice under both statutory and common law. Nurse Practice Acts, which define, regulate, and limit the practice of nursing in each state and territory of the United States, are statutory laws. However, in any lawsuit against a nurse for alleged negligence or malpractice both argument and judgment would be based upon custom, usage, and/or precedent or common law.

ACCOUNTABILITY OF NURSES

Each person endowed with an intellect and free will is held accountable for his own acts. Your intellect and your free will permit you to choose between right and wrong. As a citizen you have legally defined rights and responsibilities and you should know what they are. Once a bill becomes a law you must live within the limits it imposes regardless of your personal beliefs. Any revision of an established law requires that the democratic process for amendment or referendum be followed. You should evaluate all proposed bills and enacted laws that govern your daily and your professional life.

LEGAL STATUS—LICENSURE

As nursing practice changes, there is a corresponding change in the rights and responsibilities of nurses. The one factor that remains constant, however, is the requirement that each nurse pass a *licensing examination* before acquiring legal status. The letters RN, LPN, or LVN after a nurse's name do not indicate a degree but a legal title and possession of a certificate to practice nursing. Licensure maintains professionalization, removes nurses without proper qualifications from practice, and ensures the quality of educational preparation for all nurses. The purpose of licensure is the protection of the public's health, welfare, and safety. This protection is a function of state government under its police power as granted in the Constitution.

Licensing laws. Licensing laws or Nurse Practice Acts are laws enacted by state legislatures. They define, regulate, and limit the practice of nursing. They specify the method for obtaining the license to practice, and they establish a state board to administer the specific Nurse Practice Act.

There are two kinds of nurse practice acts—permissive and mandatory. *Permissive law* requires licensure of any nurse who desires to represent herself as a registered nurse, licensed practical nurse, or licensed vocational nurse. Permissive law protects the use of the title only. *Mandatory law* requires that any nurse engaged for hire be licensed by the state in which she is employed. Mandatory law protects the practice of nursing. By December 1970, forty-nine of the fifty-four states and territories had a mandatory Nurse Practice Act. In the remaining states or territories bills were either pending legislative enactment or being prepared for introduction by committee. It is reasonable to assume that by the end of 1971 all who desire to practice nursing in the United States or its territories must be licensed.

State boards of nursing. The state board of nursing is the agency of state government that administers the law regulating nursing as defined in the Nurse Practice Act. Membership on the state board and the board's functions are defined in the Act. Functions of state boards of nursing usually include:

1. Carrying out provisions of the law
2. Adopting rules and policies required to administer the law
3. Conducting state board test pool examinations for registration and licensing
4. Issuing and renewing certificates of registration and licenses
5. Denying, revoking, or suspending certificates of registration and licenses
6. Investigating all violations of the Nurse Practice Act
7. Prosecuting violators of the Nurse Practice Act
8. Defining minimum curricula and standards for the educational programs of schools of nursing
9. Surveying and inspecting schools of nursing
10. Approving schools of nursing or denying or withdrawing approval of schools of nursing

Process of licensure. A nurse (registered, practical, or vocational) may become licensed by *examination, waiver,* or *endorsement.*

Licensure by examination. Licensure by examination means that the nurse candidate has passed the state board test pool examination with acceptable scores and has established proof of competency to practice nursing in that state. To be eligible to take the state board test pool examination you must send to the executive secretary of your state board of nursing documentary evidence of (1) graduation from an approved school of nursing and (2) good moral character. In addition, you must pay the fee required by your state.

Licensure by waiver. Licensure by waiver is licensure in which some or all of the qualifications required by examination are waived. Waiver is customary when a permissive nurse practice law is changed to a mandatory one. When licensure by waiver is permitted, there is a time limit established for such allowance.

Licensure by endorsement. Licensure by endorsement, formerly called "reciprocity," is the granting of a license without examination to an applicant who is already licensed in another state. License by endorsement is granted only to those nurses who received their original license by examination. The nurse must meet the requirements stipulated in the Nurse Practice Act of the second state.

If you plan to move to another state and seek employment as a nurse, you will need to apply to the secretary of the state board of nurse examiners in that state. (The name and address of the secretary of the state board of nurse examiners is listed in the official directory of the *American Journal of Nursing.*) The secretary of the state board will contact your state board for verification of certification.

Annual renewal. Mandatory law requires active licensure. For a nurse to maintain legal status most states require that she renew her license annually. Review the Nurse Practice Act of your state to determine the exact dates and requirements for renewal.

Denial, revocation, and suspension. A license requires responsibility on the part of its holder; it is not a permanent right. It is granted upon stated and specified conditions and may be held only subject to these conditions. A breach or violation of these defined conditions on the part of the nurse may require the licensing board to revoke or suspend her license. To deny, revoke, or suspend a nurse's license or certificate, the state board of nursing must have proof that this nurse has been (1) convicted of a felony or a crime involving moral turpitude (shameful act); (2) convicted of violation of a municipal, state, or federal narcotic law; (3) habitually using narcotics or other drugs or alcohol which affects her professional competency; (4) aiding or abetting in the attempt or execution of a criminal abortion; or (5) declared mentally ill or not restored to legal capacity by a competent court. Before any action can be taken to deny, revoke, or suspend a license, written charges must be filed with the board by its executive secretary and a legal hearing held. As in all other cases of American jurisprudence, a person is innocent until proved guilty.

NURSING FUNCTION

Nursing is a unique and essential public service. In the practice of nursing great emphasis is placed on the acquisition of knowledge, the application of scientific principles, and the development of skills. When planning patient care, each nurse is expected by the public to use good common sense and mature judgment. Developing and implementing this plan require nurses to function both dependently and independently.

Your *dependent function* as a nurse is the traditional one of implementing the doctor's orders, but the major difference today lies in the interpretation of these orders. You are not a blindly obedient servant of the physician. You must know *why* the medication or treatment is ordered, *what* to observe, *how* to prevent an untoward reaction, and *when* to intelligently and safely intervene if a reaction should occur. Consequently, you may have occasion to question the advisability of putting the physician's written order into action. The team concept in patient care calls for a cooperative relationship between you and the doctor. To question the physician's order does not mean that you countermand the order. Such an action would be defined as *prescribing,* which falls within the realm of *medical* practice. To question means to seek clarification, thus ensuring the patient's safety. If you deem an order written by the physician a *must* order and administer it without thoughtful contemplation, you may place your patient in jeopardy. Whether you are a student nurse or are licensed by your state to legally practice as a nurse, you are obliged to bring knowledge, skills, competence, and alertness to all aspects of patient care. This obligation includes the intelligent implementation of the doctor's order. If, as a student, you have occasion to question an order, discuss the situation with your instructor first. Then under her guidance ask the doctor to clarify his order. A registered nurse should be aware of her professional responsibility and should ask the doctor herself for an interpretation of the order. If the physician is not available, the nurse should discuss the problem with the team leader, head nurse, or supervisor. Most doctors will appreciate the observations of an alert nurse, since these observations benefit both his patient and himself.

The *independent* functions of a nurse are related to three factors: (1) the limitations as defined in the Nurse Practice Act, (2) the level of competence achieved as a nurse-practitioner, and (3) what is deemed prudent and safe nursing practice according to local regulations. Independent functions in nursing include:

1. Developing, executing, evaluating, and revising a patient care plan
2. Observing, reporting, and recording signs, symptoms and/or reactions manifested by the patient
3. Developing and executing a plan to educate the patient and his family in order to ensure continuity of care
4. Supervising ancillary workers and assigning to each person only those responsibilities that the team member is capable of doing

When a nurse assigns a procedure to an unskilled worker, the bulk of responsibility is on her (*respondent superior*). However, any person accepting an assignment that he knows he cannot do safely is equally guilty of negligence. This is true of nurses as well as any other health team member.

Violating the dependent and independent functions in nursing denies the patient the safety that is ensured by the state Nurse Practice Acts. To ensure the safety of your patients and to ensure the quality of your nursing practice, follow these few rules:

1. Study the personnel policy of your hiring agency to determine the responsibilities and expectations of you as an employee.
2. Study your job description carefully to determine the scope of your responsibility.
3. Study the hiring agency's policy manual and procedure manual and follow these rules in giving patient care.
4. Be sure you clearly understand and can interpret any written orders. Check with a person in authority when in doubt.
5. Do not assume responsibility for any level of professional practice for which you are not prepared.
6. Carry malpractice insurance (available through your professional organization) as a safety precaution.

OFF-DUTY LIABILITY

You know that each nurse is responsible for her own acts, whether those acts include performance in the line of duty or measures in an emergency. Legally a nurse is not obliged to give assistance in emergencies, but what nurse could not go to the aid of someone obviously in need of help? Keep in mind, however, that once you volunteer to give assistance, your obligation to this individual remains until you are relieved by competent medical help. When you do give aid in an emergency you are expected to use sound professional judgment and to give only that care that is in direct correlation to your skill. Even with these limitations placed upon you, there are many life-saving measures that you can institute. Do keep the individual cognizant of the fact that you are giving him whatever assistance is necessary and possible during this time of emergency. Apprise him of the limitations you are placing on his care, and that you will remain with him until the ambulance or a doctor arrives. It would help, also, if you would write down the names and addresses of some of the witnesses, make notes (or a chart) about this person you have helped, and specify the care that you gave. "Good Samaritan" laws give some legal immunity in emergency situations, but there are rare instances when you may be placed in a situation as a defendant. The primary objective in all nursing care is to assist in attaining or maintaining a state of well-being. It would not be in keeping with this objective to ignore a cry for help in an emergency—as long as the assistance you give is *within the area of nursing practice.*

SPECIFIC CRIMES AND TORTS

A person commits a *crime* if he commits an act that is prohibited by law or if he fails to perform a duty that is required by law. Crimes are wrongs committed against the public. Morals, ethics, and religious tenets are not considered in defining a crime. A *tort* is a legal wrong committed against a *person* for which a civil suit can be brought (for example, an accident victim can sue the driver who caused the accident). A person guilty of a crime is fined and/or imprisoned by a court of law; a person guilty of a tort is sued for a specified amount of money.

Crimes or torts may be committed in one of three ways: (1) by *doing* something which the law forbids, (2) by *failing* to do something which the law requires, and (3) by *performing* a legal act in an unlawful manner. You could be involved in a crime or tort as a *principal,* which means that you are the one actually committing the crime. This may be by your own act, by your act produced through another, or by your cooperation in committing the crime. However, your involvement may lie in recommending or encouraging another person to commit this act, in which case you be an *accessory* to the crime. If your participation occurs before the crime takes place this would make you an *accessory before the fact.* However, if your involvement consisted of concealing the crime or in helping the offender evade punishment, you would be an *accessory after the fact.*

Regardless of your involvement, you would still be guilty in the eyes of the law.

Negligence. Classed as either an act of omission or commission, negligence implies that the person accused did not use ordinary prudence and was not guided by the usual or expected consideration for another person. The act of negligence might include inattentiveness, ignorance, confusion, or carelessness. Negligence also implies that either another person or his property has been placed in jeopardy. *Malpractice* is often used as a synonym for negligence. Malpractice is usually interpreted as the negligence of a person licensed to practice, but a student is also expected to act in a responsible and prudent manner. At all times the safety of the patient must be assured. If you as a nurse are accused of being negligent or are sued for malpractice it must be proved:

1. That you failed to do your duty. It must be proved that in a given situation you failed to perform the duties or assume responsibilities expected of you, and as a result of this failure, the patient (or recipient) was injured or deprived.
2. That you did not administer the ordinary care expected under the circumstances. It must be proved that any reasonable person would have exercised due care in a like situation.
3. That your failure to administer this ordinary care was responsible for the patient's injury. It must be proved that because you failed to use proper precautions, injury to property or person resulted.
4. That the patient is entitled to damages as compensation for the injuries that resulted from your act of omission or commission.

Assault and battery. *Assault* in law means to give the appearance of trying to inflict injury upon another person or to be menacing. There must be the implied threat to do physical harm. *Battery* in law means to actually inflict the injury that was threatened. In the normal course of patient care you may inadvertently find yourself in a situation where you could be sued for assault and battery. For example, each time you approach a patient to give him an injection, you are committing assault. If you give the injection without obtaining the patient's permission, you are committing battery. However, if you identify your patient, follow the administration method you were taught, tell him why you are there, and the patient silently acquiesces to the treatment by getting into position for you to inject the medication, he has given consent by his action.

If the physician orders a medication for his patient, but the patient refuses to accept it because it would be a denial of his religious faith you can be sued for assault and battery if you force the patient to accept this medication. You are attacking his person without consent. For safety, the patient's refusal of any medication or treatment should be accurately recorded on the patient's chart and reported to your superior and the physician. It has also been recommended that when a patient refuses needed therapy (such as a blood transfusion) that he sign a form releasing the hospital, doctor, and nurse from responsibility as a safeguard against malpractice liability.

Restraints—false imprisonment. False imprisonment means to illegally restrict the freedom of another. A nurse applying restraints to a patient without a doctor's specific order is illegally restricting the patient's freedom. The need for restraints to protect the patient from himself or to protect others from him does not give the nurse license to prescribe their application. Restraints may be applied only in an emergency. If you deem restraints advisable, consult the patient's physician and obtain his order. Orders for restraints should be written before restraints are applied.

Much has been written in recent years about the injuries patients have sustained while being restrained. Nurses and attendants can have a false sense of security when a patient is restrained, and this false security decreases the amount of surveillance given the patient. The result of this laxity on the part of the nursing personnel is injury to the patient. Use care, observe your patient frequently, and guard his safety and well being.

The isolation and restriction of a patient suffering from a communicable disease is not classified as false imprisonment. Such isolation is usually written into the local health laws as a means of protecting the general public from exposure. Not to isolate such a patient is a violation of law and would imply negligent nursing practice.

PRIVILEGED COMMUNICATION

Confidential information revealed during, or as a result of, a patient's treatment is classified as privileged information. Patients often ventilate guilt feelings, anxieties, and confidences to the nurse who is available and willing to listen. Reporting pertinent information gleaned from and about your patient to the appropriate personnel is an integral part of your nursing responsibility. However, revealing information obtained during clinical practice to any person not involved in the patient's care is unethical and illegal. Such revelation infringes on the individual's right to privacy guaranteed under both common and statutory law. Statutes in several states require a release signed by the patient involved before the nurse may divulge such privileged communication even in a court of law.

Exercise caution when giving information to others about patients. Especially use discretion when sharing interesting experiences with your friends or family. Hospital "news" or information concerning clinical nursing practice is a fascinating topic to many people. Such communication may legally be held to be libel. To avoid being judged libellous, information must be ". . . offered in good faith in the performance of duty, or where there is an interest to be upheld. . . . It must also be limited to such purpose, made on a proper occasion, published in a proper manner and to proper persons only. And it must be made without actual malice—that is, without intent to commit an unlawful act."*

*Creighton, H.: Steering clear of libel, RN 22:42, June 1959. Reprinted by permission. Copyright 1959, The Nightingale Press, Inc., Oredel, New Jersey.

Because accidents are reported by the press, accident victims may be pursued by reporters. newscasters, and photographers. Although representatives of the various communication media have a job to do, you must protect your patient, and your first concern is the patient's well-being. Refer anyone seeking information or wishing to take photographs to the hospital public relations department, the hospital administrator (or his agent), or the attending physician. Do not release any information unless you are authorized to do so. If it is your responsibility to give such information, think before you speak. Guard against defamation (unguarded derogatory remarks) of a personal nature or concerning the character of a patient, physician, co-worker, or anyone else. To be the basis for a lawsuit, libel (printed defamation) or slander (oral defamation) by the use of derogatory statements, pictures, or implications must be seen or heard *and understood* by a third person. From both an ethical and legal point of view, guard your words. Respect the confidential nature of all personal and professional information.

PATIENT'S CONSENT

Consent refers to the patient's agreement to accept tests, therapies, surgical procedures, or any other treatment deemed necessary by his physician. It is not mandatory to obtain a patient's written consent since it is not written into the law. Hospitals and medical facilities, however, obtain such consent as a preventive measure against possible lawsuit for assault and battery. Every adult deemed mentally competent has the right to be apprised by a responsible person concerning all aspects of any procedure to be done. Consent for a minor or a person declared mentally incompetent should be obtained from a parent or legal guardian. Always obtain consent before taking any action. Every institution uses its own specific consent form and has its own method for obtaining it. Since no single consent form will cover all aspects of patient care, it may be necessary to use a variety of forms. Check the policy manual of your institution for the exact method to follow and use it as your guide. When in doubt consult your instructor or supervisor.

RECORDS

All health agencies maintain complete records of their patients. You have been keeping a hospital record (chart) on each of your patients. These records should contain a complete account of all observations and care received during his hospitalization. Laws differ from state to state on whether the patient's record, especially the nurse's notes, may be submitted as evidence in litigation. It is, however, potentially a legal document. Many of the documented cases available in law libraries indicate that the chart was introduced as important legal testimony. In those cases, regardless of the amount of other evidence already presented, judge and jury carefully studied the day-by-day evidence of the caliber of care and the skill of those responsible for this care.

It is imperative that the chart be written clearly and accurately and that it be easily understood. The prevalent practice is to save time by using abbreviations and symbols, check lists, or codes. These devices can depersonalize the record to the extent of eliminating much that is pertinent and relevant concerning the patient. Also, abbreviations and symbols are sometimes misunderstood and they may obscure the true meaning. Occasionally a chart presents such an incomplete picture of the patient's treatment that the care appeared to be inadequate and carelessly given. The manner in which notations are made reflect the attitude of those administering care. The nurse's record should reflect the following:

1. The observations of the nurse doing the recording
2. The quality and continuity of patient care, including administration of medication and treatment
3. The patient's attitude toward his care
4. Any unusual symptoms of nervousness or mental stress manifested by the patient
5. An accurate description of objective and subjective symptoms
6. The exact time of medication and treatment administration, doctor's visits, birth, and death, or any other pertinent observation
7. The patient's reaction to medications and treatments administered or the results of such medication or treatment

DRUG ABUSE AND THE NURSE

Drug abuse is the nonmedical use of drugs in quantities large enough to cause uncontrollable behavioral changes. We live in a drug-oriented society, and there is a drug to meet the needs of everyone. When drugs such as tranquilizers, barbiturates, or amphetamines are used under the direction of a physician they are beneficial. Unfortunately it is a relatively simple matter for an individual to obtain these drugs and he may use them as his passport to Utopia. The indiscriminate use of drugs to shut out life's problems is not peculiar to any one segment of the population. People in all socioeconomic levels, age groups, and educational levels are seeking the same answer. Unfortunately drug abuse only adds additional problems. Passing and enforcing laws are not the final answer; such laws do not eliminate the supply of drugs, nor do they correct the cause of the dependency (physical, psychologic, or economic) which originally led to the use and abuse of drugs.

Before casting aspersions at others, nurses must first look at themselves and their own drug patterns. They are not immune to the temptations, frustrations, anxieties, or the desire for approval that entice the rest of society. Nurses have no more right to take medication without medical supervision than any other citizen. Only a physician can diagnose and prescribe and only a pharmacist can dispense drugs. It is illegal for a nurse to prescribe medication for herself or others. Some nurses do become addicted to narcotics or indulge in the use of hallucinogens and other dangerous drugs.

Drug abuse affects everyone. The role of the nurse in any drug abuse control and rehabilitation program is significant. Nurses can aid materially in tearing down the mystique about drugs. Do not take medication yourself unless it is under medical supervision. Be alert to your colleagues also. If you become suspicious that drugs are disappearing or that patients are not getting expected results from medications, report to the proper authority. This is a legal responsibility and will be handled as privileged communication. When you are giving patient care, use other comfort measures before you administer medication to relieve pain or anxiety. This does not mean that you should ever deny a patient needed medication, but you must not be a "shot happy" nurse.

Since your first days in nursing you have been told that nurses are teachers of health. As a teacher of health you have a leading role in the prevention of drug abuse. Be prepared to aid in all programs of education. Know about the drugs listed by the Bureau of Narcotics and Dangerous Drugs. Prepare yourself so that you will be able to speak authoritatively and factually to parent groups, church groups, and youth groups. Do not use "scare" techniques, but state the facts as they are. Young people are very knowledgeable about drugs and will accept only information that is scientifically based. Tell them, for example, that marijuana is an unpredictable drug used by unpredictable people and has unpredictable results. Teach that there are other answers to life's problems than drugs. Some of these answers are to be found in using one's intellect to its fullest capacity, in participating actively in a cause, or in expending time and energy in acts of love or compassion to another human being.

An individual who misuses drugs is harming himself; he is a sick person. As a nurse, can you refuse assistance to a person in need?

CONTROL OF NARCOTICS AND DANGEROUS DRUGS

As a nurse you are knowledgeable, skillful, and qualified, and are concerned with every aspect of the law when administering narcotics and dangerous drugs. You may administer these drugs by mouth, topically, subcutaneously, intramuscularly, and (in some instances) intravenously. To administer narcotics (derivatives of opium) or dangerous drugs (barbiturates, amphetamines, or any agent acting to depress or stimulate the central nervous system) there must be an order written by a doctor or a dentist. This order contains specific instructions concerning the type of medication, dosage, route, and frequency of administration. Local regulations and federal laws establish the specific time that the physician must represcribe a drug order. Under the *Drug Abuse Control Amendments* of 1965 pharmacists may refill depressant or stimulant drugs five times; the *Harrison Narcotic Act* states that narcotic orders must be written and are not refillable. The physician must write a new prescription each time the drug is needed.

Drug laws are criminal statutes. Any nurse administering a narcotic or dangerous drug after the expiration date of that order is guilty of a crime as well as negligence. By definition, drug laws are criminal statutes specifying the crime, identifying the criminals, and stating exact punishment to be meted out to anyone breaking these laws. The statute to control the manufacture, importation, and distribution of narcotics has been in effect since enactment of the *Harrison Narcotic Act* in 1914. Its primary purpose is to prevent the indiscriminate use of habit-forming narcotics. Enforcement of this law was placed with the Federal Bureau of Narcotics under the Treasury Department until 1968. A new Bureau of Drug Abuse Control (narcotics and dangerous drugs) was established in 1968 under the Food and Drug Administration of the Department of Health, Education and Welfare. The program of this new Bureau is fourfold:

1. Law enforcement—finding both pushers and users
2. Compliance with the law—preventing the counterfeiting of drugs or divergence of drugs from legitimate sources
3. Education and training—improving the health, welfare, and safety of the nation
4. Research—taking place at the Division of Drug Sciences, Institute of Public Health, Washington, D. C.

Narcotic Addict Rehabilitation Act of 1966 and Uniform Narcotic Drug Acts are currently in effect in all states. These acts also include provisions for rehabilitation of the addict. None of these laws broaden the nurse's authority. They do, however, impose additional stringent requirements in record keeping and in adhering strictly to rules and regulations for administration of drugs.

LIABILITY FOR ADMINISTRATION OF DRUGS

Nurse Practice Acts specifically state a nurse may not diagnose or prescribe medication. The nurse is an agent of the physician (or dentist) who writes the specific order. This order states what medication the patient is to receive, how much he is to have, how often it is to be administered, and by which route. You may not substitute one drug for another, and you must keep an accurate record of all drugs administered. This record is kept on the patient's chart and you also make an entry on the appropriate narcotic or dangerous drug record so that there is a constant inventory of drugs used. You must be certain that your drug order is current.

Nurse Practice Acts and local laws regulate the route of drug administration and specify which dangerous drugs may be administered by a nurse. The American Nurses' Association Committee on Nursing Practice states that delegated medical tasks or procedures as defined in Nurse Practice Acts or local laws are within the province of nursing practice. Any nurse failing to remain within the limits as established by law is negligent and guilty of a crime.

LIABILITY FOR ADMINISTRATION OF CARE

You should always determine whether the administration of a medication or treatment is defined as a "medical" or "nursing" practice. Because both the dependent and independent functions of nursing are constantly broadened, it is not possible to establish a list of nursing functions that would be applicable to all nurses. By state law or by stipulated local regulation nurses may be legally permitted to administer intravenous medications, blood transfusions, or to perform external cardiac massage and defibrillation. In other localities these therapies are classified as medical practice and outside the realm of nursing. For this reason it is extremely difficult to differentiate in a textbook between a medical or a nursing function. When in doubt, consult your instructor or supervisor.

In addition to adhering to established limits of the state Nurse Practice Act and to established local regulations, each nurse must realistically evaluate herself. Your own depth of knowledge, manipulative skills, ability to maintain safety for your patient, and ability to make mature judgments are the measures you must use in determining whether you will accept a delegated task. Every individual is responsible for *his own* acts. Performing any nursing function without adequate preparation and the proper skills can endanger your patient. If such an act is poorly executed and results in harm to the patient, it is an act of negligence and you can be sued for malpractice.

LIABILITY FOR SUPERVISION

One of the independent functions in nursing practice is the delegation of nursing functions to other nurses or ancillary personnel assigned for patient care. Each team member is expected to make a definite and specific contribution to the patient's total care based upon the contributor's level of competence. However, the nurse must use care and judgment in evaluating each person's qualifications before making assignments. The person assigning a task to other personnel is responsible for any harm or injury that results from that care. Poorly prepared or careless co-workers require that superiors maintain constant supervision to ensure safety to the patient.

The following preventive measures will ensure safety to your patient in the administration of medications and treatments and in supervising other nurses:

1. Ascertain that all orders of medications

or treatments for your patient were written by his physician (or dentist) and that they are complete in every detail.

2. Verify the order with the doctor prescribing it when in doubt. In his absence, consult your instructor, supervisor, or the head nurse.
3. Know the usual dosage, route of administration, expected effects, and any possible side effects of any medication ordered.
4. Know the treatment ordered, expected results, any possible untoward effects, and any contraindications.
5. Follow the state and local regulations of nurse functions, whether assuming active patient care yourself or assigning it to others.
6. When handling narcotics and/or dangerous drugs, follow the stipulations in the law:
    a. Administer narcotics or dangerous drugs *only* when prescribed by a *licensed* physician.
    b. Carefully maintain all records.
    c. Keep narcotics or dangerous drugs in your possession only when working directly with a patient under a licensed physician or when you are a patient yourself.
    d. Return *all* unused drugs. Never keep them in your possession.
    e. Never obtain any drugs by fraud or deceit.

BIBLIOGRAPHY

Bernzweig, E.: Liability for malpractice; its role in nursing education, The Journal of Nursing Education **8**:33-40, Apr. 1969.

Covington, R. N.: Moral and legal responsibilities of surgical nurse, Nursing Forum **4**:19-26, Mar. 1965.

Creighten, H.: Steering clear of libel, RN **22**:42, 1959.

Dolan, M. M.: Violent patients! You and the law, RN Aug. 1968, pp. 42-43.

Donahue, J. C.: Symposium on the nurse and the law, Nursing Clinics of North America **2**:115-197, Mar. 1967.

Dutresac, C.: Mind your own business, Canadian Nurse, Sept. 1969, pp. 46-48.

Hershey, N.: Perspectives on liability risks, American Journal of Nursing **70**:1511-1512, July 1970.

Hershey, N.: The changing law, American Journal of Nursing **69**:120-122, Jan. 1969.

Hershey, N.: Questions of life or death, American Journal of Nursing **68**:1910-1912, Sept. 1968.

Lesnik, M. J., and Anderson, B. E.: Nursing practice and the law, ed. 2, Philadelphia, 1962, J. B. Lippincott Co.

McKenna, F. M.: Thresholds to professional nursing practice, ed. 2, Philadelphia, 1960, W. B. Saunders Co.

Murchison, I. A., and Nichols, T. S.: Legal foundations of nursing practice, New York, 1970, The Macmillan Co.

Olson, E. V.: Needed: a shake-up in the status quo, American Journal of Nursing **68**:1491, June 1968.

Professional liability information, Occupational Health Nursing Feb. 1969, p. 23.

Reagan, W. A.: Insurance, a must for every licensed nurse, **10**:3, Aug. 1969; Nursing and the Jehovah Witness, **9**:2, July 1968; Nursing experience counts in court, **7**:7, Dec. 1967; Nursing liability for restraint accidents, **8**:6, Nov. 1967, The Reagan Report on Nursing Law.

Reagan, W. A.: The new standing orders and their legal pitfalls, RN Apr. 1968, pp. 38-41.

Sarner, H.: The nurse and the law, Philadelphia, 1968, W. B. Saunders Co.

Willig, S. H.: The nurses' guide to the law, New York, 1970, McGraw-Hill Book Co.

Booklets

Drug abuse—a primer for parents, Washington, D. C., National Education Association.

Drug abuse—a call for action, New York, American Social Health Association.

Films

Escape to Nowhere. A 16 year old girl describes her start on drugs and her hapless predicament. 25 min. for senior high through college. Professional Arts, Inc., P. O. Box 8484, Universal City, California, 91608.

Hide and Seek. Story of a young boy's introduction to drugs, continued mental and physical deterioration, his loneliness, his anguish. 14 min. black and white for junior and senior high students. Columbia University Press, Mass Communications Center, 44 W. 110 Street, New York, N. Y. 10025.

The Losers. An examination of the prevalence of experimentation and the habitual use of chemicals among young people twelve to twenty-one years of age. 31 min. color, junior and senior high students. Carousel Films, Inc., 1501 Broadway, New York, N. Y. 10036.

COMPLETE WORK SHEET ON PP. 337 AND 338

CHAPTER 18

Basic considerations for spiritual health

Religion can be defined as a belief in a Divine Power. Religion is also the practice of ritual and a system of conduct based upon a code of ethics and beliefs.

Religious beliefs are individual and unique to each person; no one can force his religious ideology upon another. However, your own attitude toward formal religious observance will influence the spiritual care you administer. It will determine whether you feel comfortable or uncomfortable when trying to meet your patient's spiritual needs.

The practice of nursing requires that each nurse be tolerant of the beliefs of others. To be tolerant of another's belief is to be capable of recognizing and respecting the ideals, opinions, or behavior of others. For you to recognize and respect the spiritual beliefs of your patient is to respect the inherent individuality of man. You cannot do everything for every patient, but you can do *something*. You can listen for the undercurrent of urgency that means that this patient wants to be noticed, to be helped, and to be cared about. When you have reached the limit of your own capability to meet a patient's spiritual needs, or when you feel inadequate attempting to meet these needs, seek the assistance of someone better prepared for this function. You may ask for help from the hospital chaplain (included as a member of the hospital health team) or from the clergyman the patient selects.

The American Nurses' Association Code for Professional Nurses states, "Professional nursing service is therefore unrestricted by considerations of nationality, creed, or color. . . . The religious beliefs of a patient must be respected." Because these beliefs deal with the basic nature of man and his search for an understanding of the meaning of life, religious beliefs are probably the most important of all the beliefs that your patient holds. What your patient believes greatly influences his mental and physical health. Under no circumstances are you to force religious consolation upon the patient not desiring it, but it is your responsibility to obtain this consolation for the patient wishing it.

MEETING PATIENTS' SPIRITUAL NEEDS

Providing for spiritual care is an important part of each patient's nursing care plan. To implement this aspect of his care is extremely difficult, since nurses often feel inadequate or embarrassed. They may lack preparation for administering this care. Spiritual care may be needed by *any* patient, not just the terminally ill. The mysteries of life and death hold deep religious meaning for most people. It is especially at times of stress that patients and their families desire to participate in the religious rites which their faith associates with the events of birth, illness, or death. It is usually the nurse who first becomes aware of the patient's need for religious consolation. In providing for this care the following suggestions may prove helpful.

1. Assess and specifically identify the religious consolation needed.

2. Keep the patient's articles of religious significance close to him.
3. Reading from the Bible or his prayer book is often a source of comfort for the patient desiring this consolation, but never force the patient to accept Bible or prayer reading—it may prove to be emotionally and mentally upsetting.
4. Furnish him with religious writings of his faith, when possible, if he requests them.
5. Provide for the appropriate rites of his faith as needed.
6. Call upon his clergyman for additional consolation, if the patient desires.

RELIGIOUS CONSOLATION

It is an accepted fact that people generally draw nearer to God and to the practice of their religion during misfortune, including illness. To assist you in offering your patient religious consolation the following information is offered.

The Jewish patient. Judaism is based upon three pillars or principles—the worship of God, the love of learning, and the practice of good deeds. This faith does not accept the doctrine of original sin. Judaism teaches that all of man's appetites are natural. It teaches that each individual is endowed with the free will that permits him to choose between good or evil and is responsible for his own acts. Every Jew is expected to observe God's commandments out of his love for God, not because he desires a reward or is afraid of punishment. Central focus is on the home, not on the synagogue or temple.

The Jewish faith is divided into three groups: Orthodox, Conservative, and Reformed. Even though philosophically divided, all Jews have a common bond through their mutual sharing of history, literature, prayer, moral precepts, and spiritual purposes. *Orthodox Jews* accept the Old Testament of the Bible and its laws as the revealed word and will of God. They follow tradition strictly and adhere rigidly to the disciplines of their faith. Dietary laws are followed stringently, men and women sit separately for religious service, men wear prayer shawls and keep their heads covered at all times, and the religious service is conducted almost entirely in Hebrew. *Conservative Jews* also follow tradition, but they have introduced some modern concepts into their religious observance. The Sabbath, Holy Days, and dietary laws are traditionally followed and prayer shawls and head covering are worn; but men and women worship together. Both English and Hebrew are used in prayer and ceremony. *Reformed Jews* follow only those customs that they believe adapt to the ideas of modern civilization. They accept those moral Biblical laws and follow the religious rites they believe elevate and sanctify the life of man. Services are conducted primarily in English, head covering and prayer shawls are not worn, and instrumental music is used in the temple.

Since Judaism does not accept the doctrine of original sin, or that the story of Adam and Eve reflects man's fall from grace, *no Jewish patient is ever baptized.* Male infants are circumcized and named through ritual observance on the eighth day after birth; this rite may be postponed if the infant is in poor health. Girl babies are named in the synagogue with appropriate prayers on the days that the Torah is removed from the Ark and read. For the terminally ill or dying patient, a rabbi's visit and reading of prayers will bring solace and consolation for him and his family. When a Jewish patient dies his rabbi will offer comfort to the family, call the committee of congregants who take care of the deceased, and notify responsible persons concerning his burial.

The Sabbath, observed from sundown Friday to sundown Saturday, is the holiest of days for observant Jews. For the patient in a hospital, the scheduling of any diagnostic or surgical procedure during this holy period should be postponed, unless such postponement would be harmful. The Holy Scriptures (Old Testament) and a Hebrew-English prayer book should be available for the patient to read.

Observant Orthodox and Conservative Jewish patients will follow dietary rules, called the rule of "Kashruth." They will eat only Kosher foods, which are ritually prepared and ritually served:

meat and milk dishes are kept and served at separate meals.

Spiritual care of the Jewish patient must be planned individually depending on how closely the patient adheres to the traditional disciplines of the Jewish faith. Assess the patient, listen for his expressed wants or needs, and when you are uncertain as to the correct action to take, seek assistance from his rabbi in developing a plan for spiritual care.

Christianity. Christianity is based upon belief in the Trinity of God—the Father, the Son, and the Holy Spirit. Christians accept both the Old and New Testaments of the Bible. Jesus is the "Christ"—the Saviour and Redeemer. Most Christian groups believe in original sin and salvation. The Christian ethic is rooted deeply in the three elements of faith, hope, and charity (love).

Within the realm of Christendom there are many denominations, but all Christians seek a state of grace through prayer and through receiving the sacraments of their individual creeds.

Roman Catholic patient. Since 1962 there have been many changes in the Catholic Church, including the use of English instead of Latin during the Mass and less stringent rules for fasting. These changes are resisted by many Catholics, especially the elderly. Therefore, the wishes of the patient should be respected regarding any aspect of his practice of religion.

Spiritual consolation to the Roman Catholic patient requires that the nurse become familiar with the sacraments of baptism, penance, Communion, and anointing of the sick. To a Roman Catholic sacraments have the power to assist him in attaining a state of grace so vital for his salvation.

Baptism, which gives absolution of sin and signifies birth into the life of Christ, is the first sacrament received by the Roman Catholic. Since church doctrine teaches that from the moment of conception an infant has a soul, and that all Catholics must be in a state of grace at the time of death, any infant born of Catholic parents who is in danger of death must be baptized. If a priest cannot be present before death occurs, anyone, whether or not he professes the Catholic faith, should perform the baptism. Pour water on the infant's head, and as the water flows say: "I baptize you in the name of the Father and of the Son and of the Holy Spirit." Make a record of the baptism on the chart and fill out a card, which should include the following information:

1. Name of the baptized infant (Baby Boy Jones)
2. Parents' name
3. Your name
4. Names of witnesses to the baptism
5. Date of birth
6. Date of baptism
7. Place of baptism
8. It is helpful, also, to include the name of the parish to which the parents belong

You should also inform the parents (usually the mother) that the infant received baptism before death. Such information provides consolation to the grieving family.

Penance is a means of being forgiven for sins of omission and commission by confessing to a priest and performing the exacted penance. The only preparation the nurse must provide is to arrange for complete privacy for the patient and his priest.

Communion is offered to patients daily in a Catholic hospital and at any time in hospitals or at home for terminally ill patients. The exact procedure followed in the hospitals where you serve will be discussed with you. Preparation of your patient includes the creation of an environment of cleanliness and order. If permitted, elevate the head of his bed. To prepare for an individual communion service for the patient cover a table near the bedside with a clean white cloth, and place a glass of water, spoon, crucifix, holy water, and two candles on it. After your patient is ready for the priest's visit, allow him the privacy to prepare himself.

Anointing the sick, a sacrament offered to any Roman Catholic patient, has also been called Extreme Unction, Last Rites, and Viaticum. Sacraments of penance, Communion, and anointing of the sick are always offered to a dying Roman Catholic patient by a priest. Preparation includes a neat environment, with the bed clothes loosened at the foot for anointing. Cover a table with a white cloth, and place a crucifix, holy water, two candles, and six small cotton balls in a dish on this table. These cotton balls are to be burned separately from other waste materials after the patient has been anointed. The priest will bring the oil which has been blessed by the bishop, and anoint the patient's eyes, ears, nostrils, lips, hands, and feet while chanting the appropriate prayers.

The Protestant patient. One of the three main divisions of the Christian church is Protestantism. There are many denominations, each with its own particular beliefs and practices. However, all Protestant sects believe that man gains his salvation through the life he lives.

Baptism is an accepted sacrament of most Protestant churches, but the age of the recipient and the manner in which this sacrament is performed varies. It is expected you will call a minister, in the event this rite is to be performed, but in the event an infant may not survive, anyone with proper intent may perform this ritual. Pour water on the infant's head and say while water is flowing: "(Name), I baptize you in the name of the Father, and of the Son, and of the Holy Spirit. Amen." Record the baptism and report this information to the clergyman of the church to which his parents belong. Baptism, once performed, is valid. Most Protestant denominations do not observe any sacraments for the acutely ill, terminally ill, or dying patient. Patients and their families, however, may derive solace and comfort from prayer and a visit with their minister.

Communion, although not offered by all Protestant churches, should be made available to the patient who requests this sacrament. Notify the patient's minister, when possible, that the patient desires to take Communion, and he will tell you what to prepare. Provide a neat and clean environment, a quiet and private corner, a table covered with a white cloth, and whatever else the minister requests.

Dietary regulations may be specific to the Protestant sect to which the patient belongs. Your patient will be happy to explain these restrictions to you. Do not hesitate to ask him. If your patient is unable to provide this information, consult his clergyman or a responsible member of his family. To many patients this aspect of care is as important as any therapy.

Remember, some patients do not follow any formal religious doctrine. They are entitled, however, to the same consideration and respect shown to patients professing a religious faith. Never force spiritual consolation on any patient. Just as this aspect of care will assist those patients with an expressed need, forcing spiritual care if he does not wish it will create a situation that is harmful to your patient.

THE DYING PATIENT

Woven into the pattern of every culture is the thought that as mortal beings each of us will ultimately reach the end of his time on earth. In spite of this reality, the customs of the various ethnic cultures demonstrate that fear of death is ever present. Maybe this fear is based upon the superstitious belief of "an eye for an eye or a tooth for a tooth," retribution for sins of omission or commission, or is simply based upon a fear of the unknown. Reaction to the fear of death, either expressed or felt, may give rise to one or more of the defense mechanisms that a person may use to combat any situation disturbing his emotional and mental equilibrium.

Scientific and technologic developments have not altered the fact that death is feared. The basic difference in the attitude of today's society lies in the fact that science has developed many techniques for prolonging life, and in critical situations the medical profession is expected to use these devices. In attempting to prolong life through the use of either ordinary or extraordinary means the patient may be denied the right to die with dignity, and he may die without the preparation for death that his faith teaches him is necessary. It may deny him the right to prepare his affairs properly. Medicine and nursing are caught between technocracy on the one hand and the humanity of man on the other. Even with the realization that the ultimate end of life is death, no one is ever prepared to face this separation from a loved one.

As a nurse, you must first face your own attitude toward death before you can begin to help meet the needs of your patient, his family, and his friends. Adjustment and emotional reactions usually follow a pattern described by many authorities as the "stages of grief and mourning." No two authorities agree on the period of time each stage lasts, but if you feel they are lasting too long and may prove harmful, seek the assistance of your instructor or the hospital chaplain. In order to increase your understanding of this pattern of grief a brief description of the stages a patient or his family follows is included here.

1. The first stage is called the freeze or denial stage. The ill person cannot believe that the illness he is now suffering may be terminal. He concludes it must be a case of mistaken diagnosis: it just cannot happen to him. Even though he is among family and friends, he must face this situation alone. Because he is alone, he is in a state of induced shock or freeze. This is nature's way of allowing for "rest of part," for a beginning stage in emotional healing when not prolonged.

2. The second stage is called the thaw or melting period. It is during this time that emotional expression occurs. This thaw may be expressed as crying, as depression, or as rebellion. It is a time when the individual reaches the depths of depression and isolation. The expression of any emotion is often difficult for those in listening distance, since our English heritage seems to conspire against such expression. Allowing for ventilation of feelings by the patient frequently has a calming effect.

3. The third stage is one of repair or restitution. This stage is characterized by both external and internal manifestations. External manifestations include somatic factors believed to be an "attention-getting" mechanism. Internally, the individual is in a panic while externally there may be a tendency to self-pity. When the patient begins to accept the situation, the person has indeed made a beginning toward resolution. It is not easy to understand and to work through grief; it is an extremely difficult task. It is during this stage that the assistance of your hospital's chaplain or the patient's own clergyman will have the greatest effect.

4. The fourth stage is one of the patient's returning interest in life, picking up the threads, and carrying on the will to live until peace and hope are attained. It is during this stage that each person faces the reality that nothing will ever be quite the same again; the realization that this experience can and will result in strengthening individual character. This is a time for you to be available to listen, to read the Bible or a prayer book, to pray, or to help arrange for the patient to receive the sacraments of his church if the patient wishes.

Your role as nurse is many-sided. Nurses are frequently privileged to assist in the patient's cure; to help the patient, his family, and his friends adjust to the inevitable facts of life or death; and at all times to give the comfort and assurance that only a nurse in constant attendance can administer. Your role cannot be assumed until you have looked into yourself and built up the necessary inner strength to assist others. It is important, therefore, for nurses to understand the place of grief as a normal part of life, and for them to acquire the knowledge and skill to help the patient and his family face this crisis.

Keep in mind that there is no short road to achieving your objectives of care for the terminally ill. It will require using all of your knowledge of the sequence that the reaction to grief follows. It will require the application of this knowledge in the utilization of your skills to meet your patient's needs, and it will require you to summon up all of your resources for personal strength—only then can you help the patient, his family, and his friends meet this crisis in their lives.

BIBLIOGRAPHY

Aldrich, C. K.: The dying patient's grief, Journal of the American Medical Association **184**:329-331, May 4, 1963.

Bachman, C. C.: Ministering to the grief sufferer, St. Louis, 1964, Concordia Publishing House.

Cushing, Cardinal Richard: The Christian ideals for nursing, Hospital Progress **42**:68-70, June 1961.

Heschel, A. J.: The insecurity of freedom, New York, 1966, Farrar, Straus & Giroux, Inc.

Jackson, E. N.: Understanding grief, Nashville, 1962, Abingdon Press.

Kubler-Ross, E.: On death and dying, New York, 1969, The Macmillan Co.

Pelikan, J.: The shape of death, St. Louis, 1961, Concordia Publishing House.

Phillips, C.: Meeting your patient's religious needs, RN **29**:61-71, Apr. 1966.

Reed, E. L.: Helping children with the mystery of death, Nashville, 1967, Abingdon Press.

Sister Mary Hubert: Spiritual care for every patient, The Journal of Nursing Education **2**:9-11, May-June 1963.

Smith, H. L.: Ethics and the new medicine, Nashville, 1969, Abingdon Press.

Sudnow, D.: Passing on, Englewood Cliffs, N. J., 1967, Prentice-Hall, Inc.

Westberg, G. E.: Good grief, Rock Island, Ill., 1961, Augustana Book Concern.

White, D.: Dialogue in medicine and theology, Nashville, 1969, Abingdon Press.

COMPLETE WORK SHEET ON P. 339

CHAPTER 19

Looking ahead

ACCOMPLISHMENTS TO THE PRESENT

You are advancing to a level in your nursing education where, presumably, you exercise the kind of judgment and administer the quality of patient care that reflects growth and maturity in your nursing practice. Take the time, however, to pause and look back over the path that has brought you to the present.

You selected nursing with great expectations and high ideals, and you are fulfilling the educational requirements of your nursing education program. There are times of discouragement and certainly times of elation. Hopefully, you look forward to each new educational experience with eagerness. Your educational achievements, your social developments, and your emotional maturity have all united to make you the person you are. You accept the present *you* as a matter of fact, and you surely have the full realization of all that has gone into the process of your maturing in nursing. The present you is of value only as you profit by the experiences of the past and prepare for the experiences that the future holds for you.

The purpose of the following pages is to tie your past to your present. By being fully aware of the present and its potentialities, you can direct your future. Just as it is not possible to clearly visualize the entire horizon from a distance, so it is not your privilege to see all of the future that lies before you. As long as you have life and hope, you seek to broaden your horizon and to reach the unknown that lies just beyond your view.

Time spent in consideration of your preparation for your chosen career should serve to stimulate your thinking about the future and what you wish to do with it. Your expressed interests will guide you and your stated goals will inspire you. You may choose to accept the helping hand of those who direct you, or you may choose to follow in the footsteps of those who have preceded you. Whatever your choice, you must move steadily on into the future increasing your knowledge. Certainly you will want to discover new and better ways of fulfilling your responsibilities both to the public and to those who provide you with the opportunity for service. This ability to discover new ways is your challenge for the future.

YOUR STRENGTHS AND LIMITATIONS

Before you select the specific area of nursing in which to practice, it is wise to determine whether you are fitted to follow your particular choice. To evaluate your strengths requires two types of realistic analysis—self-analysis and occupational analysis. Self-analysis means to evaluate your ability to interact with others and your attitude toward the people to whom you will give care. Occupational analysis includes the identification of your area of interest and evaluation of your competence in nursing practice, your ability to apply knowledge to patient care, and your ability to meet the health needs of your patients. You have been periodically evaluated by your instructors. Your proficiency, ability, and attitude were noted carefully, and, hopefully, objective opinions were recorded in a variety of formats. Most of you have been evaluated by a rating scale that attempted to exclude any subjectivity. It is expected that you have seen your various evaluations, and as a student have had the opportunity to identify areas of both strength and weakness, and have had the opportunity to strengthen areas of weakness.

The objectives of your school of nursing will identify the expected behavioral changes for graduates of your school. These statements will also determine the level of nursing practice you will be prepared to assume upon graduation and the areas of nursing practice that will require additional educational preparation. No single program can prepare its graduates to assume all positions available.

Take a look at your experience as a student nurse. The type and quality of education you have received, the grades you achieved, and the areas of practice that were challenging and interesting should influence your realistic evaluation of your strengths and limitations of nursing practice. Other factors to consider include your age, aptitude, physical condition, emotional stability, and ability to adapt to new and traumatic situations. All of these should be factors for consideration in a self-analysis.

Through such self-evaluation you should be able to identify your strengths realistically, and by studying the objectives of your school of nursing you can identify the limitations imposed upon your nursing practice. However, the final determination of your specific choice of an area of nursing practice rests with you. Use every resource available, study the results of your analysis carefully and objectively, and base your decision upon intelligent evaluation, not emotion. Just as it takes all types of people to make a world, so it takes a variety of nurses prepared to function in a variety of situations to meet the needs of an ever-changing society. Douglas Malloch presented a valuable basis for selecting your future professional career:

If you can't be a pine on top of the hill,
Be a scrub in the valley—but be
The best little scrub at the side of the rill;
Be a bush if you can't be a tree.

We can't all be captains, we've got to be a crew,
There's something for all of us here;
There's big work to do, and there's lesser to do,
And the task you must do is near.

If you can't be a highway, then just be a trail,
If you can't be the sun, be a star;
It isn't by size that you win or fail—
Be the best of whatever you are.

HALLMARKS OF PROFESSIONAL PRACTICE

Because you possess certain rights it is assumed that you have complete awareness of the duties and obligations that accompany these rights. You should recognize your moral, personal, and civic responsibilities. Some hallmarks of professional practice expected from you as a graduate are reviewed here for your benefit.

ADMINISTERING PATIENT CARE

In the administration of patient care, you will concern yourself with responsibilities to both the patient and to nursing. They include responsibilities to yourself and to others.

To yourself. Remain true to yourself and your principles. Carefully protect your own health. Endeavor to live a life that upholds your own self-respect and in turn commands respect from those with whom you come into contact.

To others. You have the responsibility of applying your knowledge for the well-being of others. Apply this knowledge in the care of the sick, in the promotion of health principles, and in the advancement of social welfare. Pay particular heed to your professional conduct concerning the following.

Duties to your profession. Your profession has the right to expect from you the conscientious fulfillment of nursing practice, the acquisition of increased knowledge required for professional development, the upholding of the standards of professional practice, and the prudence to maintain ethical practice at all times.

Duties to your patient. Your patient expects you to administer quality care and to consistently respect him as a person. You have the responsibility to do all that you can to maintain his life and to avoid anything that may cause him injury. Your professional status places you in a position of trust, and matters involving the patient's personal life are treated as confidential information.

Duties to the physician. The physician expects from you the intelligent implementation of his orders directed toward patient welfare. He believes you will not only administer quality nursing care but also will carefully observe the patient's condition and report information that will assist him. He also expects loyalty to himself and to his reputation.

Your responsibilities extend to others of the health team as well. They expect coordination of health services, diligence, cooperation, kindness, sincerity, and the conduct becoming to a member of a service profession.

PROFESSIONAL CONDUCT IN PUBLIC

Your professional conduct in public should reflect credit to you as a person and a nurse. Any behavior that causes you to become unnecessarily conspicuous or detracts from your good name can be classed as unprofessional.

Traveling with a patient. When traveling with a patient, be considerate and stay within his financial means. Have an understanding of the traveling expenses needed and the provisions that have been made to meet them. It may be advisable to obtain Travelers Cheques from a local bank or the American Railway Express to assure protection from inadequate funds or loss of money.

Make all necessary plans for the trip if this is expected of you. Preferably, members of the patient's family will make reservations, obtain tickets, notify all who are to cooperate in transporting the patient, and verify the plans for receiving him upon arrival at the destination.

Assume the responsibility for preparing all necessary baggage. Take care that necessary articles of clothing are included and that everything is neatly packed to conserve space. Determine whether or not trunks should be sent in advance or baggage checked. Keep articles for immediate care of the patient in a separate case with you.

Remain with the patient throughout the trip. You may obtain aid from those designated to furnish necessary assistance. Remember to compensate them for their services if it is socially correct to do so. If you have received many favors and assistance over and above that required in usual circumstances, a gift or contribution of money may be in order for services rendered to assisting personnel at the end of the trip.

Accompanying a patient in public. You may be asked to care for your patient in a hotel, accompany him to a health center or hospital, or act as a companion.

In a hotel. You may or may not wear a uniform when caring for a patient in a hotel, depending upon the nature of the illness. Remember that the manager of the hotel is your host and he deserves consideration. Notify him of your presence and your patient's illness. Request assistance from him when additional care, food, or changes are needed. This will assure willing cooperation and acceptance.

In a new hospital or health center environment. Make all plans for the admission of the patient in advance. Notify the admission clerk of the time of arrival, the patient's condition, and the doctor's expectations. Be prepared to supply all necessary information concerning the patient upon arrival. Be pleasant and cooperative in helping the patient to make the new adjustment. Report to the director of nursing. Offer your credentials, acquaint yourself with the regulations, and proceed as a guest in the new location. Remember that both mandatory law for nursing practice and courtesy require this action. Abide by the rules established for members of the nursing profession in the hospital or agency. Express gratitude for courtesies extended to your patient and to yourself, especially when you prepare to leave.

In a companionship capacity. You may accompany the patient into his own home, and in this instance you will adjust to his environment. It is assumed that you accept this role because you possess professional knowledge that can be utilized should necessity demand it. However, the major portion of your time is expected to be spent in forms of occupational or recreational therapy while in the company of the patient. Your social poise, your pleasant personality, and your understanding manner can contribute to the comfort of the patient as should your contacts with those who comprise his household.

You may also accompany the patient into a place for designated therapy, particularly for recuperation. If you assume these duties, you will be expected to partake in the forms of entertainment supplied for the patient's welfare. As a companion for this type of patient your duties frequently relate to the restoration of spiritual, emotional, mental, or social health rather than of physical health. Therefore, it is up to you to make use of your social knowledge under these circumstances with a proficiency that will reflect credit upon you. This type of experience could help one to develop the characteristics of a good listener and a quiet observer with the manner of a gracious hostess and the eagerness of a confirmed socialite.

BIBLIOGRAPHY

Allison, E. W.: Changing the climate for nursing care, The Journal of Nursing Education **8**:3-5, Aug. 1969.

Bennis, W. G., Benne, K. D., and Chin, R.: The planning of change, New York, 1964, Holt, Rinehart & Winston.

Director of Vocational Counseling Agencies, Washington, D. C., 1969, National Vocational Guidance Association (published annually).

Goldsborough, J. D.: On becoming nonjudgmental, American Journal of Nursing **70**:2340-2343, Nov. 1969.

Moore, M. A.: A point of view on evaluation, Nursing Outlook **16**:55, Jan. 1968.

Olson, E. V.: Education—for what? American Journal of Nursing **70**:1508-1510, July 1970.

Schwier, M. W., and Gardella, F. A.: Planning, orienting, and preparing for a new kind of nurse leadership, Nursing Outlook **18**:42-45, May 1970.

Toward quality in nursing: needs and goals, Washington, D. C., 1963, U. S. Department of Health, Education and Welfare, Government Printing Office.

COMPLETE WORK SHEET ON PP. 341 AND 342

CHAPTER 20

Building for economic security

PERSONAL ECONOMICS

When you begin to plan for your own economic security you are really looking at your ability to earn money and how you can use this earning power to best advantage.

Assuming you will be employed following graduation, let us look at your present capacity for earning money, at the ways in which you will be expected to use money, and at the responsibility you will have for managing money to your economic benefit. In our society a worker receives payment from his employer for performing specified functions or services. The salary paid for each job, as well as other job-associated benefits, depend on many factors; but generally speaking, these wages and benefits should provide the employee with sufficient resources for daily expenses and savings against future needs.

The desire to build for economic security and to plan for the future is inherent in most people who realize the importance of using their earning power efficiently.

Some students have already had experience in handling money. Some have helped to put themselves through school or have contributed to the support of their families. Others who have received an allowance have had some experience in "making ends meet" according to their needs and desires. But all students, regardless of their previous experience in managing money, should seriously consider a plan for the sound management of their personal finances to achieve the dual goal of meeting current needs and saving for the future.

MANAGEMENT OF PERSONAL FINANCES

Throughout your nursing program you have seen the need to budget your time in order that you will have adequate time for study, rest, relaxation, and personal needs. The budgeting of money is similar to the budgeting of time in that it requires you to manage the financial resources you have at hand in order to meet both immediate and future needs.

If you receive an allowance regularly during your nursing program or if you have received a scholarship, you know this money is intended to provide for your needs and wants until the next payment is received. If you receive money on an irregular basis for meeting these needs, you must still develop a plan for spending these amounts.

A budget is a plan for allocating and using money to meet specific purposes. A budget will help you to manage your money effectively and comfortably and will also keep you informed about the amount of money you have at a given time, what you will probably have to spend during a given period of time, and what adjustments must be made to balance income and expenses. In other words, a budget will tell you how much money you have, how much you need, and how you have used the money that you spent.

Budgeting. Let us assume you are interested in developing a budget that will give you an accurate picture of your present financial situation and what you will need to make for present needs and future desires. This decision requires that you take these basic steps: (1) make a determination of your total income, (2) estimate your total expenses, and (3) adjust your expenses to meet your needs within the limits imposed by your income. Of course, in order to do this you must set up an accurate system of record keeping and accounting of income versus expenses in order to figure out your financial status.

Once you have developed a budget you must put it into practice and give it a chance to work. No sample plan or example of budget development can possibly apply to everyone. The budget you prepare as a student will differ from the one you prepare as an employed graduate nurse, but the purpose of a budget remains the same—to make a plan for spending that fits your income and your way of life.

In order to maintain a workable budget, you must know the fixed expenses that must be paid annually, such as insurance premiums, auto licenses, taxes, and professional dues. List the yearly total and the total monthly average of each item. If an amount equal to this monthly average is put aside as savings, you will have

Week of January 1-7

Budget Items	Expenditures	
Health and Personal " "	Jan. 1 Shampoo $.75 Tooth paste .49 Cleansing tissues .75	$1.99
Miscellaneous	Jan. 2 Crossword Puzzle Book (Paper-back)	.53
Recreation	Jan. 3 Bowling Fee	.50
Clothing	Jan. 4 Duty Shoes $12.00 White hose 2.25	14.25
Recreation " " Miscellaneous	Jan. 5 Movies $1.25 Bus fare .30 Snack .75 Stamps (postage) 2.00	4.30
Gift-Contributions	Jan. 6 Mother's Birthday Gift $5.00	5.00
Gift-Contributions	Jan. 7 Church collection $.25	.25
	Total	$26.82

Income-Allowance $12.50 (1/4 of $50.00 Monthly Allowance)

Expenditures 26.82

Amount over/under income $-14.32

A STUDENT'S RECORD OF ONE WEEK'S SPENDING BASED ON A MONTHLY PERSONAL ALLOWANCE OF $50.00.

the money necessary to pay these bills as they come due. The smooth operation of this fund is an important step in effective money management.

Other expenses include such items as rent and housing, installment payments on large items such as appliances or a car, transportation, and tuition fees and books. These commitments may vary in amount or not extend throughout the year, but you should estimate the total and find the average monthly amount. When you subtract the fixed expenses and other commitments from your income, the remaining amount is available for food, clothing, recreation, other miscellaneous expenses, and savings.

Your budget is an incentive to apply self-discipline. Careful accounting for all spending tells you where your money goes. As daily expenses are recorded you will become aware of the need to reorganize or readjust your spending habits so that you can stay within the limits of your income. An accurate spending record

Spending Record January 1971

Budget Plan:	Health and Personal Needs	School Activities and Supplies	Recreation Snacks Fares	Clothing and Upkeep	Miscellaneous	Gifts and Contributions	Savings	
Budget Allocations	$10.00	$7.00	$8.00	$10.00	$7.00	$6.00	$2.00	Total $50.00
Week of January 1-7	1.99	–	2.80	14.25	2.53	5.25	—	
8-14	1.92	2.35	.95	—	4.22	.25	—	
15-21	2.67	1.05	1.05	—	.25	.25	.75	
22-31	1.92	2.60	2.20	—	—	.25	.50	
Total	8.50	6.00	7.00	14.25	7.00	6.00	1.25	$50.00

Monthly Summary

Income (allowance) $50.00

Total Spent 50.00

Amount over/under income 0

SUMMARY OF WEEKLY EXPENDITURES ACCORDING TO BUDGET CATEGORIES AND ALLOCATIONS BASED ON A $50.00 ALLOWANCE PER MONTH.

can identify unnecessary "leaks" that may be eliminated so that the money is available for other purposes. If you reduce your expenses by 10 cents a day for a year, you will save $36.00 for Christmas gifts or other special occasions. Twenty-five cents saved daily for 5 years will mean $500.00 exclusive of the interest that builds up if you deposit it in a savings account.

You can keep track of daily expenditures in an ordinary notebook, lining it to include information for a week at a time on one sheet. You may want to divide each weekly record sheet with a line down the center to list each daily expenditure on one side and the categories you have devised for identifying each expense opposite it as shown in the figure on page 193. Transfer your weekly records of expenditures to a summary sheet, which provides an overview of your financial situation at the end of the month in terms of your income, expenditures, savings and/or deficits (see figure on page 194). At the end of each month transfer the *totals in*

Monthly Spending Record	January		February		March		October		November		December	
	Planned	Spent	Planned	Spent	Planned	Spent	Planned	Spent	Planned	Spent	Planned	Spent
Health and Personal	$10.00	$8.50										
School Supplies School Activities	7.00	6.00										
Recreation Fares Snacks	8.00	7.00										
Clothing and Upkeep	10.00	14.25										
Miscellaneous	7.00	7.00										
Gifts Contributions	6.00	6.00										
Savings	2.00	1.25										
Total	$50.00	$50.00										

A MONTHLY SPENDING RECORD SHOWING THE BUDGETED (PLANNED) ITEMS AND THE AMOUNTS OF MONEY ACTUALLY SPENT IN EACH CATEGORY.

each category to a monthly spending record. This will give you a comparison with last month and the year so far. You can see where you are spending more or where you were able to spend less than you estimated (see figure on page 195). In this way you can adjust your spending plan as you go.

Wise spending. When you begin earning your own salary you should have a clear understanding of the difference between gross pay and take home pay, so that when you are considering a budget plan, you can immediately mark off the amount of salary that you will never actually see. This will include amounts withheld for various federal taxes, possibly state and local taxes, insurance plans, and credit union obligations. The remainder is yours to spend as you wish. It is the income on which your budget plan is established.

Your salary should, of course, be used wisely, and you should continue the good practices of money management established during your student days so that earnings meet both current commitments and long range goals. The following figures are suggested allocations for expenses that may be helpful when you plan your budget, although naturally your personal circumstances may mean that alterations are in order. The following is a suggested distribution of a salary check.

Items	*Suggested percentage*	*Your plans*	
Housing (not to exceed 25%)	15 to 25	__%	$______
Food	20 to 30	__	______
Clothing	10 to 20	__	______
Operating expenses (laundry, utilities, transportation)	15 to 20	__	______
Savings	5 to 20	__	______

Everyone should pay some attention to information about the cost of living. It is reported monthly in the press and on television and radio. Detailed information is also available through the United States Bureau of Labor Statistics. When the Consumer Price Index shows either an increase or a decrease in the cost of goods and services, such information may serve as an indication to either postpone nonessential purchases and conserve savings, or to plan on buying an essential item before its price is increased.

Each month you should compare the amount of money spent with the amount set aside for each category in your overall budget. By keeping records for several months and evaluating them in terms of the goals set forth in your budget, you can make adjustments to achieve more efficient personal economics or to adjust the amounts of money necessary for a realistic budget plan. When you start a budget, stick with it. Evaluate it carefully each month and learn to anticipate certain types of expenditures. Prepare for these expenses while adjusting the allocation of your money to your benefit. Remember that you don't cheat a budget—only yourself.

Housing. Deciding whether to live at home and contribute to your family's general maintenance or to rent a room or an apartment must be your own decision, but you should remember that budgeting allotments for shelter, including garage rental and home furnishings, should not exceed one-fourth of your monthly income. When housing plans involve sharing expenses with others, it is suggested that a clear understanding be established beforehand about the plan for dividing financial responsibility among the parties concerned and evidences of its acceptance as a mutual obligation.

Food. The money budgeted for food should provide for purchase of the following:

1. Lean meats, fish, poultry, and eggs
2. Milk and cheese
3. Bread, flour, cereals
4. Fats, sugars, accessory seasonings
5. Fruits and vegetables

Caution should be used in spending money budgeted for food on gourmet items or snacks and other things used in the entertainment of guests. It is preferable to include these items in your budget for recreation expenses.

For most effective usage of your food dollars you can:

1. Plan meals beforehand to avoid unnecessary purchases and possible waste.
2. Compare prices and patronize shops where values are obtained.

3. Watch for sales for staples, canned goods, and foods used in quantities that can be satisfactorily stored until used.
4. Select your own fruits and vegetables.
5. Purchase fresh foods in season in amounts that eliminate spoilage before use.
6. Learn to prepare and serve appetizing left-overs for some meals.

Clothing. An adequate and well-cared-for wardrobe is an essential requirement for all who work and are otherwise active in today's world. Acquiring a suitable wardrobe takes time and money, so it is necessary to use care in selecting each item. The following suggestions may be helpful as you plan your clothing budget:

1. Buy quality materials in styles and colors that you will not tire of through repeated wearing.
2. Dress to make the most of your attractive features.
3. Use accessories that complement your basic outfits and keep abreast of fashion.
4. Know the better shops in your community that offer clothes that suit you.
5. Watch for sales. Add scarves and other small accessory items to your wardrobe at minimum cost.
6. Avoid buying sale items on impulse. If it doesn't meet your needs, the purchase is no bargain.
7. Take care of your wardrobe. Keep articles mended and cleaned. Patronize a reliable dry cleaner.
8. From time to time take inventory of your wants and your needs. Plan ahead for major clothing you intend to buy, such as a winter coat.

Operating expenses. Your daily expenses include such items as laundry and housekeeping services, telephone, babysitting fees, and transportation fares or the costs of maintaining and servicing a car. Costs for any of these items should be identified within your budget and carefully reviewed to determine if each item is serving its intended purpose. In meeting your automobile expenses, you may have to decrease the mileage you drive, to drive more carefully, and, in some instances, to rediscover the joys of walking.

Recreation and vacations. The change of pace provided by rest and recreation is a necessary part of your life. Doing something that is different from your daily routine is important if you are to maintain a balance in your point of view, but recreational activities may require careful planning if your desires involve expenditures of money that comes out of a budget. Diversion and rest from a routine should be planned within each day's assignments as well as within your weekly schedule, but the type of recreation pursued and its cost should be faced realistically.

Free or relatively inexpensive recreation, such as a day in the country, a visit to an art gallery, or a trip to the beach serve the purpose of change. These inexpensive outings allow you to save for a special treat such as a play, a shopping expedition, or a skiing weekend with friends. It is easy to spend more money than you intended on recreation if you do not establish limits. Discipline in spending is an individual responsibility, and nowhere in your budget plan is there greater need for more careful supervision than in recreation.

Vacations are a special kind of recreation because they usually involve a distinct change in your style of living for a period of at least one week each year. Planning ahead for an annual vacation and saving a definite amount of money for it each month is the best way to ensure this treat. A vacation need not be expensive to be enjoyable, but if you plan to see new places and meet new friends, you must make a financial outlay. Items such as vacation clothes, luggage, hotel accommodations, and transportation need to be kept in mind as extra items apart from those included in your usual monthly budget categories. It is much better to tailor vacation plans to the money available and make up your mind to enjoy a vacation that stays within your budget than to succumb to the salesmanship that encourages "playing now and paying later."

Debts and loans. A debt is usually a sum of money owed by one person to another. A loan in terms of economics refers to a sum of money given to one person (debtor) for a specified period of time to be repaid (to the lender) with interest. When a person obtains a loan he becomes indebted to the lender and is responsible for abiding by the specific obligations agreed upon for repayment.

Anyone may face circumstances that require a sum of money that can be obtained only by taking out a loan. A prospective borrower's chances for obtaining a loan are enhanced if he has a good employment record, a good credit rating, and, depending on the amount of the loan, the legal collateral he needs to provide assurance that the loan will be repaid according to the terms.

Some hospitals or health care agencies have funds available for loan to employees, or a credit union may serve as a resource for the convenience of qualified personnel who need loans. These services are usually described to employees during their pre-employment interview. Other sources of financial aid include commercial banks, mortgage companies (if the prospective borrower owns property), and life insurance companies (for holders of certain types of policies).

A bank will check on a borrower's credit ratings and personal references. It will also expect assurance that repayments will be made in accordance with the contract signed by the borrower and his co-signer, if one is required. Finance companies exact high rates of interest for money they lend. They do not investigate as extensively as banks, but because these companies are in business to make a profit, the borrower pays more for the use of funds.

If you are considering borrowing a large sum of money, you should be sure to obtain accurate information about interest rates, carrying charges, and other costs in effect on various types of loans. You should also know the time plan for repayment, and should investigate to discover the best sources of loans for specific purposes. Whether the type of loan repayment is based on discount or on installment repayments, you should remember that you pay the stated rate of interest on the total amount borrowed for the period of time for which the loan is made, even though the principal is reduced by regular monthly payments.

In spite of printed advertisements and radio and television commercials urging the public to "buy now and pay on easy credit terms," this service is often more expensive than it is worth. *There is no such thing as easy credit when it is associated with repayment of a financial obligation.* If you plan to borrow money you should carefully consider the "work insurance" that will necessarily accompany it. "Work insurance" means the requirement that you place on yourself to continue working over a period of time in order to pay back the money you borrowed plus the interest. Again, evaluate the object you plan to buy against the debt you are assuming. If the happiness you expect to derive from your borrowing overbalances the interest you will pay, you have convinced yourself that you are wise to assume this obligation.

Educational grants and loans. Today there are many scholarships, grants-in-aid, and loan funds. Nursing students are especially fortunate, because national, state, and private agencies concerned with the state of health care have made a broad range of financial assistance available. Inquiries about these resources and the qualifications required of applicants can generally be directed to high school guidance counselors, deans or directors of financial aid in colleges and universities, directors of diploma and practical nurse programs conducted in hospitals, or to the Committee on Careers, National League for Nursing, 10 Columbus Circle, New York, N. Y. 10019.

We mention these kinds of financial resources at this point in order to emphasize the importance of taking full advantage of the educational opportunities that such resources make available, and also to stress the importance of repaying grants and loans in strict accordance with the terms agreed upon when the aid was offered to you.

If you have received a grant or a loan that has enabled you to become a nursing student, you have a good idea of just what this assistance means to you in allowing you to pursue your chosen career. When it is time to repay this money, think of those who will follow in your footsteps as nursing students. Remember how important this assistance has been to you, and repay these funds so that future students will have this same opportunity.

Credit ratings and charge accounts. Credit rating refers generally to the status of a person's finances and the method used for keeping money available for use, such as savings deposits in a bank. It also refers to the manner in which a person plans to meet financial obligations when they are due. Your ability to obtain credit is based on your financial assets (capital), your ability to pay your debts and meet other responsibilities from your current income (capacity), evidences of your former payment habits (character), and what you might offer as security (collateral). We mentioned earlier that your credit rating is checked when an application is made for a bank loan. It is also checked by stores and other business establishments when you apply for a charge account. A credit rating indicates your ability to plan and save, and it furnishes to members of the Retail Credit Association information on how you meet obligations of paying for services or goods purchased on credit or through the use of charge accounts. The credit rating you establish follows you wherever you go. A sound credit rating can be one of your most valuable personal possessions.

The use of credit is important in our national economy. Industries are built, governments maintained, and business ventures established and operated on credit ratings. This means that those involved give evidence that they are capable of meeting their obligations when their creditors expect payment. In a more personal sense you use credit in the form of checks drawn against money deposited in a checking account and in your use of charge accounts, which may also draw payments monthly from money deposited in your bank account. However, you must exercise caution and common sense in using credit, either through checks or charge accounts, so that these remain a convenience and do not become a trap.

There are so many kinds of credit plans available that sometimes even experienced shoppers become confused. For example, you will find that you can pay for purchases through such diverse methods as credit cards, check credit plans, installment sales, or a revolving account. It is up to you to make certain that the different types of payment plans are explained in detail, so that if you wish to make a purchase on credit, you can select the plan that is best for you. Certainly you want to avoid paying for expensive items with long-term payments because the purchase was made to appear painless through the use of "easy credit."

Remember that charged purchases for which you must pay over a stated period of time will cost more than the original purchase price. This cost may be called a service charge, interest, carrying cost, or finance charge, and it is often more than you may realize. It may be calculated as a percentage return on the balance owed after the down payment. Additional fees may also be included in this cost. The cost is added to the original amount of the article prior to deciding on the amount of the monthly repayments for the period during which credit charges are in effect. The following is an example of this application:

Television set	Cash price	$400.00
	Down payment	75.00
	Balance owed	325.00
	Finance charge or dollar cost of credit	32.50
	Total	357.50
Monthly payments	(12): 11 of $29.79, 1 of $29.81	
	Plus down payment	75.00
	Total amount paid using credit	$432.50

In the example above, the finance charge (10% of the balance owed after down payment) represents the dollar cost of credit. Finance companies and businesses that extend credit use a formula to determine the amount of true annual interest paid for use of credit. Over a twelve-month period this interest is estimated at 18%.

There are times when credit buying is indicated and payment for the service is worth the use of the item purchased, since it will provide benefits lasting beyond the termination of payments. The decision is yours. When you plan to buy on credit you may wish to take the following steps to reduce the finance charges: (1) make the down payment as large as possible, (2) borrow the smallest amount of money possible, and (3) pay off the contract within the specified time period.

Wise use of credit privileges requires that you manage your money to meet payments when they are due. It requires knowledge about the kinds of credit plans available and the amount of credit to seek. It requires an understanding of the terms of any contract you are asked to sign. In some instances an awareness of how credit usage is applied will cause you to have second thoughts about whether the purchase merits use of your credit, whether it is better to pay cash, or whether it is advisable to postpone making the purchase for the time being.

Savings. The emergencies in your life that call for financial aid may vary from an illness in your family, an opportunity to take an unplanned trip, or an economic slump that requires revised living plans. Generally, it is wise to have savings equal to at least one month's salary for immediate use in case of any emergency. To supply this economic security, savings accounts should be considered.

General savings accounts. General savings accounts are usually established with a bank or a savings and loan association. Even a small amount of money deposited each month builds economic security. Small amounts consistently saved accumulate more rapidly than you realize, and there is the added advantage of interest being entered on the account at regular intervals. This method of planning provides a source of ready cash that can be withdrawn for use in case of necessity. The establishment and maintenance of a savings account also help to reinforce your credit rating.

The important thing about saving is to get started. You should deposit a definite amount in a savings account each month, increasing the amount as your earnings increase. The earlier you start the saving habit, the better are the chances to gain advantage of interest earned and added to the principal. If, for example, you set aside $10.00 a month in a savings account for twenty years, the principal of $2,400.00, plus the compounded interest, could bring your total savings to $3,877.00. If you saved $20.00 a month for 10 years, the principal would be the same, but the accumulated interest would total $3,028.00. By starting the savings habit early the same amount of total principal would have earned an additional sum of $849.00.

Special savings accounts. These savings may revolve about a variety of patterns such as Christmas club or vacation fund saving, Government Savings Bonds, or investments in a credit union.

Club or special fund savings. This type of savings account usually takes care of particular events that occur annually and provides money for definite expenses such as Christmas presents or vacations. These special accounts can be established at most banks or savings and loan associations. Any cashier or officer of the financial institution will be glad to explain the plan in effect for this purpose.

Definite amounts are deposited for each week or month, ranging from one dollar to several dollars for approximately a year. Deposits may be made weekly, monthly, or annually, but they are not available for withdrawal prior to a given date. When that time is due, a check is sent to the depositor for the amount and the savings fund is closed for that year. Usually the establishment of another club fund is encouraged by the bank for the coming year.

Government Savings Bonds. This is a safe form of saving, since the bonds are backed by the federal government. They are obtained in either series E or H. E bonds are available in smaller denominations (less than $100.00); H bonds are used for investments of $500.00 or more. Bonds may be obtained directly from a local bank or through a payroll savings plan. They have a relatively high rate of interest and can be cashed before maturity if necessary. The price paid for a Series E bond is 75% of its maturity value, so that a bond yielding $25.00 at maturity costs $18.75; a $50.00 bond costs $37.50 and a $100 bond is purchased for $75.00. Series E bonds are best suited to long-range savings plans. They are dated to begin bearing interest from the first day of the month in which payment is received by the issuing agent. They may be held jointly by two or more persons with right of survivorship, so that if one account holder dies or becomes disabled, the funds are available to the others.

Credit union membership. Some hospitals, health agencies, industries, and school departments have established credit unions for the benefit of their members. Those eligible may deposit a definite amount monthly in the union's savings plan. Should a need arise to borrow money, one may do so from the credit union. If the privilege of credit union membership is yours, it would be worth your while to investigate the plans developed for saving and/or borrowing money under its sponsorship.

Investments. Additional ways to build up savings may be through investing part of your income in stocks, bonds, mutual funds, or by purchasing real estate. However, these particular methods for putting your money to work should not be used by the beginning wage earner. In fact, experts in investment fields agree that these kinds of investments should not be used until a reserve fund has been built up in a savings account to take care of living expenses for several months and life insurance protection has been obtained.

A potential investor in stocks, bonds, and mutual funds should first seek out a responsible securities broker and obtain the information and advice on the objectives that can be achieved through these particular kinds of investments. For example, it is necessary to understand the differences between issues of common stock and preferred stock, growth stocks and income stocks, and to have some basic knowledge about the different types of bonds and mutual funds available as investments. A securities broker can offer assistance and guidance tailored to individual resources and expectations for returns on an investment. He can also explain how to figure out the income taxes levied on dividends and the methods of reporting capital gains and profits from the sale of stock or similar holdings.

An investment in real estate, particularly a home—is something almost everyone considers during their earning years. Ownership of your own home can provide many personal satisfactions in addition to being an investment. A well maintained home in a desirable neighborhood usually increases in value. However, monthly mortgage payments, interest payments, and taxes are part of the upkeep expenses to be included in a monthly budget.

Because the purchase of a home usually represents the largest single investment a person makes in a lifetime, it merits careful consideration. This investment of savings and earnings should be based on an examination of all facts relative to your financial status, with assistance, as needed, from qualified people whose objective advice contributes to the final decision.

Insurance. The general state of the economy in the United States is better today than it has ever been. At the same time, costs of living are higher and larger sums are required to obtain both necessities and luxury items. Suppose you have $1,000.00 in your savings bank account. At today's prices, how far would this money go in paying for a prolonged illness, an extensive emergency, or in providing for your needs after you stop working?

To prepare for these types of emergencies, most people establish and maintain an insurance protection program soon after becoming wage earners to provide for meeting circumstances that may develop in the course of everyday living. In one sense insurance is a type of social security. It provides the basic protection associated with health insurance; it is a way of assuring an income for dependents; it provides for protection of property against fire, theft, and other losses; it protects you from liability for injury to others or liability for damages to their property; and, after death of the insured, it provides essential financial assistance to meet final expenses.

Because of many varieties of insurance coverage that are available, it is helpful to consult an insurance specialist for advice in determining the kinds of insurance programs that will meet your own particular insurance needs. It is also recommended that you ask your insurance representative to explain the distinction between such classifications as ordinary life insurance, term insurance, limited payment life, casualty insurance, health insurance, endowment, and retirement and annuity income plans. With an understanding of the benefits these types of plans provide and knowledge of your financial obligations, it is reasonable to assume that you will choose the best type of economic security.

Because you are a nurse, your insurance program should also include protection against lawsuits for malpractice. In Chapter 17 the legal aspects of clinical practice were presented as a special topic. You should be fully aware of the legal responsibilities that you have in acting within the framework of instruction and the practice of your professional role. Doubtless your instructors have discussed and demonstrated, by their example, the practicing nurse's legal obligations. Specific information about malpractice insurance is available from state nurses' association offices. Request information about this type of security when you apply for district and state membership in your official nursing organization after you receive your license to practice.

Taxes. You will be required to pay federal income taxes, and perhaps state and city taxes. In addition, most wage earners must pay Social Security taxes.

Federal income taxes. Every person in this country whose gross income during the calendar year is $600.00 or more is required to file a federal income tax form. As an employee you may authorize your employer to withhold stated amounts from each salary check you receive. These amounts are applied against the tax you will have to pay at the end of the year. Your employer will give you duplicate records (W-2 forms) of these withheld amounts covering the previous year's employment. If this tax is not withheld from your salary, you must plan to pay the entire amount in one lump sum. Any additional income you receive during the year from other sources in excess of $10.00 will also be recorded on W-2 forms by the agency issuing the money. This form states that the Department of Internal Revenue has been informed of the amounts paid to you. When you file your income tax return, one copy of each W-2 form received should be attached to your return; you retain the other copy for your files.

Those with annual incomes of less than $10,000 may use the "short" form (1040A) to report their federal taxes. The "long" form (1040) is used to show a person's salary, investments, and other monies, which yield a return of $10,000.00 or more. The form also provides for reporting of donations, refundable expenses, and other information the government requires. Receipts or other acceptable records verifying deductions must be available and they should be kept with the tax report copy for future reference. Detailed instructions are included with tax forms each year and the staff members of local Internal Revenue offices are available to answer questions or clarify the meaning of the statements. Information about deductions allowed to members of the nursing profession is also reported in nursing publications, or it may be obtained by consulting an attorney or a reliable accountant.

State and city taxes. The state and sometimes the city in which you live or work may levy special taxes. Since you are earning your living within a definite locale you are expected to contribute to the area's services and needs by paying the tax authorized by law. As a member of a profession and as a member of the community, you are expected to know about these taxes. The amounts you are to pay are based on your income and will be indicated on the reports to be filed with the state and/or city in accordance with stated regulations.

Social Security. Old-age and survivor's insurance was created in 1937 when the Social Security Act became effective. Under this act employer-employee plans were established, which provided for the employee's retirement at 65 years of age. However, few nurses were eligible for benefits under this act. Subsequently, the American Nurses' Association made provisions for the development of an Economic Security Program for nurses and recommended that more nurses be made eligible for Social Security benefits. In August 1950, a bill known as the Social Security Amendments Act was signed into law by President Truman. This law gave nurses self-employed in private practice or employed in state and nonprofit institutions the opportunity to benefit from old-age and survivor's insurance.

Social Security provides an income based on the amount of money received from the worker during his working years. Social Security benefits may also be paid to the family of the wage earner following his death. Everyone who works must have a Social Security card and number, which may be obtained from the Social Security office in your community. Your Social Security number is assigned for your exclusive use and must be indicated on tax returns, memberships in professional organizations, applications for employment, and various other records.

If you are classified as an employee, you and your employer share the cost of Social Security and both are taxed equally. Your tax contribution is deducted from your salary check each pay day and matched with funds paid by your employer. If you are a self-employed (for example, a private practice nurse) with net earnings of $400.00 or more a year, you pay the entire tax yourself (7.5% on earnings up to $7,500). The tax for Social Security is payable when you file your federal income tax return.

Because new laws pertaining to elderly persons and survivors are constantly being enacted, it is not possible to include current information here. Therefore, it is wise to check with the Social Security Administration or the personnel director at your place of work for up-to-date information about how Social Security regulations affect you as an employee.

Social Security alone does not provide absolute financial security, nor will it offer the financial independence in retirement you may desire. You need to make additional plans during your working years to provide for an adequate retirement allowance that can cover expenses incurred during illness, hospitalization, or disability in order to ensure more complete security during this period of your life.

Care of valuable papers and documents. Your personal papers and documents are of great importance, and you should become familiar with their contents and organize them and keep them safely. Such a procedure makes it possible to know what is available for use in an emergency and what resources are to be used when help is needed.

Ask yourself the following questions: Could I immediately obtain facts about my personal affairs or legal matters in case of an emergency? Are papers and documents I consider valuable readily available to other members of the family? Do I know the content of the various papers I have? Have I made a will? Have I indicated clearly the names, addresses, and phone numbers of those people who are familiar with my goals and wishes? Hopefully, as you develop plans for your chosen career and for your personal life you can answer these questions in the affirmative. If you are married, you and your spouse share the responsibility for safeguarding essential documents so that you both know the contents of these documents and where they are kept.

Papers should be checked periodically so that you can be certain that they are current and complete. You should also prepare a summary including the most important information about them. They should be assembled and filed under appropriate headings to include personal, insurance, real estate, and contracts, investments, benefits, debts, and so on, and then stored where they are accessible and safe.

Summary record booklets are available to help you in listing essential information. Many banks and insurance companies issue such booklets to their clients, or they may be purchased at certain stationery supply stores. The important thing is that you take the time to assemble such information and make any necessary revisions to keep this information as current and clear as possible for those who might need it in case of emergency.

We hope that your efforts to build for your economic security can succeed in making your dreams a reality, so that you achieve the goals which you establish. Through persistent and systematic planning, wise spending and savings, you can experience many satisfactions and the happiness that comes from knowing you met your responsibilities and have provided for your own financial independence.

BIBLIOGRAPHY

Building a second income (pamphlet), Francis I. duPont & Co.

Hathaway, B. H.: Your life insurance, Garden City, N. Y., 1962, Doubleday & Co., Inc.

How to live on your income, Pleasantville, N. Y., 1970, The Reader's Digest Assn. Inc.

Novatny, M.: Your money to manage, to spend, to invest, to protect, Davis, California, 1964-1965, University of California, Agricultural Extension Service, (four booklets: Make your money count; Use credit wisely; Building financial security; Your valuable family papers).

Proven and practical ways to handle money better, Changing Times, the Kiplinger Magazine **24**:25-29, July 1970.

U. S. Department of Health, Education and Welfare: Your Social Security, Washington, D. C., The Department.

Understanding the modern securities market, New York, 1967, Walston & Co., Inc.

COMPLETE WORK SHEET ON PP. 343 TO 345

CHAPTER 21

Keeping up to date

SOCIAL AND PROFESSIONAL RESPONSIBILITY

You have been told by many people the importance of preparing properly to assume your place in society. As a citizen and nurse your role and responsibilities are, and will continue to be, vital, but no one can foresee the specific part you will play in the drama of life. However, there is one universal constant which all are destined to experience—change. Resistance to change is common to most people, but there have always been some who have dedicated their lives to change through research. The great difference between the scientific, technical, and social developments since 1950 and those of preceding centuries lies in the speed of change. The rate is so rapid that discoveries of today become obsolete tomorrow. What will be the implications of change for nursing during each year that you practice? No one can prophesy exactly what will happen, but nursing practice must keep pace with the changing world. Nursing has always reflected its social setting and has been subject to the pressures exerted by social, technical, and scientific developments. This will and must continue.

How can you prevent professional stasis? How will you remain a contributing citizen? One suggested method of accomplishing this objective is to become a lifetime learner—a person interested in self-development. Quality patient care is your goal, and to administer this kind of care requires an awareness of the needs of your patient—both those needs that are specifically his and those he shares with his peers. The public considers each nurse to be an expert. The term "expert" implies competency and the ability to provide the highest caliber of nursing care. A competent nurse utilizes all related knowledge and skill for her patients' benefit. To consistently administer quality patient care is a monumental task requiring the nurse to conscientiously keep pace with changing nursing practice.

As Alexander Pope, eighteenth century English poet, said in his *Essay on Criticism*:

> A little learning is a dangerous thing;
> Drink deep, or taste not the Pierian spring;
> There shallow draughts intoxicate the brain,
> And drinking largely sobers us again.

A contributing member of the nursing profession never ceases being a student. To meet the needs of the society in which you live, you must add both depth and breadth to the knowledge you have already acquired. In psychology you learned that one of the most prolific sources for learning is the learner himself. To achieve fulfillment of this continued learning it is important to establish a program of self-enrichment and continuing self-improvement.

MEANING OF A CULTURED PERSON

Culture is defined in many ways. Sociologically this term refers to the way of life characteristic of any society comprised of a homogeneous group of human beings. The word "culture" also implies breeding or refined taste acquired by esthetic and intellectual training. This personal refinement is accompanied by characteristics such as fine feelings, good taste, polished manners, and consistently correct behavior, which are the result of contact with the very best offered by society.

A cultured person is one who utilizes every available opportunity to acquire this sensitivity, taste, and social awareness, which in turn enhances his understanding, empathy, and sympathy for the people who inhabit his world. A cultured person seeks knowledge with the same energy and urgency that he uses to gratify any other hunger. He has the ability to identify his reactions to art, literature, or music, and the discrimination to select those stimuli most meaningful to him. Since art forms reflect a specific historical period (either the time developed or the time depicted), they offer important clues concerning the people for whom or about whom the picture was painted, the book was written, or the music was composed.

The above is not new to you, but we do recommend that you continue to utilize the resources available in your community for continued self-improvement, such as art museums, the theater, concerts, and libraries. Contacts such as these will enhance your understanding of the world in which you live (including its sociologic and psychologic implications) and assist you in gaining variety in self-expression, becoming a more interesting person, and realizing your potential.

THE ROLE OF BOOKS IN PERSONAL DEVELOPMENT

Francis Bacon, in his *Essays on Studies,* says that "Some books are to be tested, others to be swallowed, and some few to be chewed and digested." Whether these books are tomes, texts, or ones written for the sheer pleasure of reading, it is expected that some of each classification have already been an integral part of your life. One facet of your self-enrichment program will depend, in part, on whether you continue to spend enjoyable hours in the world of books.

When reading for pleasure, begin with books that interest you the most. You can select books that motivate you to read more and more about more and more. If your interest lies in historical novels, biographies, or autobiographies there is a wide variety and a large number from which to make your selections. Both history and biography help you to learn about people. These books help you to understand how people thought and lived in other periods. As you read, ask yourself such questions as, "What message is the author trying to convey?" "What was happening in the world at the time this story took place?"

You may find more pleasure in so-called escape literature: books of science fiction, mysteries, or success stories. Selection of these kind of books is often based upon a reader's liking for a particular author's writing style, or identification with the main character depicted, or upon being stimulated to read for further information on a particular topic. Aside from gaining satisfaction from reading, your appetite will be likely to increase for learning and lead you to become familiar with even more books. When you read and *think* about what you read, your appreciation of your own world is likely to deepen.

As a lifetime learner, it is imperative that you keep informed. Each year new and excellent nursing texts are published, but it is impossible for you to read them all. It is possible, however, for you to select those texts that hold special interest for you. Reviews of current texts can be found in each issue of nursing publications. The Educational Services Division of the American Journal of Nursing Company is currently publishing a series of paperback books on contemporary nursing practice. The first issue titled *The Clinical Nursing Specialist* appeared in November 1970, and contains selected articles relating to the book titles which were first published in the American Journal of Nursing Company's publications. These publications should assist you in keeping pace with current nursing practice.

OFFICIAL PUBLICATIONS OF THE NURSING PROFESSION

Of inestimable value to the nurse wishing to keep well-informed and well-qualified are the many professional journals. We assume that you are already familiar with many of them, and have probably found it valuable to subscribe to some of those that relate to nursing and the nursing profession. The American Journal of Nursing Company publishes the *American Journal of Nursing, Nursing Outlook,* and *Nursing Research.* The company is owned by the American Nurses' Association.

The *American Journal of Nursing,* the first official journal for nurses, began its publication in 1900. The story of the development of the company and its journal may be found in its publication, "The Story of the Journal—1900-1960." The *American Journal of Nursing* is the official publication of both the American Nurses' Association and the National Student Nurses' Association. Editorial content and articles promote and attempt to clarify purposes, programs, and developments within the nursing profession. The *Journal* offers clinical material valuable to all nurses and contains information concerning national and international health care, current events, new publications, and indications of "things to come." Each issue features the "Student's Page" and information of general interest to students. Twice a year the *Journal* publishes the names and addresses of nursing and related organizations, and the list of approved registries of state nurses associations' districts. Annually it publishes a cumulative index, and every five years a cumulative index is also published. Each monthly issue includes classified listings of employment opportunities available in nursing practice.

Nursing Outlook, published monthly by the American Journal of Nursing Company, is the official journal of the National League for Nursing. Prior to January, 1953, the *American Journal of Nursing* served as the official publication for the National League of Nursing Education while *Public Health Nursing* was the official journal of the National Organization of Public Health Nursing. When the first issue of *Nursing Outlook* was published in January 1953, it became the official journal of the National League for Nursing into which both former organizations were consolidated at the official convention of the national nursing organizations in June, 1952.

Nursing Outlook promotes the organization's programs and contains articles of interest to public health and occupational health nurses, material stressing methods for improving nursing skills generally, articles and reports of concern to all nursing education programs, and classified information regarding opportunities for employment. Each year three of the monthly issues of *Nursing Outlook* include an official directory of nursing and health organizations, nursing education programs accredited by the NLN, and an annual index.

Nursing Research did not begin as an official journal. Originally it was sponsored by the Association of Collegiate Schools of Nursing, which, with another organization, merged to form the National League for Nursing in 1952.

Nursing Research, first published in June 1952, is now co-sponsored by the National League for Nursing and the American Nurses' Association. It is a quarterly publication devoted to research related to the profession and includes many valuable abstracts of studies in nursing and allied fields. Included also are reports and articles intended to inform members of the nursing profession of scientific studies being conducted and to stimulate continued interest in research in nursing.

There are many other nursing publications, which you should find valuable. Your own state nurses' association publication will supply you with data concerning your immediate professional activities. You are urged to acquaint yourself with the content of these resources, since they serve your regional area and state and enable you to give better service to your community and state.

The International Nursing Review is the official journal of the International Council of Nurses. It is published six times yearly. Articles are written in English, German, and Spanish. Content concentrates on nursing practice throughout the world and the journal is read by nurses in many countries. Reading and studying this publication is recommended as one way you can broaden your scope of nursing knowledge and your understanding of the universality of nursing needs.

In addition to official publications there are

others dedicated to the general welfare of nurses, nursing preparation and practice.

The Journal of Nursing Education is published by the Blakiston Division of the McGraw-Hill Book Company, Inc. The first issue was published in January 1962. It is issued to nurse educators and to school of nursing libraries free of charge. *The Journal of Nursing Education* emphasizes changing trends in nursing education. It serves as an excellent sounding board for ideas and for the presentation of useful information concerning teaching trends and methods. This publication attempts to stimulate ideas, revisions, experimentation, and evaluation by personnel in nursing education toward improving the caliber of nursing education and preparing better nurse practitioners.

Nursing Forum is published quarterly by Nursing Publications, Incorporated. It was introduced in January 1962. Its primary purpose is to promote more creative nursing skills and techniques in the cause of better patient care. The magazine is not affiliated with a national nursing organization.

RN is a monthly magazine. It has a wide circulation and contains information of interest generally to nurses in areas of both professional and technical practice. It is published by Medical Economics, Inc., and is available to any registered or licensed nurse.

OTHER PROFESSIONAL JOURNALS AND PERIODICALS

Libraries in hospitals and schools of nursing contain many other publications that can serve to enrich your background of knowledge. Listed below are a few of these resources.

Two publications that will aid nurses in meeting the psychologic and emotional needs of patients with physical problems, as well as the needs of patients with psychiatric problems are the *Journal of Psychiatric Nursing and Mental Health Services* and *Perspectives in Psychiatric Nursing*. The *Journal* includes original and stimulating articles written by authorities in all areas of psychiatric practice. *Perspectives in Psychiatric Nursing* is prepared primarily for those who administer care to the mentally ill. Nursing leaders in the field of psychiatric nursing serve on the editorial board. Utilization of mental health principles can aid the nurse serving in an intensive care unit, coronary care unit, or a medical or surgical unit to meet the traumatic situations that may arise for a patient during both the acute and convalescent phases of his illness.

World Health, the magazine of the World Health Organization with headquarters in Geneva, Switzerland, contains articles and information concerning health conditions throughout the world. Special issues are often devoted to specific phases of international health care and include the identification of the role and responsibilities of the nurse in a participating capacity.

Another excellent resource is *Facts About Nursing*, an annual publication of the Research and Statistics Department of the American Nurses' Association. This book includes in statistical summary information such as the education, preparation, and distribution of registered and practical nurses; the economic status of registered nurses; data on related health information; and functions and purposes of nursing organizations. Several pharmaceutical houses also supply up-to-date materials concerning diseases, medications, and treatments. For one's professional development this information may prove extremely valuable, and the illustrations included also help to clarify the discussion of the topic.

Newspapers, popular and news magazines, television programs, and radio offer information for you to evaluate, accept, or reject. It is hoped that you will not be influenced by incomplete, inaccurate or slanted information. You are charged with the responsibility to cultivate your thinking ability so that you may be able to select authentic information and formulate views which contribute positively toward the development of your scientific background as a nurse and your personal happiness as an individual. Formulate your own conclusions and opinions only after you have given careful consideration to the pros and cons of the ideas of others. Pride yourself on being among the twenty-five percent of the people who appreciate what they read and prepare to use it along life's way. Continue to strengthen your foundations of nursing and to fortify your purposes in living by continuously seeking knowledge from the wealth of information available.

CONTINUING EDUCATION

As health care improves nursing practice becomes more complex. The increased patient load, emphasis on prevention, and the addition of intensive care, coronary care, mental health, rehabilitation, and extended care units require nurses to learn and apply new skills. The American way of life, with expectations for improving the health status of the nation, encourages all nurses to participate in continuing education. A basic education only forms the foundation on which the nurse can grow and develop.

Quality nursing care requires that each nurse keep up with current health practices. Many sources of continuing education are available to you. Among these are in-service education, workshops, institutes, extension courses in colleges and universities, and enrollment in a college for a baccalaureate or advanced degree (see Chapter 24).

In-service education in the institution in which you are employed apprises you of the procedures and policies of that organization. Education in-service is directed toward keeping nurse employees aware of changes and, hopefully, skilled in the use of new techniques so that patients will receive the benefit of these improvements.

Workshops and institutes on nursing skills, knowledge, and its implementation are conducted usually by national, state, and local nursing organizations and allied organizations such as colleges or universities. The dates on which these programs are offered and an application for enrollment will be available through the publication of the sponsoring group. There are so many programs offered that nurses can usually find a workshop or institute that will benefit them in their nursing practice. Attending is not enough, however. It is necessary to practice and apply what you have learned, to evaluate what you have gained from participation, to share this knowledge with co-workers and to adapt this new learning to the improvement of nursing in your institution. Your education at the basic level does not automatically prepare you for acceptance of leadership roles, but potential leadership qualities will be evident to your superiors through your participation and utilization of the information gleaned through continuing education.

Still another facet of continuing education is enrollment in courses offered through extension in universities and colleges. Through such courses you may further develop latent interests in areas other than nursing. Some courses offered through extension can be taken for transferable college credit. Since this aspect of your self-development program can hold great promise for you, you should not misuse this opportunity if it is available to you. The courses offered on an extension basis are varied, thus offering you specific opportunity for broadening your personal and professional horizons. Many universities offer short term courses also, which are intended to enrich your background of professional knowledge and your ability to strengthen and deepen your skills in nursing practice.

Last, but certainly not least, is the continuing of your education to earn either a baccalaureate or higher degree. Select your university or senior college carefully with an eye to whether you will be offered the opportunity to pursue your desired major field of study, and whether you will qualify for admission.

To become a leader in nursing, you must diligently persevere until you have acquired the knowledge and skill commensurate with the position you desire. Then you must continue to follow a path of self-development and self-enrichment.

Pursue one of the suggested paths for continuing as a lifetime learner. By adopting the methods or ideas presented in this chapter, it is possible for you to prevent becoming professionally static. You will continue to function as a contributing member of the society in which you live.

BIBLIOGRAPHY

Abdellah, F., and Levine, E.: Better patient care through nursing research, New York, 1965, The Macmillan Co.

Alford, H. J.: Continuing education in action, W. K. Kellogg Foundation, New York, 1968, John Wiley & Sons, Inc.

Avenues for continued learning, New York, 1967, American Nurses' Association.

Editorial: The cultural lag in nursing, Nursing Outlook **16**:19, Aug. 1969.

Georgopoulas, B. S., and Mann, F. C.: The community general hospital, New York, 1962, The Macmillan Co.

Howard, E. R.: Developing student responsibility for learning, Washington, D. C., 1966, National Association of Secondary School Principals.

Long, L. D.: The evaluation of continuing education efforts, American Journal of Public Health **59**:967-970, June 1969.

Marshall, M. J., and Ruhn, J. G.: Refresher courses and the reactivation of nurses, Nursing Outlook **15**:51-61, Jan. 1967.

Osgood, G. A.: Dimensions of involvement, Nursing Outlook **17**:53, Sept. 1969.

Piepgras, R.: Obsolescence of nursing skills, American Journal of Nursing **66**:1980, Sept. 1966.

Popiel, E. S.: The many facets of continuing education in nursing, The Journal of Nursing Education **8**:3-13, Jan. 1969.

Price, E. M.: Learning needs of registered nurses, New York, 1966, Teacher's College Press, Columbia University.

Smith, D. M.: From student to nurse, Nursing Outlook **11**:735-736, Oct. 1963.

Tait, E. A.: Art appreciation and the nurse, The Journal of Nursing Education **9**:29-33, April 1970.

Wooley, A.: Inactivities, American Journal of Nursing **66**:2661-2663, Dec. 1966.

COMPLETE WORK SHEET ON P. 347

CHAPTER 22

Health and nursing legislation

HEALTH LEGISLATION

Traditionally the people of the United States have prided themselves on their "rugged individualism," shying away from any changes or controls that were remotely suggestive of socialism. However, in 1935, because of the pressures of the Depression, widespread unemployment, enforced retirement of the elderly, and the needs of the disabled, Congress passed the *Social Security Act of 1935*. The health provisions of this law established a program of grants-in-aid to states with matching funds for health services. Direction of these services was kept in state and local agencies. Passage of the *National Cancer Act of 1937*, the *Venereal Disease Control Act of 1938*, the *Hospital Survey and Construction Act of 1946* (Hill-Burton Act), and the *Mental Health Act of 1946* vastly expanded the federally directed health care.

The Social Security Act has been amended many times since its original passage, and with each amendment coverage and benefits have been more broadly identified and extended. The passage of the 1965 Amendment to this Act included guidelines for programs of health care and disease prevention of children, maternal and child care, rehabilitation programs for the disabled, and for old-age and survivors insurance, medical assistance, and a Health Insurance program for the aged (Medicare).

By 1970, over 100 million Americans were enrolled and insured under the Old-Age, Survivors, Disability, and Health Insurance Program (OASDHI) of Social Security and were eligible for the benefits of this coverage. To be insured an employee and employer share the payment of the social security tax equally; a self-employed individual must pay 1½ times the amount ordinarily assessed an employer. Tax assessment is based upon a percentage of the employed person's salary. Before any claim in order to obtain awards and benefits from Social Security can be made, the insured must have been covered and paying into the fund for a minimum of six quarters. The current law provides that the insured may choose to retire at age sixty-two with a plan of reduced benefits; if he elects to retire at age sixty-five, he receives full and maximum benefits. Specifically written into the law are (1) the amount of income a retiree may earn and continue to receive his monthly benefits, (2) his monthly payment upon retirement, (3) the benefits dependents and/or survivors will be paid, (4) the amount of financial assistance toward funeral expenses of the insured to be awarded to his survivors, (5) the schedule of payment to the disabled, and (6) the requirements for eligibility and the amount of assistance given the insured unemployed. To receive any Social Security benefits, the individual must file a request for them. No one receives benefits automatically. This law is not static, and it is wise to visit your local Social Security office for exact and current information.

Administration of Social Security (OASDHI) is the responsibility of the Department of Health, Education and Welfare, a federal department created in 1953. The Secretary of the Department of Health, Education and Welfare appoints a commissioner of Social Security to direct the activities of this important program. Fees are collected by the Internal Revenue Service, benefit checks are issued by the Treasury Department, and the Secretary of the Treasury manages all of the trust funds accrued.

The 1965 Amendments to the Social Security Act took cognizance of growing social problems and related health needs. Some aspects under consideration were social mobility from rural to urban to suburban areas; slum development in crowded cities and the need for urban renewal; air and water pollution; and the population explosion added to the lengthened life-span, which has resulted in overcrowding of health facilities. The Amendments of 1965 placed greater emphasis on the development of programs in preventive pediatrics, health care for preschool and school-age children, organized community activities for the health care of low income families, and the strengthening of medical assistance programs for the aged, the blind, and the disabled. The most controversial provision in this Amendment was the passage of Health Insurance for the Aged (Medicare).

MEDICARE

Medicare is a health insurance plan for people age sixty-five or older. This program was established to ensure health care for the person who is old and no longer working. Since 1968 only those senior citizens who have worked under the Social Security law are eligible. Medicare offers two kinds of health insurance—*Plan A, Hospital Insurance,* and *Plan B, Medical Insurance.* To qualify for either plan an application must be filed at the local Social Security office three months prior to the month of the individual's sixty-fifth birthday. Protection under Medicare is then in effect immediately upon the birthday, otherwise there may be a waiting period with no coverage.

Plan A, Hospital Insurance helps defray the expenses of hospitalization. Provisions for payment of skilled nursing care, post-hospital extended care facilities or home health services, and for outpatient hospital diagnostic services are included in this plan. Financing for this program is derived from the Social Security taxes paid by employers and employees with one-half the cost paid from federal funds. Hospital Insurance payments are collected with the regular Social Security deductions and are placed in the Hospital Insurance Trust Fund from which all benefits and administrative costs are paid. At age sixty-five the individual enrolled in this plan will be issued a health insurance card. He is to present this card to the health agency or person administering his care in order to facilitate payment for this service.

Hospital Insurance, Plan A, covers the following:

1. *Hospitalization* is paid for up to ninety days in each spell of illness. A "spell of illness" begins on the first day service is covered by this basic plan at a hospital. It ends when no benefits are received under hospital insurance for sixty days. If the patient is rehospitalized before the expiration of these sixty days, it will be considered the same "spell of illness." There is a schedule of contributory payment for each spell of illness.

2. *Post-hospital extended care* payments are made for care in a nursing home unit or in the extended care facility of a hospital. Admission with insurance coverage is granted following three days hospitalization. The program pays for twenty days in the facility during a spell of illness and all but $5 per day for an additional eighty days.

3. *Post-hospital home health care* payments are made for services of nurses, physical therapists, and other health workers (excluding doctors), if their services are supplied under an approved plan. The cost of up to one-hundred visits by these approved health workers in the 365 days following discharge from a minimum three-day stay in a hospital or health care facility is paid by the program.

4. *Outpatient hospital diagnosis services* payments are made under Plan A for eighty percent of the cost for any diagnostic services rendered to an outpatient of a participating hospital during a twenty-day period. The first $20 for each twenty-day period is paid by the patient.

Plan B, Medical Insurance, requires that the insured pay a small monthly premium (automatically deducted from his Social Security benefits). The law requires that premium rates be examined nationally every two years to determine whether the premium rate plus the government's share covers the cost, or whether an increase in rates is necessary. Regardless of cost, the government will continue to pay its share of one-half the cost. Plan B is not an automatic plan, but requires that the person who is sixty-five or older enroll during the last three months of any odd-numbered year. Once enrolled, the health insurance card will include both Plan A and Plan B. This medical insurance plan supplements the coverage in Plan A by including:

1. *Physician's and surgeon's services* wherever these services are rendered.
2. *Home health visits* up to one-hundred health visits per year under an approved plan without the necessity of prior hospitalization.
3. *Other medical and health services* wherever these services are given. Such services as diagnostic studies, x-rays or radiation therapy, surgical dressings, some ambulance services, the cost of prostheses, and rental of needed medical equipment are covered.

Additional information concerning Medicare can be obtained through contacting the local Social Security office and requesting *Your Medicare Handbook.*

OTHER LEGISLATION

Any legislation concerned with the safety, health, or welfare of the American people is important to you as a citizen and a nurse. Some examples of the legislation which influences you daily are:

Manpower Development Training Act of 1962, which offers the unskilled the opportunity of training in technical skills, including many of the paramedical fields.

Vocational Education Act of 1963, revised in 1968, which opens the door of vocational preparation to all.

Civil Rights Act of 1964, with its provision for equal opportunity for every American citizen.

Voting Rights Act of 1965, which attempts to remove the onus of second class citizenship from minority groups.

Immigration Law of 1965, which removed the quota restrictions that had been in effect for over one-hundred years.

Wholesome Meat Act of 1967, which President Lyndon Johnson signed in the presence of Upton Sinclair, who had first exposed the meat packing industry in his book, *The Jungle* in 1906.

The Child Health Act of 1967, revised in 1969, which is the government's attempt to offer every child the opportunity to fulfill his promise in life.

Drug Abuse Control Amendment of 1965 (see Chapter 17).

Community Mental Health Centers Act of 1963, which provided the funds to create mental health care centers.

Community Mental Health Centers Staffing Act of 1965, which provided the funds to staff these centers.

The list could go on and on. Watch the section of your monthly *American Journal of Nursing* magazine titled, "Off the Press," for current and vital information concerning health legislation.

NURSING LEGISLATION

As previously stated, all legislation affecting health care reflects upon the life and practice of nurses. Specific nursing legislation for many years was confined to the development and passing of state Nurse Practice Acts. As a result of growing social awareness and the shortage of nurses, the *Health Amendments Act of 1956* was passed. This was the first time that members of the health professions were eligible to receive financial aid. This aid, in the form of traineeships, made it possible for nurses to prepare themselves academically for positions in nursing education, administration, and supervision. Renewed annually, this traineeship program effectively prepared nurses from 1959 to 1963.

Following the publication of the report of

the Surgeon General's Consultant Group on Nursing, *Toward Quality in Nursing: Needs and Goals* in 1963, the need for increasing the number of nurses at all levels became very apparent. Also evident was that this increase would not be possible without some program of financial assistance. *The Nurse Training Act of 1964* was signed into law by President Lyndon Johnson on September 4, 1964. This law authorized matching grants for new construction of schools for diploma, associate degree, baccalaureate, and higher degree nursing education; authorized five-year grants to eligible schools for strengthening and expanding their programs; provided financial assistance to students in hospital diploma programs; continued the program of professional nurse traineeships; and established loan funds for students wishing to enroll in any type of nursing program (the individual school was responsible for determining the amount of the loan and for collecting payment).

The Nurse Training Act of 1964 was revised, and became Title II (Nurse Training) of the *Health Manpower Act of 1968*. Extending and broadening the scope of the provisions of the 1964 Act, Title II changed the schedule of funds available commensurate with the rising cost of education. The student nurse loan program was designed to assist qualified applicants achieve careers in nursing by providing long-term, low interest loans. Federal funds for this loan program are allocated to accredited schools of nursing, and the school is responsible for determining the amount of financial aid a qualified applicant will need. The applicant may borrow $1,500 or less for each academic year, the total amount borrowed not to exceed $6,000. When the borrower makes the initial loan, a schedule for repayment is selected. Repayment may be deferred, however, if the nurse enters the Armed Forces or the Peace Corps. Cancellation of loans is possible on the basis of selected employment. For example, loans may be cancelled 100 percent at the rate of fifteen percent per year under specific conditions. This cancellation is possible for a nurse employed full-time in a public or nonprofit hospital designated by the Secretary of the Department of Health, Education and Welfare as having a substantial nurse shortage.

The opportunity for nurses to continue their education through federal grants or loans is expected to continue. Quality in nursing—the study of the needs and goals of nurse-power is not just a report to be filed, but achieving "quality in nursing" is the responsibility of every practicing nurse. The opportunities for you to reach this goal are limitless—take advantage of this funding program and continue to learn so that you will meet the needs of society.

BIBLIOGRAPHY

Bowen, O. R.: The medico-legal conflict in drug usage, Journal of School Health **39**:165-168, Mar. 1969.

Hershey, N.: Abortion and sterilization. Status of the law in mid 1970, American Journal of Nursing **70**:1926-1928, Sept. 1970.

Legislation, Journal of American Association of Nurse Anesthetists (monthly column).

Mensel, F.: The new government comes to Washington, Junior College Journal **39**:11-14, Feb. 1969.

The effect of Medicare on two hundred agencies, Nursing Outlook **16**:42-45, Jan. 1968.

Vocational Education Amendments of 1968, American Nurses' Association Subscription Service, May, 1969.

Your Medicare handbook, pub. no. 1348, U. S. Public Health Service (available from local Social Security offices).

For further information regarding Student Loan Programs, write to:

U. S. Department of Health, Education and Welfare, National Institutes of Health, Bureau of Health Professions Education and Manpower Training, Division of Health Manpower Educational Services, Student Loan Scholarship Branch, Bethesda, Maryland, 20014.

COMPLETE WORK SHEET ON P. 349

CHAPTER 23

The graduate nurse's first job

As graduation day approaches it is only natural that students in the senior class start thinking about the first job they will have as graduate nurses. Some students may have determined their goals when they began their nursing program and have used their learning experiences to achieve these goals. Others may not be certain their original choice was the right one, for they have worked in and liked several different clinical areas of nursing service. Still others have not decided how they want to apply their nursing education to advantage as beginners in the nursing profession.

Students' career goals can change during the course of their nursing program. Naturally, as students become more aware of career opportunities and the prerequisites for career choices that interest them, they recognize the possible importance of additional formal study or concentration in a specific area. Personal circumstances may require that a student adapt or change her goals either temporarily or permanently. The student's sense of values may change, causing in turn a revision of the patterns for achieving personal goals.

As graduation approaches, you are nearing the completion of your preservice educational program. You have an obligation to yourself to seek the kind of job that will not only provide an adequate salary, but also will serve as the logical step into the area of nursing practice for which your educational program has prepared you. As a beginning practitioner you are expected to use your background as a foundation for continuing personal and professional growth as you develop and strengthen your competence in using those nursing skills that you, as a beginning practitioner, are expected to have.

SELECT THE JOB YOU ARE PREPARED TO DO NOW

When nursing students think about the career they have chosen and recognize the importance of participating as part of the health care team to provide quality patient care, they should feel a sense of satisfaction and accomplishment because they are actively involved in acquiring the knowledge and skills they will need to pursue their chosen careers. Because increasing numbers of nurses are needed, there are many opportunities for employment following graduation, and this is an additional incentive to the student who is looking ahead and planning for her experience as a member of the nursing profession.

What does it mean to be a beginning nurse practitioner? What should the new graduate be prepared to do? Think for a moment of the requirements for admission to your nursing program and recall the stated purposes of your program and the patterns of instruction, clinical assignments, and supervision of your learning experiences as a student. Each of these items is relevant to your preparation as a beginning worker in the profession.

If you are to graduate as a practical/vocational nurse, your nursing career will involve giving nursing care to designated types of patients under the direct supervision of a registered nurse (or licensed physician) within a framework of activities legally identified as your scope of practice. If you are to graduate from either a hospital school or a community college associate degree program, your activities as a practitioner are expected to center on performing the technical aspects of nursing care under the supervision of a physician or experienced professional nurse. As technically proficient nurses your responsibilities include the performance of "nursing and other therapeutic measures with a high degree of skill, using principles from an ever expanding body of science."* In using measures and techniques for the relief of a patient's distress, in checking a patient's responses and reactions to therapeutic aids, and in applying prescribed treatments exactly and with good judgment, you are responsible for guiding and supervising others who will assist you with some of the technical aspects of patient care.

The new graduate of a baccalaureate degree program is a beginning practitioner able to assume the direct care of patients under appropriate supervision. Her skills and knowledge in the administration of nursing techniques is complemented with a broad familiarity with, and understanding of, the social sciences and humanities, which serves as a foundation for making independent decisions and demonstrating leadership potential abilities.

Each educational program prepares its students so that, as graduates, they are able to practice those basic skills and apply the information acquired during their studies. In this manner graduates increase their proficiency and competence as they develop their skills and self-confidence through practice.

Graduate nurses who are looking for their first professional position should look for jobs that their nursing program has prepared them to perform. As students look forward to graduation and that first pay check, they should also consider whether a specific position will offer the opportunity for maximum personal and professional benefits.

We assume that every eligible graduate plans to take a state board examination for licensure as soon as possible following graduation. We also assume that students will persist until they pass the examination and qualify for a state license either as an RN or as an LVN/LPN so that their nursing careers can begin with proper legal identity within their profession (see Chapter 17). Think for a moment about beginning your practice of nursing and what this new role means to you. How do you plan to use the time spent in your first position to become adjusted to your new status? What goals do you intend to set for yourself for the first year or two following your graduation?

THERE WILL NEVER BE ANOTHER FIRST JOB

After your supervised course of study has prepared you for your chosen career, you will need a period of time to learn to apply these skills in practical everyday situations. During this time you will develop assurance and expertise. Just as doctors spend the years following graduation from medical school as interns and residents learning to apply their knowledge and skills, so graduates of nursing programs need at least a year under the direction of experienced nurses in service to apply the knowledge and skills they have learned as students. During this time they have the opportunity to develop the self-confidence and proficiency they will need as competent nurses. This period encourages new graduates to test their knowledge and ability, and they will gain confidence in their ability through the daily routine of using their present knowledge and gaining new skills in applying it. In other words, this work experience for new graduates is providing opportunities for them *to become,* with guidance and on-the-job supervision, *expert* in their practice of nursing.

Your director and instructors will no doubt review the areas in which you are prepared to work. As a beginner in the world of nursing practice, it is important that you select the kind of nursing position you are prepared to fill *now.* New graduates with potential for great profes-

*American Journal of Nursing, 67:1378, July 1967.

sional growth and advanced formal training often disregard the fact that they are, after all, beginners. Sometimes these graduates pass up positions that would allow them to strengthen their fundamental skills in favor of a more advanced assignment for which they are not truly prepared. Nurses who allow themselves to be trapped in this way damage their own careers as well as perform a disservice to the nursing profession.

Beginning at the beginning can have a number of very positive results. One is the assurance that you will have time to adjust to the work situation and to become familiar with the policies and channels of communication operating in the work situation. (It is taken for granted that orientation programs and in-service training will be available to help you in the institution you have chosen for employment.) Another result is your own awareness of the basic knowledge and skills you possess as a beginner and of your obligation to test them as you learn through working to develop proficiency and competence in ministering to the needs of patients. In your first job as a nurse practitioner you will learn that different skills and roles are expected of you than when you were a student. Hopefully, as a beginning staff nurse you will participate with others in a team relationship and you will be given opportunities to coordinate your efforts with those of others who are also responsible for meeting the needs of the sick.

Your first job will test not only your present knowledge, but also your capacity for learning and using new information. Your initial experiences and the variety of assignments you receive in clinical areas can serve as background for your increasing competence and as a basis for your ultimate choice of a particular branch of nursing service.

There will never be another first year as a beginning practitioner. There will never be another first job in which you can establish a pattern for continuing growth and achievement in your chosen career. That is why you should consider the effects of your first experiences as a worker. All successive jobs can be affected by the learning experiences obtained in the first position you take after graduation from your basic preparatory program.

APPLYING FOR A POSITION

Today, there are employment opportunities in hospitals, clinics, convalescent and rehabilitation units, doctors' offices, and other types of health care facilities. In addition to positions in local hospitals, hospitals and health agencies across the country publicize their needs for new staff members and request that graduating classes be informed of these opportunities. The position sections in professional journals and want ad sections of daily papers indicate the variety of work opportunities for nurses throughout the country. Representatives of placement agencies, hospital personnel departments, physicians, friends, and classmates may also serve as sources of information about available jobs. There is no lack of jobs—the real problem lies in selecting the most desirable job for you and in making application for it. Assuming that you have considered the position you can fill as a beginning nurse, that you have discussed with your director or instructors your strengths and the areas in which you could use further training, and that you have considered opportunities presently open to you, it is appropriate to review in broad terms the process of applying for your first position.

FINDING THE RIGHT JOB

When seeking employment there are some decisions that only you can make. These involve choosing the locale in which you would prefer to work. Important considerations are community services such as transportation facilities and other situations to which you must adjust. You must also consider the way in which you will go about finding the right job and applying for it to change your status from that of applicant to that of new employee. As an applicant, it is to your advantage to check on all available job resources. Make specific inquiries by either a letter or a telephone call and then follow up by requesting a personal interview.

If you are seeking a position in another city or town, you will probably want to write a letter to express your interest in a prospective position and report your qualifications. If you are interested in a local job, a telephone call to the director of nursing or the agency's personnel department will introduce you, allow you to briefly discuss your interests and qualifications, and to schedule a personal interview. It is advisable to make inquiries about employment prospects at several agencies so that your final choice of a job is a good one, based upon a broad range of information. You will then have the satisfaction of knowing more facts about the positions available before selecting the one that is best for you.

As a job applicant, you should have an honest and positive attitude toward yourself both as a person and as a prospective member of the health team. You should know the limit of the responsibilities you are prepared to undertake and be aware of those areas in which you need additional knowledge and supervised practice. While you are working and becoming more skillful, you are still expected to perform your job to the best of your ability in exchange for your salary, on-the-job training, and the supervision you receive.

As an applicant, it is important that you think for a moment about the importance of the first impression you give to your prospective employers. Your educational preparation has been grooming you to meet this challenge. Your sincerity and honesty in presenting information, the completeness of your statements, and the general impression created either by letter or telephone, and your ability to be at ease during an interview should all work in your favor. You are, in effect, selling yourself as a valuable future member of the staff.

WRITING A LETTER OF INQUIRY AND APPLICATION

Your written letter of inquiry concerning a position is significant in conveying an image of you as a person and as a member of the nursing profession. It should present a positive and favorable impression, because it introduces you personally to your potential employer. It serves as a valuable public relations aid. As a student you have doubtless had experience in letter writing. Nevertheless, you ought to give some thought to the format and contents of this very important letter.

1. Use white, squarely cut unlined letter paper. Never use the stationery of a hotel, business, or other institution.
2. If the letter is handwritten, use black or blue ink. If typewritten, black or blue ribbon is preferable. In either instance the signature is always written.
3. The heading consists of your street address, the city, state (country), zip code, and the date of communication.
4. A letter should be addressed to the person who will consider your request or, if the name is not known, to the title of the position—Director of Nursing Service followed by the salutation "Dear Madam" or "Dear Sir." Never use the phrase "To Whom It May Concern."
5. Provide margins on the letter, space between paragraphs and express your thoughts in a concise, courteous, tactful manner.
6. Correct English (or other language), correct spelling, correct abbreviations when use is indicated, and proper punctuation are essential.
7. A letter is concluded with your signature and the proper title—Miss., Mr., Mrs.—in parentheses before the name.
8. When enclosures accompany a letter the notation "Encl" may be added in the lower left hand corner of the letter sheet followed by the number of sheets enclosed. This serves as a check on the contents of the envelope in which the letter is mailed.
9. For return of enclosures and assurance of a prompt reply, a stamped, self-addressed envelope should be included.
10. A letter should be folded to fit neatly into the envelope. The envelope is correctly addressed, sealed, and mailed with

5821 Holloman Street
Elmwood, Ohio 50921
April 16, 1970

Miss Alice Shipwell, R.N.
Director, Nursing Service
Florence Nightingale Hospital
990 Satellite Drive
Los Angeles, California 98236

My dear Miss Shipwell:

My father will be transferred to a position in Los Angeles so I expect to move to California with my parents at the end of this month. I am interested in obtaining a position as a staff nurse in your hospital.

My choice of Florence Nightingale Hospital is based on two sources of information: one, the advertisement on page 193 in the March 1970 issue of the American Journal of Nursing indicating opportunities available for continued education as a member of the staff and two, a statement by a family friend about the excellent nursing care she received while a patient in the hospital.

In August, 1968, I graduated from the Henry County Hospital School of Nursing, Elmwood, Ohio. My Ohio registration (#999739) by state board examination was awarded September 30, 1968. Since November 15, I have been employed as a staff nurse on the surgical division of Santa Maria Hospital in Elmwood.

My application and other credentials for registration in California have been sent to the office of the Board of Nurse Registration and Nursing Education in Sacramento, California. I expect to have my California R.N. license before starting to work in that state.

As for personal information, I am 22 years old, single but engaged and planning to be married next year. I am healthy, interested in sports, music, drama and life in general. A passport photo taken recently is enclosed for your inspection.

The following persons have indicated their willingness to provide references for me:

Mrs. Janet Cooper, R.N.
Director, School of Nursing
Henry County Hospital, Elmwood, Ohio 50921

Sister M. Irene, R.N.
Director, Nursing Service
Santa Maria Hospital, Elmwood, Ohio 50923

James Scheff, M.D.
Chief, Surgical Service
Santa Maria Hospital, Elmwood, Ohio 50923

I would appreciate receiving information about policies and regulations concerning employment in effect at the hospital as well as an application form. Should you wish a personal interview I shall be available at your convenience after May 1. A stamped, self-addressed envelope is enclosed and I shall look forward to hearing from you.

Very truly yours,
Elisabethe McCloud
(Miss) Elisabethe McCloud, R.N.

Encl (2)

SAMPLE LETTER OF APPLICATION FOR POSITION.

with sufficient postage to assure prompt delivery.

11. In a letter of application you should make the following points:
    a. Your purpose in writing the letter (first paragraph).
    b. Why you are writing to the particular agency or institution.
    c. Your qualifications and significant work experiences.
    d. Complete names, addresses, and positions of three persons who know about you and your preparation as a worker and who have agreed to submit references in your behalf.
    e. The availability of additional information, your willingness to appear for a personal interview, and specific requests for additional information (see sample letter).
12. It is recommended that you keep carbon or other exact copies of letters submitted to prospective employers for future reference.
13. Educational transcripts, records verifying work experiences, and the name of the placement agency where your professional biography is on file may be submitted in follow-up letters if you are being seriously considered for employment.

When an applicant begins her inquiry with a telephone call, it is helpful to find out from the hospital switchboard operator the department and, if possible, the person with whom she should speak. The applicant identifies herself, states the purpose of her call and then makes certain she is speaking to the correct person. It is a courtesy to make certain how to pronounce and spell the person's name as well as to verify her correct title. The same points that you would include in a letter should be used as an outline for your telephone presentation as the conversation progresses. Arrangements can be made for a personal interview at this time, or you may be asked to write to the director for an interview appointment, at which time information pertinent to the filing of an application may be discussed. Remember that everything you do to organize and implement your activities in applying for a position should reflect favorably in your behalf.

THE PERSONAL INTERVIEW

A personal interview is an important part of looking for and securing employment, from the point of view of both the applicant and the prospective employer. Ideally, both parties involved in this relationship have an opportunity to exchange information in greater detail than is possible by either correspondence or telephone. This face-to-face exchange permits clarification of specific questions and allows for the establishment of rapport to the mutual satisfaction of each participant. In effect, this personal interview should enhance the employer's opinion of the applicant's qualifications for a position, since presumably it affirms the impressions already gained through a review of credentials and references submitted earlier. As an applicant, you should regard the interview as an opportunity to strengthen the positive image previously created. An interview personalizes your formal record and serves to strengthen your identity in the mind of your prospective employer. The following points are listed as guides for you to review as part of your preparation for a personal interview.

1. Make an appointment for the interview and be certain about the time, the place, and the name and title of the person with whom it is scheduled.
2. Be on time. It is advisable to give yourself a few minutes grace if parking a car or seeking directions is necessary.
3. Your personal appearance should be neat, clean, and appropriate for the occasion. Omit no detail that will contribute to making a favorable impression.
4. Be poised and at ease while waiting and during the period of the interview. This is an occasion to practice the social courtesies you have practiced when meeting others.
5. Refer to your prospective employer by

name and identify yourself when you meet.

6. Permit your interviewer to initiate the conversation and to determine what you have to offer as a prospective employee. It is expected that you will be frank and factual in response to questions and will, in turn, ask any questions you wish about the position.
7. If you have prepared notes to help you remember questions you wish to ask, ask for permission to use them as a guide for your comments. You might ask about the following:*
   a. Responsibility and authority for nursing care policies?
   b. Is it employment in nursing or for some other area?
   c. Orientation program?
   d. Staff development program?
   e. Professional salary with planned incerements and advancement?
   f. Time off for educational programs?
   g. Job description? Nursing care plans? Nursing resources?
   h. Written personnel policies?
   i. Letter of appointment? Or contract?
   j. Responsible to whom? For what?
   k. Position title? Vacation? Sick Leave? Retirement? Insurance?
8. Be prepared to give evidence of your registration or the legal status of your identity as a nurse practitioner, if you have not submitted it previously.
9. Questions about salary and fringe benefits identified with the position should be considered after both the qualifications and functions of the position have been discussed. The salary should be in line with the responsibilities of the position and meet the standards established by the state's nurses' association.
10. Should you decide you are not interested in the position, say so frankly but tactfully and give your reasons. This gives the interviewer an opportunity to terminate the appointment and to consider other applicants.
11. If you wish additional time to think about the position before making a commitment, you should inform your interviewer accordingly. If you wish to be considered as a formal applicant, make certain your application form is completed and presented for review. A final answer on your selection should not be requested before you leave the interview.
12. When this appointment is terminated thank the interviewer for her time and courtesy. A follow-up note of appreciation is also suggested whether or not the position is available. At some future date you may wish to reapply for another position.
13. Following your notification of acceptance as an employee it is advisable to write your employer expressing your appreciation, stating the terms of your employment and verifying the time you report for duty. This letter, together with the one offering you the position, constitutes evidence of mutual understanding of the conditions of employment and serves, in effect, as a written contract.

*From What you need to know about your first position in nursing. Reprinted with permission, Ohio State Nurses Association, Columbus, Ohio.

THE JOB APPLICATION FORM

In Chapter 10 the significance of the application for admission to the nursing program was reviewed. Similarly, the application you submit when applying for a position serves as a source of information for employers and assists them to evaluate your qualifications to fill the assignments they seek. Directions for completing an application should be read and scrupulously followed; handwriting, printing, or typing should be legible, spelling correct, and terminology properly used. All requested information should be provided completely and accurately. This record can serve as an effective spokesman for you when it conveys a positive impression to those who study its contents.

A completed application becomes an essential part of your employment file. It implies your understanding and acceptance of the obligations identified with the position in return for the salary and other related benefits resulting from your employment.

HANDLING YOURSELF AND YOUR JOB

When you decide to accept a position, a new opportunity is created for you to continue your growth and development. Moving from the status of student to that of employee or staff member will require adjustments in your pattern of activities and responses so that you are able to accept those responsibilities associated with your newly acquired identity. Your new role will require you to apply knowledge learned in previous experiences in a work setting that will further challenge your development of nursing skills and your interpersonal relationships. Your employer will look for tangible evidences of your growth and development as you become oriented to your new job.

If you have selected the job that is right for you, your interest and enthusiasm will convey to others your personal satisfaction and pleasure in the work you do. Your job should provide opportunities for both learning and practice that will serve as a foundation and a steppingstone to future advancement. The experiences associated with your first position can affect the way you function in all subsequent assignments.

You bring to your job the personality, characteristics, and knowledge demanded in the practice of your role. When you use your talents and abilities to effectively meet the demands of daily interpersonal exchanges, you will be recognized and appreciated as a valued member of the nursing service staff.

During the period of your employment you are urged to keep abreast of new ideas and to take advantage of every opportunity to become more efficient and effective in your job. Welcome the chance to participate in continuing education courses designed to improve the quality of your nursing and your interactions with others. Prepare to accept assignments that will test your ability to use your new knowledge by serving in different nursing areas and clinical divisions. It is by growing in the job and working as a member of a team that you measure up to the ideals you set for yourself. In this way, too, you can establish your identity as a valued employee and prepare yourself for the next step forward and upward in your career.

WHEN YOU LEAVE A POSITION

Some authorities say that an employee should remain in a position for three years in order to be certain that opportunities for growth and learning are exhausted before another job is sought. This time period will vary depending on the nature of the job, the responsibility it involves, and the policies enforced by the employer. However, your professional interest virtually demands that you remain in a position for at least one year. Generally speaking, it will take a year for you to adjust to the demands of a given job situation and to evaluate your prospects for growth on the job. On the other hand, a person who decides to change jobs after a few months of employment may not have had time to demonstrate a pattern of work and relationships that can be objectively evaluated. The applicant who changes jobs frequently establishes a reputation for being flighty or tending to move from one position to another. This kind of image will not favorably impress prospective employers with the applicant's dependability or sense of responsibility.

Nevertheless, there are several reasons why a person might wish to leave a position. Some of these include promotion, marriage and family responsibility, relocation in another city, or the opportunity to continue education on a full-time basis. Also, an employee may recognize her inability to meet the requirements of the position. All the factors relative to vacating a position must be carefully reviewed, and the advice of more experienced persons should be considered so that the decision to leave is based on reason rather than on a momentary whim.

A position is vacated either through resignation or dismissal. Resigning is generally accepted in the business and professional worlds as the privilege of an employee who wishes to leave a position. The procedure requires that the employee notify the employer in writing of his intention to end the working agreement on a given date. The letter should also state the reasons for the employee's decision. Sometimes it is possible to give an employer advance notice in a personal conference of probable or impending factors that may make a resignation necessary, but the actual decision to leave should always be communicated to the employer in a written communication (letter of resignation).

When you obtain a position, your letter of inquiry and application constitute a contract. If you resign, the letter terminating your affiliation with your employer also becomes an important part of your professional file. It will be retained for future reference, together with a record of your employer's response to it. If you decide to submit a resignation from your position, the following suggestions will assist you to observe the customary procedures:

1. Inform your employer of your intentions before you tell others.
2. Give your employer sufficient notice of your intention to leave so that efforts to find a replacement may be initiated. At least one month's notice is indicated unless the agency's personnel policies state otherwise. Notice of two weeks or less should not be considered adequate unless an emergency arises and it is necessary. Never leave a position without notice. This so-called French leave is a violation of the nurse's professional code. It is also a black mark in your employment record.
3. State the reasons for your resignation in a clear, unemotional manner. Throughout your letter retain the element of dignity and avoid reference to any unhappy experiences.
4. Express regret for leaving and appreciation for the kindness and consideration shown to you.
5. State the specific date on which you wish to terminate your employment. Indicate your willingness to participate in a terminal conference at the convenience of your employer.
6. Organize, follow through, and complete your duties until the day you depart. Leave records and equipment in good order; leave those with whom you have worked in the most graceful and professional manner possible. You have finished one learning experience and you are taking a step forward to new learning experiences.

Occasionally a person is dismissed from his position or his resignation is requested by his employer, thus terminating employment in accordance with the employer's policies and the regulation affecting the position. The employee usually receives all salary due him to the time of discharge. However, circumstances may require review by a grievance committee, which will make a final disposition of the problem. Dismissal is usually the result of misconduct or malfeasance that requires the employer's immediate intervention and action.

Your success as a nurse depends on the position you fill and upon the quality of your performance on the job. Knowledge and maturity gained during each position you hold will prepare you for the next step forward in your practice with professional competence. When you have met the challenge of one position, take your assurance and knowledge forward to new opportunities and additional challenges. At the same time you should recognize that every job experience will be evaluated and recorded for future reference. Do your best to see that each report provides a favorable addition to your record as a member of the nursing profession.

Frances McKenna summarizes this fact in the following statements:

> When the nurse leaves a position she does not burn her bridges or close a chapter. The reputation she made will go with her. Her old employer will be asked many times for comments on her performance, on her profes-

sional and social conduct, on her character and integrity. Her contribution in the nursing group and in the community will be scrutinized and evaluated and her readiness and ability to take over a new appointment will be judged largely in terms of what she did in the old one. Did she leave in a huff? Was she difficult to get along with? Or did she fill a difficult spot capably and is she missed? No greater compliment can be paid a person than to say that the agency concerned not only regrets her leaving, but would be glad of an opportunity to re-employ her.*

*McKenna, F. M.: Thresholds to professional nursing practice, ed. 2, Philadelphia, 1960, W. B. Saunders Co., p. 78.

BIBLIOGRAPHY

Hamburg, A. Z.: Evaluation before employment, Nursing Outlook **13**:45-47, Mar. 1965.

Loden, Evelyn C.: Some tips on landing that new job, RN **26**:37-42, Nov. 1963.

Major, D. M.: Career planning begins with the beginning student, Nursing Outlook **9**:534-537, Sept. 1961.

McKenna, F. M.: Thresholds to professional nursing practice, ed. 2, Philadelphia, 1960, W. B. Saunders Co.

Sleeper, R.: When you apply for your first position, Nursing Outlook **9**:230-231, Apr. 1961.

Stevens, L. F.: Look at your own practice, American Journal of Nursing **65**:106-107, June 1965.

Theis, C., and Harringtin, H.: Communications, assignments, attitudes, American Journal of Nursing **68**:1478-1482, July 1968.

Wilkins, M. C.: Fitting the individual to the job, Nursing Outlook **11**:291-293, Apr. 1963.

COMPLETE WORK SHEET ON PP. 351 AND 352

OPPORTUNITIES FOR THE PROFESSIONAL NURSE—WITHIN THE HOSPITAL SETTING

FORMAL TEACHING IN A BASIC PROGRAM OR IN NURSING SPECIALTY FOR THE R.N. (O.R.)

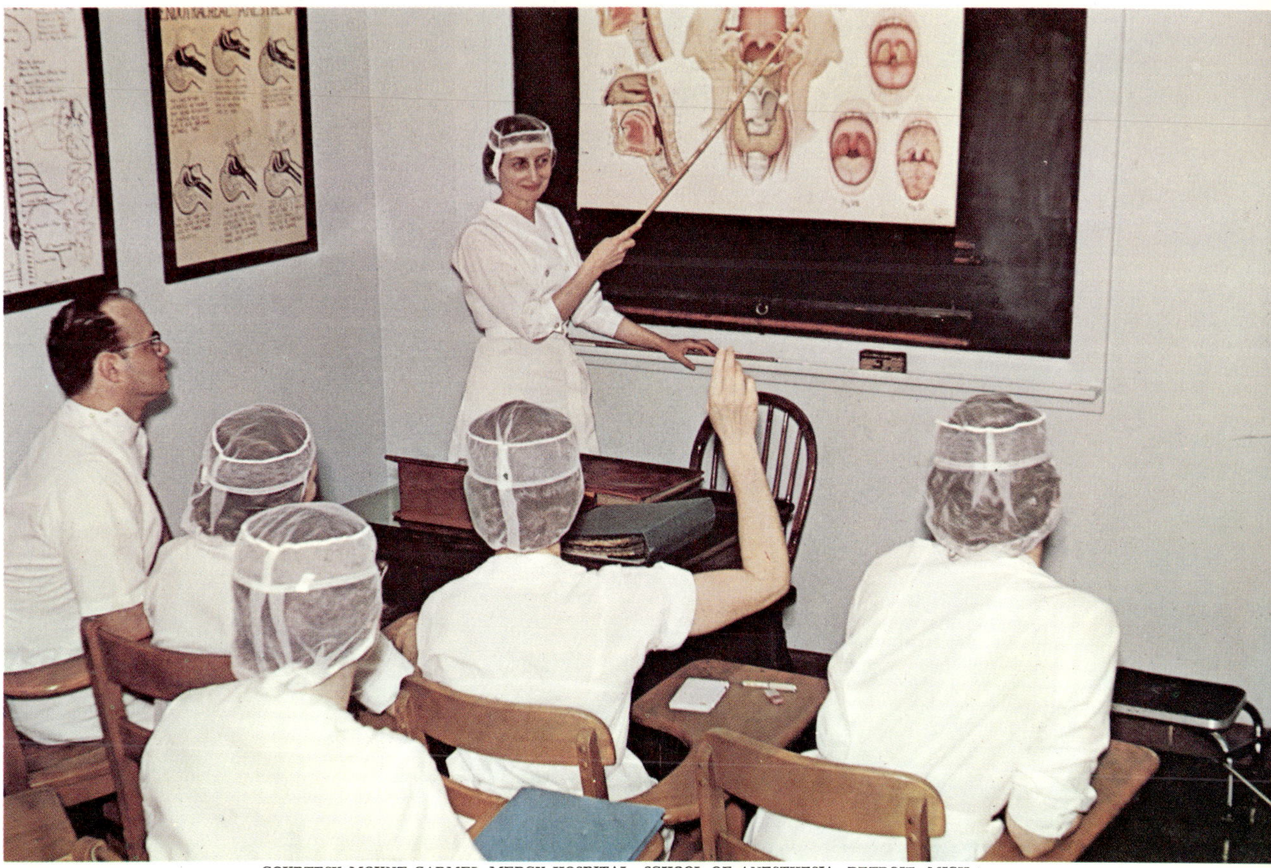

COURTESY MOUNT CARMEL MERCY HOSPITAL, SCHOOL OF ANESTHESIA, DETROIT, MICH.; PHOTOGRAPH BY DOROTHY M. SELVES, DETROIT, MICH.

NURSING SUPERVISION INVOLVES CHECKING ON
PATIENTS' NURSING CARE AND TREATMENTS

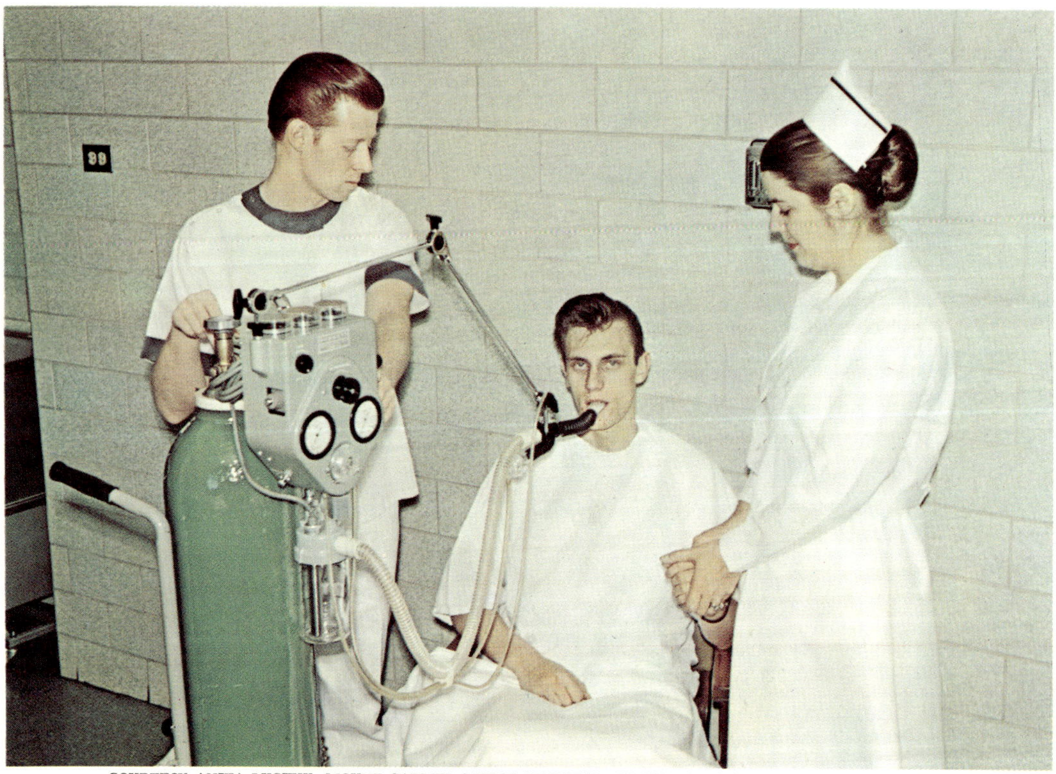

COURTESY ANITA LUCIEW, MOUNT CARMEL MERCY HOSPITAL, SCHOOL OF ANESTHESIA, DETROIT, MICH.;
PHOTOGRAPH BY DOROTHY M. SELVES, DETROIT, MICH.

THE VISITING NURSE GOES TO THE HOME TO GIVE HEALTH INSTRUCTION OR TO DIRECT NURSING CARE

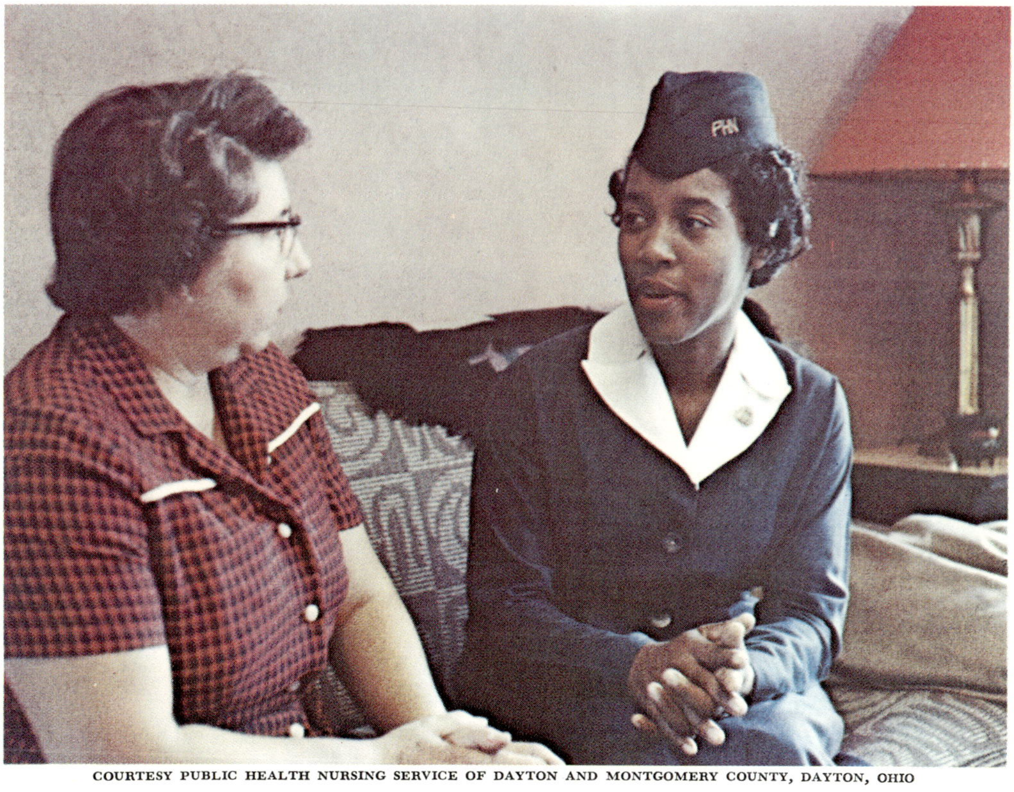

COURTESY PUBLIC HEALTH NURSING SERVICE OF DAYTON AND MONTGOMERY COUNTY, DAYTON, OHIO

COURTESY PUBLIC HEALTH NURSING SERVICE OF DAYTON AND MONTGOMERY COUNTY, DAYTON, OHIO

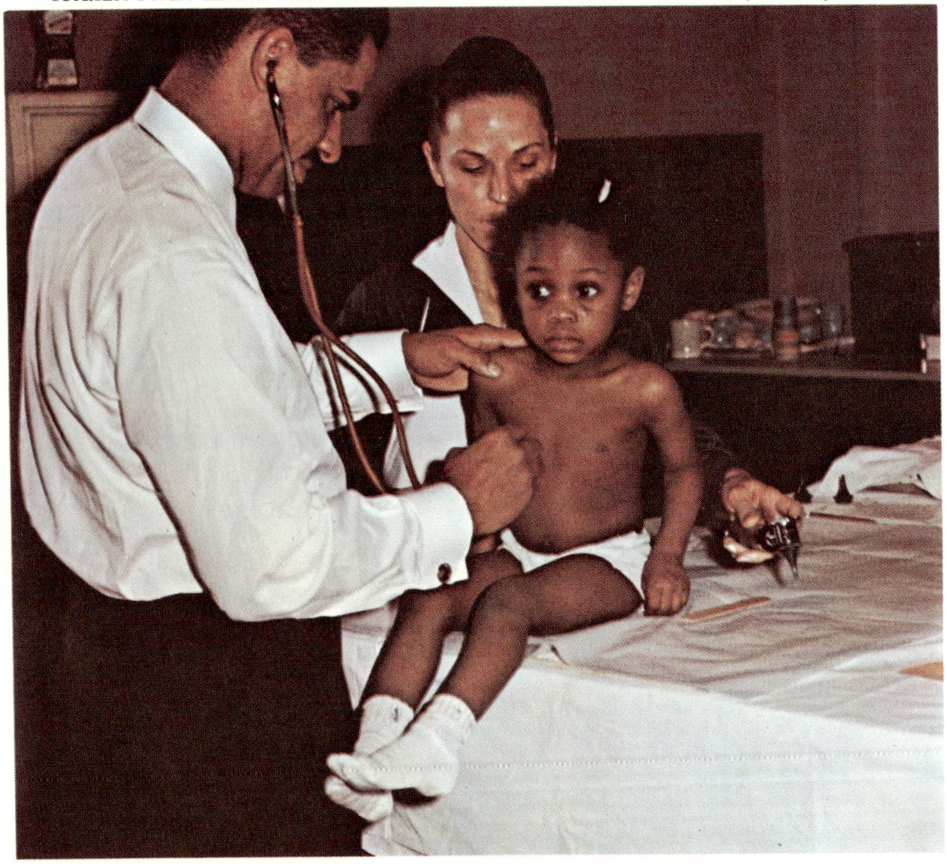

THE PUBLIC HEALTH NURSE SERVES IN A PRESCHOOL CLINIC AND/OR IN SCHOOLS AND IN INDUSTRIAL SERVICES

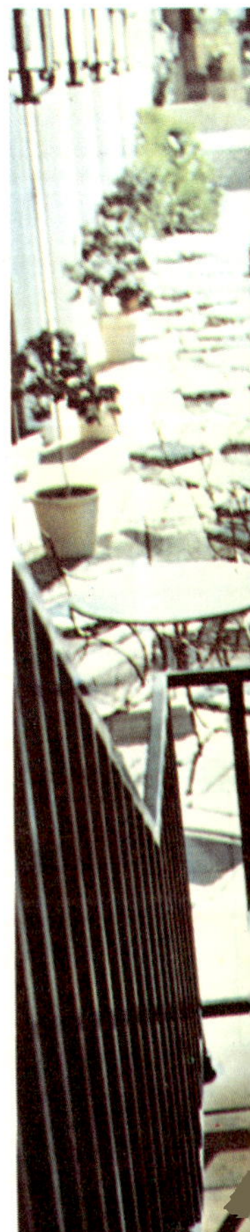

OFFICIAL U. S. AIR FORCE PHOTOGRAPH

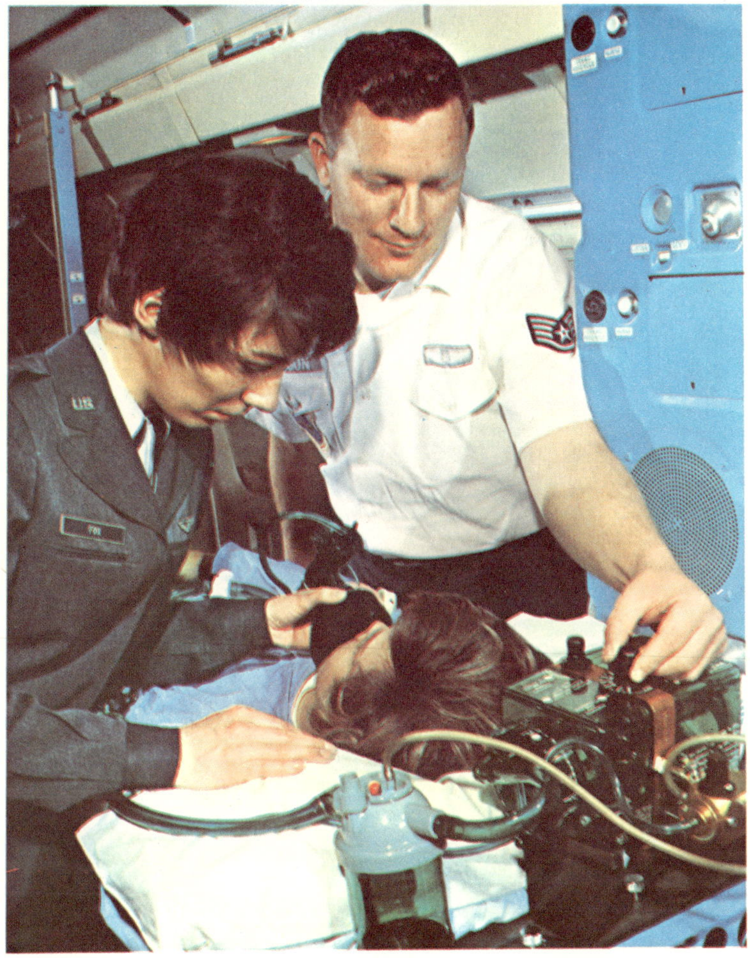

THE AIR FORCE OFFERS OPPORTUNITIES FOR EXPERIENCE IN A VARIETY OF CLINICAL SPECIALTIES

"OFF DUTY" OPPORTUNITIES FOR TRAVEL—AN ADVANTAGE OF THE AIR FORCE

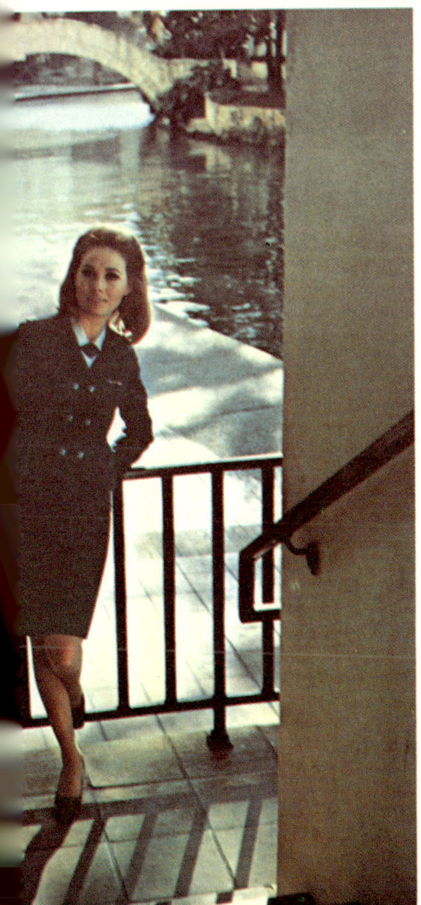

OFFICIAL U. S. AIR FORCE PHOTOGRAPH

RED CROSS NURSE ASSISTING IN DISASTER CONTROL

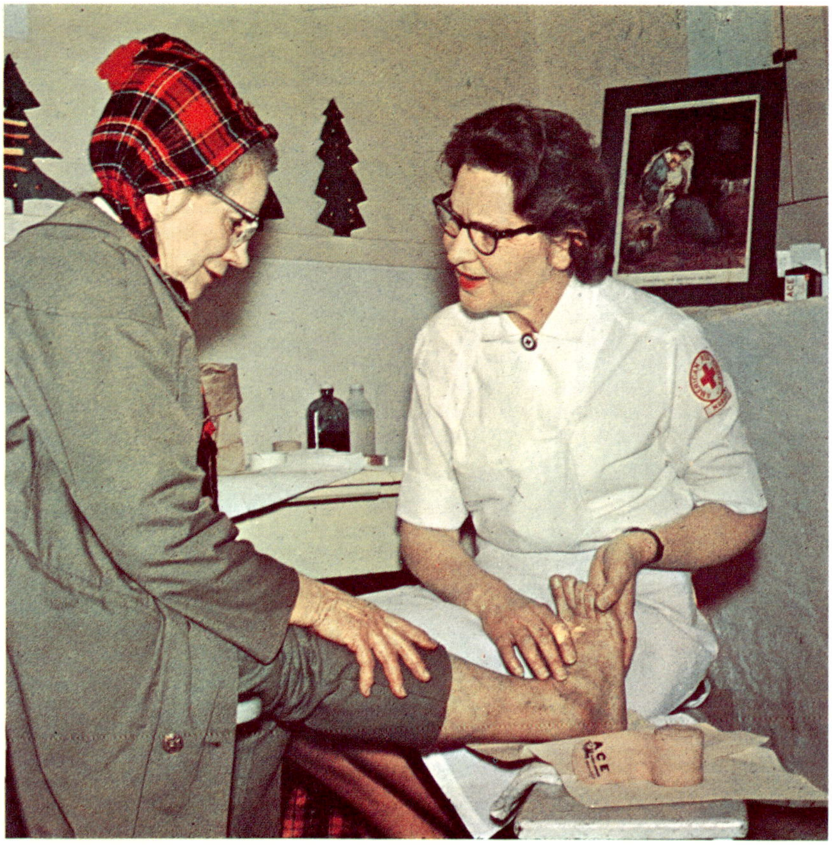

COURTESY AMERICAN RED CROSS NURSING SERVICES

COURTESY UNITED STATES PUBLIC HEALTH SERVICE, DEPARTMENT OF HEALTH, EDUCATION, AND WELFARE

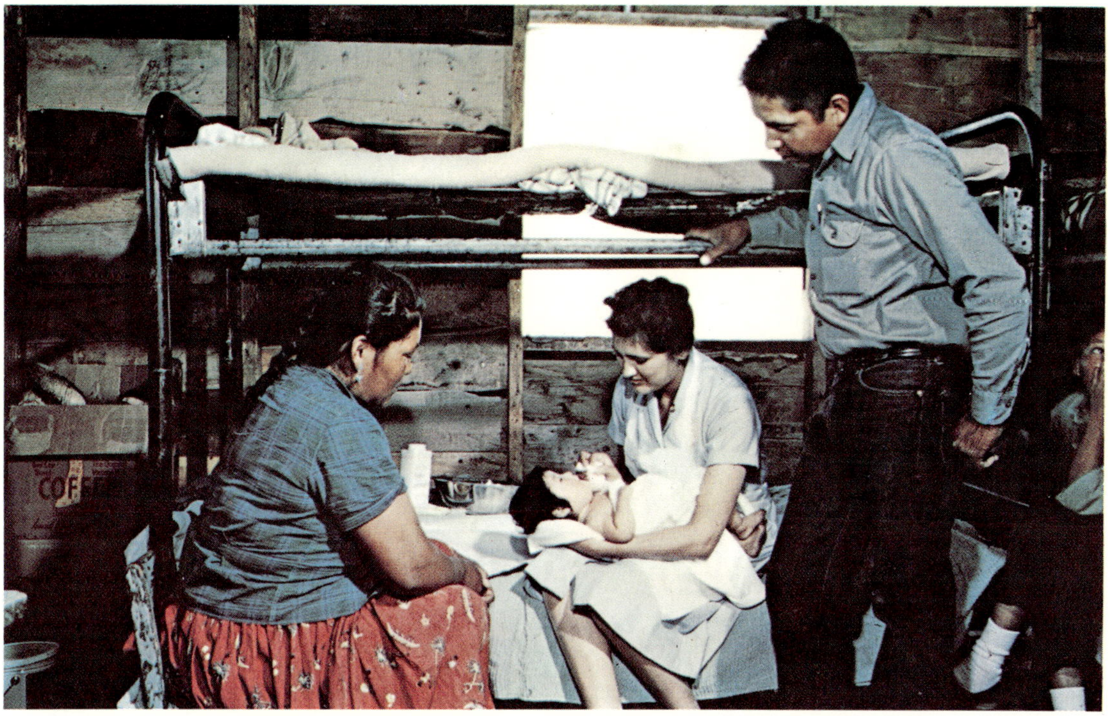

NURSING AMONG THE AMERICAN INDIANS—PREVENTIVE AND THERAPEUTIC NURSING

NURSING AS A MEMBER OF RED CROSS NURSING SERVICE—TEACHING CHILD CARE

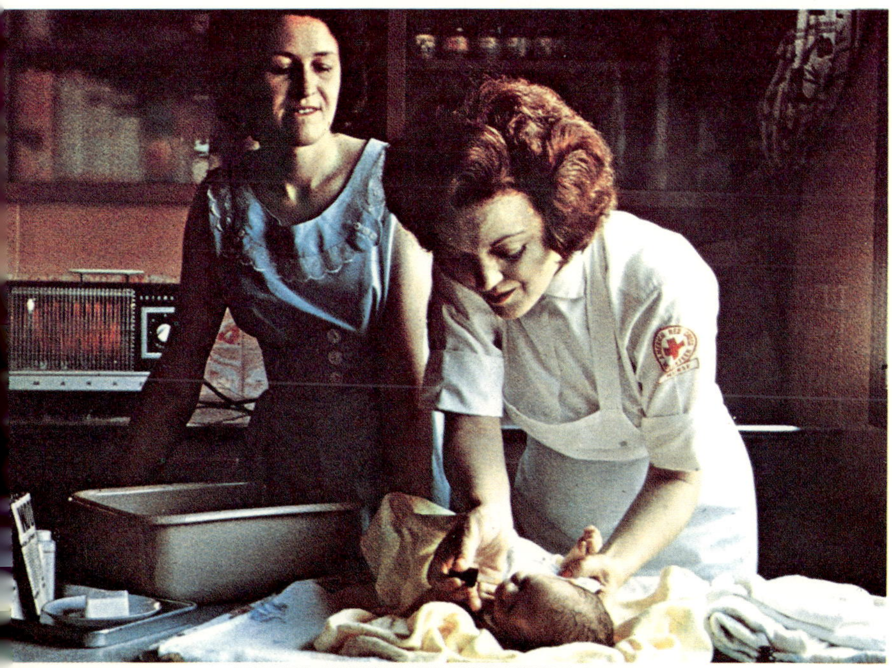

COURTESY AMERICAN RED CROSS NURSING SERVICES

NURSE FOR CAMP, SENIOR CITIZENS, AND GROUP PROJECTS

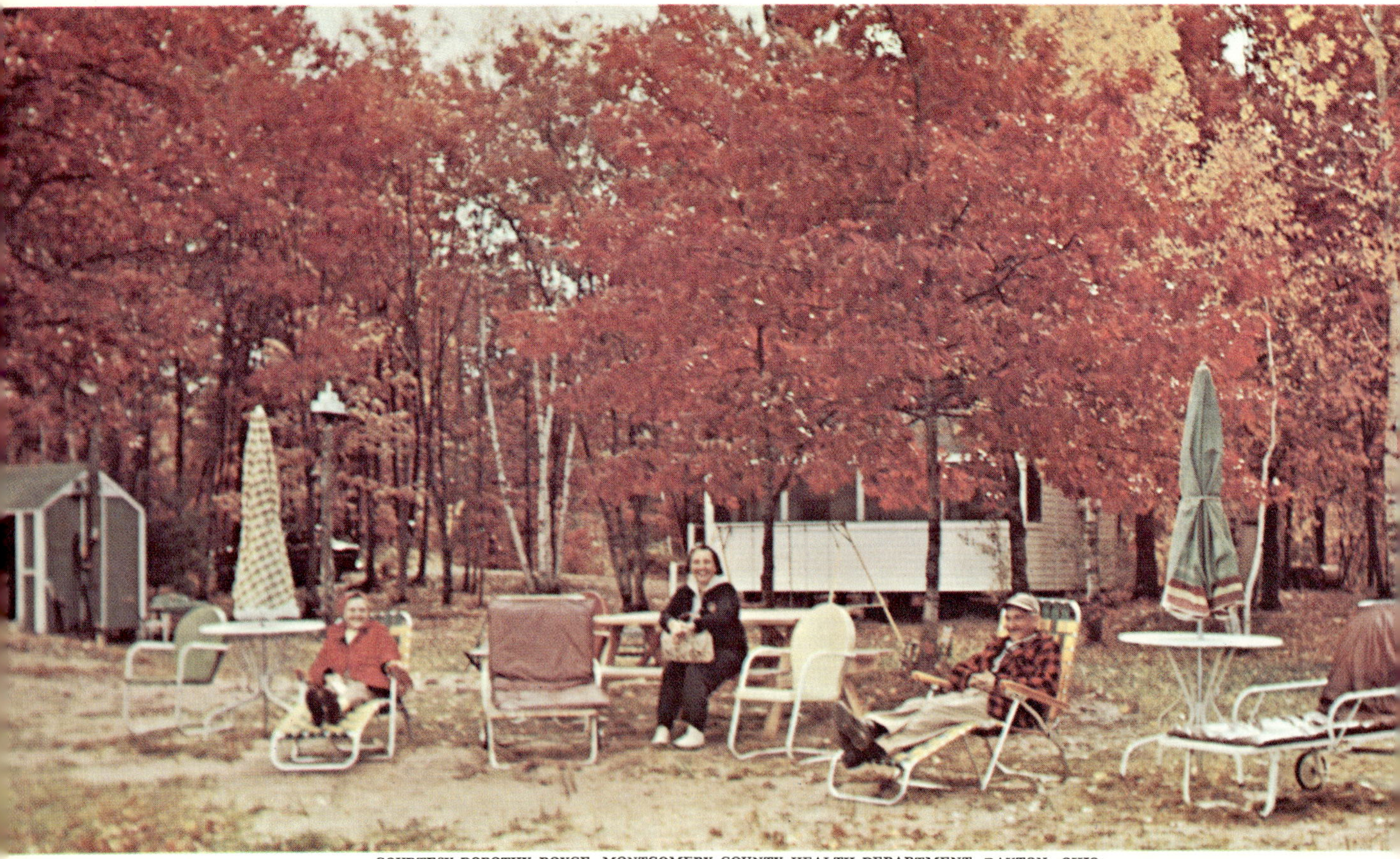

COURTESY DOROTHY ROYCE, MONTGOMERY COUNTY HEALTH DEPARTMENT, DAYTON, OHIO;
PHOTOGRAPH BY VERNON ROYCE, FAIRBORN, OHIO

CHAPTER 24

Opportunities for pursuing a career in nursing

HOSPITAL NURSING

Approximately 67 percent of all active nurses in the United States and its territories are employed in hospitals. It is the belief of many nurse educators and professional leaders that hospital experience after graduation serves to enrich the knowledge and skill the nurse acquired as a student. They also believe that such an experience facilitates the transition and adjustment from the role of student to the role of registered nurse. Assignment to a specific therapeutic area in the hospital is usually dependent upon the qualifications of the new nurse graduate as they correspond to the hospital's need; salary is usually commensurate with the nurse's qualifications.

Expansion of hospital and other medical care facilities, together with the preparation of increasing numbers of people in paramedical areas of patient care, broadens the scope of responsibilities that must be assumed by the registered nurse. When these ancillary workers become part of the health care team in hospitals, clinics and other nursing care units, clear limits must be established to define those tasks that their training has given them the competence and ability to perform. In this way patients are protected, and a chain of responsibility is set forth to provide for harmonious relationships under nursing supervision.

Increasing numbers of nurses, as well as personnel trained in some paramedical specialties, will be needed to staff present as well as proposed nursing service areas in any hospital's postoperative recovery rooms, intensive care, coronary care, convalescent care, and long-term care (chronic/geriatric) units. The majority of new graduates will most probably begin their nursing careers as staff nurses in hospitals. These new professionals should plan to spend time working in these positions so that they may enrich and build on their knowledge and simultaneously develop and refine their nursing techniques.

Staff nursing is the first rung on the ladder of work experience. It provides the foundation on which future assignments are built; it contributes to the nurse's professional growth. As a staff nurse you will have direct contact with the patient and with his family, and the opportunity to practice and develop your skills in patient-centered care. As a staff nurse in a variety of clinical services, you can acquire a broad experience so that you can choose assignments best for you in a specialized clinical area.

Staff nurses are valued members of the hospital team. They "make the wheels go 'round" as far as nursing services are concerned. The job performed by staff nurses benefits them as the first step in their professional career and also has enormous effects upon the quality of patient care (and hence upon the reputation of the institution which employs them). In short, several advantages can accrue to new graduates who begin their careers as staff nurses. The following are some of the advantages of hospital nursing:

1. As a beginning practitioner you will receive supervision from more experienced nurses who are responsible for guiding you.
2. Your learning needs and skills as a beginning team member will be recognized and provided for.
3. The work load and planned in-service instruction are adjusted to your needs as a beginning nurse.
4. Nursing care assignments and in-service instruction allow you to develop your potential as you demonstrate your effectiveness as a member of the health care team.
5. You lay the groundwork for your advancement in the profession to positions of greater responsibility.
6. You will work under a regular and stipulated pay schedule.
7. Income tax and social security payments are withheld from your check.
8. Many fringe benefits are offered, such as paid vacation, sick leave, retirement plans, and group health insurance.
9. Working an eight-hour day, forty-hour week, offers days of leisure which you can plan and enjoy.
10. You will have the opportunity to work into a higher position.
11. Increments, usually based upon the merit system, serve to motivate you toward self-improvement.

As with any job there are disadvantages associated with hospital nursing as well as advantages. Some disadvantages are:

1. A tendency to "get into a rut" if you are a person who readily becomes enslaved by routine and administrative problems. (This disadvantage can be listed in any area of nursing practice, however.) Establishing a program of self-enrichment is a positive means of avoiding this disadvantage.
2. "Status seekers" have a tendency to underestimate the hospital staff nurse. Keep in mind your own goals as a member of a nursing staff and remember that people who do their assigned jobs cheerfully and competently are always essential. As a member of the nursing staff in a hospital that meets the needs of its community you are truly attaining the objectives which brought you into nursing in the first place.

ADMINISTRATIVE POSITIONS IN HOSPITAL NURSING SERVICES

You will find many opportunities for advancement in hospital nursing service after you have taken time to find yourself and have become oriented to administering nursing care to patients competently and with self-assurance. With experience in giving nursing care, in-service education, and evidence of your initiative and interest in your work, you may qualify as a nursing team leader, assistant to the head nurse, or you may begin to concentrate your efforts on specializing in one area of clinical nursing.

Head nurse. The position of head nurse is basically administrative. It requires knowledge about, and commitment to, all activities associated with the operation of a clinical unit, including administration of personnel and supervision of all care provided in that unit. The head nurse is in charge, and this means she is primarily involved in managing through directing, planning, organizing, and coordinating the operation of her particular unit. A successful head nurse must demonstrate knowledge of these activities, and must be able to apply her knowledge on demand as supervisor, teacher, practitioner, personnel manager, and housekeeper in relation to her area. Above all she must be able to deal with people and be efficient and effective in establishing and maintaining good interpersonal relationships. The head nurse's position is an important one. It is not a beginning position. It is vital to the general morale of a nursing staff that head nurses qualify for their positions by having successfully worked on a beginning staff level, so that they have learned and demonstrated their abilities to meet the standard that they, as head nurses, are expected to enforce.

Supervisor, assistant director, director of nursing service. Such positions as section supervisor, assistant director and/or director of nursing service in a hospital or related agency require preparatory experience and a work record that confirms that the individual is competent to fill the particular position. In many cases, evidence of additional academic work, together with an advanced degree, may be required. These positions demand a broad range of knowledge and ability in the administrative functions as well as nursing skills identified with the particular job. Generally, new graduates of basic programs do not qualify for administrative positions. However, such positions are among areas of nursing service toward which you may wish to direct your future plans.

If eventually you should decide to enter the areas of supervision and administration in nursing service, learn everything you can about the exact qualifications for the position you choose, including necessary educational background. Also be sure you understand exactly what responsibilities you will be expected to assume. Try to get a complete job description. Steer your course accordingly and persevere in your efforts to attain your goal.

PREPARATION FOR NURSING IN SPECIAL CLINICAL AREAS

Nurses wishing to deepen and broaden their professional knowledge and skills in special areas of clinical practice have many opportunities to to so. Over the years colleges and universities have offered courses for advanced preparation in such clinical areas as medical, surgical, maternal-child, and pediatric nursing. Courses in the care of the mentally ill, orthopedic nursing, respiratory disease nursing, operating room techniques, and nursing in diseases of the eye, ear, nose and throat are also available to nurses for specific preparation. More recently, courses have been developed for nursing in coronary care units, intensive care areas, outpatient services, rehabilitation, and geriatric nursing.

Special preparation in these clinical areas consists of advanced classroom studies together with supervised practice work on clinical units. Usually the program is part of a collegiate curriculum that offers a degree with a major in clinical nursing. Specific information acquired in these courses prepares the nurse for more effective administration of a specialized clinical unit. Some programs also offer courses in administrative work associated with the operation of such specialized clinical units. Courses may also be available to provide basic techniques and skills for those interested in teaching nursing students and staff. Prerequisites for such special course work may be experience in basic clinical nursing as well as course work beyond the baccalaureate degree.

Your instructors will probably be able to give you current information about courses, seminars, institutes, and workshops related to continuing education in clinical areas of nursing. You may also wish to check the education section in both the *American Journal of Nursing* and *Nursing Outlook* for information about the location, length of time, and content of supplementary courses offered to graduate nurses working in clinical areas. You may obtain information about colleges and university programs by writing directly to the Department of Nursing or the Admissions Department of the institution in which you are interested. Just as you evaluated schools of nursing before selecting the one you wished to attend for your basic nursing program, so you should select the school that best meets your needs for additional education so that you may effectively work toward the future security and success of your career.

OFFICE NURSING

The nurse who selects office nursing should expect to combine nursing functions with many nonnursing responsibilities. The office nurse works under the doctor or doctors who employ her. The exact qualifications and responsibilities are dependent on the needs of the employer and on the services rendered to patients.

You will need an outgoing personality and

must enjoy meeting the public. You may fulfill the duties of a receptionist when necessary. You should possess a knowledge of secretarial duties such as making appointments, filling out insurance forms, writing statements, and recording the payment of fees. Technical competence in the various nursing skills required is essential. These skills may include preparing for and assisting with specialized examinations and treatments, assisting the doctor with hospital duties, or serving as his representative in community health relations. You will need a willing attitude and a flexible manner in order to be of service to the doctor and to the community.

The opportunities in office nursing include (1) the one-doctor office, in which the nurse is receptionist, nurse, and secretary-clerk; (2) the group-practice office, in which the nurse may also assist in x-ray technology, diagnostic testing, and the teaching of subordinate employees; and (3) the specialist's office, in which a nurse with special skills (for example, pediatric or orthopedic nursing) is needed.

Both the advantages and disadvantages of office nursing can be identified from the requirements just mentioned. The salary will depend primarily upon the amount of professional nursing administered, the locality of the office practice, the clientele of the doctor, and the responsibilities assumed by the nurse.

PRIVATE DUTY NURSING

Private duty nursing is one of the oldest fields of nursing practice and offers opportunities to the new graduate. In the 1950s and 1960s it was believed that coronary care, recovery, and intensive care units (with their specially prepared nurses) would replace the private duty "special" nurse. However, there is still a need for nurses with the desire and the qualifications to administer this kind of individual patient nursing care.

Some of the avenues by which you may enter private practice include local professional registries, direct calls, and enrollment with outside agencies.

Local professional registries. Professional registries are maintained in cities, districts, or states and are available to members of the state and district nurses' association. The names and addresses may be secured from the state nurses' associations or from the Registries section in the *American Journal of Nursing.* Application for placement on the registry may be made in person or by letter. You must comply with the established policies of the agency.

Direct calls. Direct calls may be made for your services by physicians who have previously observed the type of nursing care you administer. Calls may also be made by former patients with whom you have established an excellent reputation and who, in turn, tell others of your abilities.

Enrollment with outside agencies. These may be commercial agencies, which provide for employment on a service fee basis or public health agencies, which utilize nurses for hourly duty or rural nursing plans.

The successful private duty nurse must be especially qualified for the performance of her duties. She should have a pleasing personality and the ability to teach by carefully explaining and demonstrating procedures. Because the nurse is with one patient for eight hours, she must possess qualities of adaptability, ingenuity, tolerance, and understanding. She will find it necessary to provide for some type of self-education in order to keep current in nursing practice, since she is accountable to the physician, the head nurse of the hospital unit, and to her patient for the quality of nursing care administered. She must also display tact, consideration, and cooperation to her patient, his relatives, and visitors.

A few words concerning the professional conduct of the independently employed nurse may be helpful.

1. Follow the rules of the hospital in which you are employed. Fulfill the expectations of the family.
2. Show consideration for the customs of your environment, particularly when you are employed in a variety of hospitals or in the patient's home. Conserve supplies, avoid being demanding, and be willing to

do your part for the benefit of all who are in any way associated with your patient's welfare. Register in and out of the hospital in accordance with established policies for nurses in private practice, and express appreciation for kindnesses shown to you.

3. Observe the professional and legal aspects of private duty, which include: remaining in the employ of the patient, once you have accepted a case, until you are relieved of the assignment; and requesting assistance via proper channels when you need help in caring for your patient.

Some advantages of private duty nursing are listed below:

1. You are your own boss to a great extent. You have the freedom to accept the case and to plan your patient's care. You cooperate with all who are concerned with the patient's welfare and enjoy the satisfactions derived from instructing the patient and his family in the prevention of illness and the restoration of health.
2. You establish contacts and make friends through your association with the patient and his family.
3. You are not tied down to routines and daily duty. You may have variety in nursing environment and patient conditions. You can remain off duty after completing your services on one case until you wish to resume your practice.
4. You receive a salary based on professional standards for services in accordance with the locale and the type of case.
5. You are challenged to give your best in nursing care and experience the satisfaction of seeing the results of it.

As in other fields of nursing, private practice also has disadvantages which need to be weighed along with the advantages. All of the disadvantages of hospital nursing can develop in private practice. You may become bored with the routine. You may also be working overtime, particularly if a relief nurse is not available and you believe the patient needs additional care. You may become dissatisfied because of the competition presented by other fields of nursing and may become critical of the private practice section of the state nurses' association in the development of private duty nurses' interests.

Lack of steady income is another disadvantage. You are responsible for presenting your own statements and for collecting fees. Should the patient be unable to pay or should there be a delay in your receiving payment you must rely on your savings until payment is made.

Provisions are *not* made for sick leave, vacations, or for withholding income tax and social security deductions. You will need to plan your finances carefully to get benefits comparable to the nurse employed in other types of nursing positions.

You do not share in the satisfactions of periodic raises or merit increases in salary accorded nurses employed in other types of nursing; you are responsible for utilizing opportunities for in-service or educational programs to keep abreast with medical and nursing advancements.

Because you are an independent contractor, you assume the total responsibility for your nursing, and you are legally liable for your administrations or omissions.

You are subject to call once you have registered for duty. The type of case for which you will be responsible may be uncertain. Unless you are prepared to care for patients with all types of diseases, you may experience a sense of insecurity in your professional abilities as a private duty nurse.

OPPORTUNITIES IN NURSING EDUCATION

Instructors are responsible for providing sound, detailed instruction in the various courses and for demonstrating the most effective application of nursing skills in patient care. This responsibility is as challenging as it is important, for the lives of patients will depend upon the quality of the instruction a nurse has received. Today's demand for nurses has created an equally urgent demand for instructors in the different types of nursing education programs. In fact, the shortage of skilled nursing faculty members is critical. Obviously, if this shortage of teachers is not corrected, there will also be a shortage of skilled nurses. The solution, of course, is to increase the number of nurses who will devote themselves to teaching.

Father Nicholas H. Wegner, the present director at Boys Town, Omaha, Nebraska, says:

> A good teacher is also a good salesman. He knows how to sell himself. He knows how to sell his subject. He knows how to stimulate the mind, how to arouse enthusiasm, how to quicken the imagination, how to awaken ambition. This is not always an easy thing to do. But the easiest way is not always the best or the wisest way. Resourcefulness, infinite patience, understanding, confidence and perseverance are needed to be a good teacher. But to be a good teacher is one of the highest accomplishments one can hope for.*

After you complete your nursing program and gain some practical working experience, you may wish to consider the challenge of a career in teaching. If this is your decision you should plan to strengthen your foundation of nursing experience in the clinical areas of your choice. You should also plan to continue with your academic training so that you can acquire scientific knowledge and teaching techniques demanded by this career. Information about the educational preparation basic to a teaching career in nursing is available from the National League for Nursing and from the office of admissions of any college or university that offers nursing education programs. Earning a baccalaureate degree is the first step, and a master's degree is required for most teaching assignments in accredited programs and for appointment to a college or university faculty.

Teaching in a school of nursing offers advancement within the profession and the privilege and pleasure of assisting students to become skilled members of the profession. Teachers in nursing may have the opportunity for advancement to positions in the administration of nursing education programs, in research in nursing education, or in shaping the future of nursing education as a consultant with a state, regional, or national agency. Graduate nurses who are interested in the area of education have chosen a field of nursing that provides vast opportunities of rewarding professional contributions and personal satisfactions for a long time to come.

*From Wegner, N. H.: Boys Town Times 34:2, April 10, 1953.

NURSING IN PUBLIC HEALTH

There is a continuing demand for more nurses educated and qualified by experience to work in official public health and community health agencies, to meet not only present needs but also those created as these agencies expand the range and scope of the care they offer. Industries and agencies such as school systems also require nurses prepared to meet specialized health care needs. The need for nurses in public health is especially acute because of the increased number of paramedical personnel who need professional supervision in this field.

The Public Health Nurses' Section of the American Nurses' Association has prepared a list of minimum qualifications to serve as guidelines for nurses who wish to specialize in this area of nursing. (Similar guidelines have been prepared for those interested in occupational health or school nurse positions.) A baccalaureate degree is the minimal education requirement for positions in these areas.

Dr. Ruth Freeman, an educator in this field, has summarized her ideas concerning the skills required:

> 1. The work of public health nursing is done largely in an uncontrolled situation. The equipment, human resources, and predictability of the home situation are quite different from that in the hospital. The person who likes things 'just so' might find it hard to adjust to this.
>
> 2. The work is largely in a non-crisis situation. For some nurses the opportunity to see and know people over a long period of time, to help in simple situations in which the decisions must be made by the family itself, to see individuals and families grow in ability to cope with health problems is immensely satisfying. But the excitement and glamor of the operating room or of the emergency room are rarely found in public health work.
>
> 3. The work of public health is done largely through others. Because the family controls the environment, and because most of the health decisions that must be made can and should be made by the family itself, the importance of working through others is paramount. The school nurse works through the teacher; the occupational

health nurse works through management personnel and foremen.

4. Because public health operates on a broad front, changes occur with great frequency. The family changes its physician, and so the nursing plan must also change; the hospital institutes a new policy in relation to obstetrical care, and public health nursing must support the change; the community changes from a solid, middle-class neighborhood to a near slum or from a quiet village to a teeming suburb, and the nursing program must change as well. If change seems more a chore than a challenge to the nurse, public health nursing is probably not a good career choice.

5. Public health nursing is extraordinarily dependent upon interpersonal relationships for its success. Relationships with individuals, families, special groups, and with many co-workers from different occupational fields may make or break the nursing program. Cultural and social values, social behavior, and the values and ways of behaving of the group being served will differ from those of the nurse in many instances, and require that she adapt her own behavior so as to create a suitable climate for her work. In addition, she may differ with others with whom she works in her values and ways of doing things—the health officer or epidemiologist, the community leader, and the midwife—and these differences must be handled so that they do not interfere with the work. 'Knowing with the heart' as well as knowing the facts is important; trust and confidence may be required under the most unlikely conditions. If managing others or being in control is a great source of satisfaction to a nurse, public health work may prove a disappointment to her.

6. Public health situations are rarely reproducible experiences, and the practitioner must be a constant learner as well as a skillful teacher. She must be able to take advice as well as give it; she must be able to accept help from others with grace.

7. Public health is not a solitary pursuit. The rural public health nurse in particular must declare herself as a part of the community, and must in some measure identify herself with its concerns. Few of the problems of public health are solved individually; the health officer helps to decide how well the tuberculosis nursing visits served their purpose, the sanitarian helps with the problems of the school lunch or accident prevention on the playground. If 'going it alone' attracts the nurse, public health work may prove unrewarding.*

Opportunities for personal growth and professional satisfaction in the area of public health nursing are almost unlimited. If you are truly interested in this field and are psychologically oriented toward the demands of the work you can be certain that your services are needed and that you will find many satisfactions and rewards.

Public health nursing offers the opportunity to practice community nursing. Public health nursing provides a continuity of care for the patient following discharge from the hospital. Nursing under the auspices of a public health agency provides new challenges.

Public health nurses function under one of three types of agencies identified as *nonofficial*, *official*, or *combined agency*, depending on whether the funds for their operation derive from (1) private, voluntary, non-tax-supported resources; (2) tax-supported resources such as those that maintain city, county, state or federal agencies; or (3) a combination of both tax funds, individual donations, and private enterprises.

The insignia on p. 240 identifies one type of public health nursing agency. The insignia was commissioned by Lillian D. Wald* who founded the famous Henry Street Settlement in New York in 1893—today the Visiting Nurse Service of New York. Miss Anna Fillmore, former executive director of VNSNY and a leader in professional nursing, has generously shared the story behind this insignia, the meaning of its symbols being reported by some nursing students from China.

"When Miss Wald was in China, she noticed that members of the same family wore the same insignia on their clothing. She liked the idea of having something to signify that we were 'all one family.' However, she was in Japan before she decided to have such an insignia for the Henry Street Nurses. An artist in Japan developed it from Chinese symbols . . . it means the following: the two outer lines surrounding the pin signify the chorion and the amnion which surround the unborn baby; the three little dots signify grains of protoplasm; the symbols mean we are all of one mother and father, or we are all broth-

*From Freeman, R. B.: Public health nursing practice, ed. 3, Philadelphia, 1963, W. B. Saunders Co., pp. 400-401.

*Miss Wald was enshrined in New York University's Hall of Fame for Great Americans in 1970. She was the first nurse to be so honored.

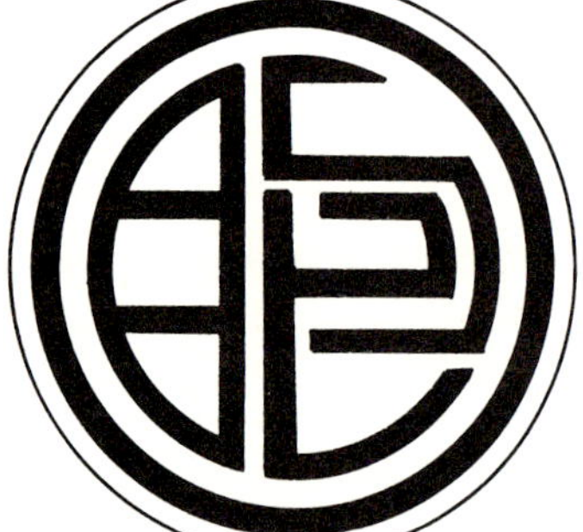

THE INSIGNIA OF VNSNY, BESPEAKING OF A UNIVERSAL BROTHERHOOD

ers—this has been shortened to mean universal brotherhood."*

SCHOOL NURSING

The position of school nurse is closely aligned with functions and responsibilities of nursing based on public health preparation. This area of nursing activity developed from Lillian D. Wald's recognition of the importance of the health of children in schools and the health aspect of the school's environment on their learning.

The nurse who enters the public health area as a school nurse must be interested in the preventive aspects of patient health and welfare and, in addition, must be aware of the trends and expectations of education in the guidance of students.

The duties of school nurses are similar, regardless of type or level of the school. School nurses are expected to correlate their nursing assignments with the teaching activities of the faculty and to function as a liaison with the faculty in planning student health programs, teaching health principles, counseling with students and with parents as indicated, and in meeting the variety of emergencies associated with students' illnesses and injuries.

In some school districts the school nurse is not a member of the official public health agency but is appointed directly by the board of trustees of the school or college. Some states require, in addition to registration and experience, evidence of the prospective applicant's possession of a health and development credential which meets the state board of education requirements, or be eligible to receive a teaching certificate.

The assignment of service and the salary pattern of the school nurse coincides with the established school year and the teachers' pay schedule. It may be necessary for school nurses to attend summer school sessions to meet policy requirements for continued employment.

If you wish to consider school nursing as a career area you should find out whether you should apply to the local board of education, the school or the college in which you are interested, or to the department of public health nursing in the community. Detailed information about requirements for applying and the functions of school nurses will no doubt be discussed by your instructors or by school nurses who are invited to speak to your class group. Opportunities for serving, learning, and growing in professional stature as a school nurse are unlimited.

OCCUPATIONAL HEALTH NURSING

The opportunities for nurses in industry are many and varied. Although some plants or working establishments employ nurses without public health background, the trend is to require public health nursing preparation. The importance of this field of patient care has extended beyond the confines of the plant itself and may include programs of preventive and therapeutic measures to maintain the workers' health.

Originally this area of nursing service was called "industrial nursing." The first nurse was employed in industry in 1895. Over the years

*Permission to reproduce the VNSNY pin and the story of it has been granted by Anna Fillmore, former Executive Director, Visiting Nurse Service of New York.

industries have become aware of the importance of sound health and working conditions for their employees and have added nurses to their working staff.

In 1958, during the convention of the American Nurses' Association, the name "industrial nursing" was changed to "occupational health" to more accurately identify the expanding scope of this type of nursing. The purposes and role of the nurse in occupational health nursing is to meet the needs of the worker and to develop and maintain the highest level of health and efficiency through: (1) prompt care of the ill and injured, (2) maintenance of health and safety educational programs, and (3) cooperation with other health and welfare agencies.

If you are interested in this field of nursing, you should attempt to gain an understanding of the general qualifications and type of experience required. You may also need additional skills such as secretarial talents, including typing and filing procedures. You will be expected to have a broad knowledge of first-aid principles and skills and be able to utilize them with maturity of judgment. You must be able to work directly under the supervision of the plant's medical director in accordance with the policies established.

A good understanding of psychology and its usage in the performance of the job will be beneficial, and a good supply of common sense is a "must." In this field of nursing practice maturity of judgment and a calm soothing demeanor are particularly essential. It is essential, also, that every precaution is taken to avoid any possibility of malpractice claims or legal involvement. Under all circumstances it is expected that the nurse who serves the needs of people in industry shall establish and maintain positive interpersonal relations with fellow employees and be aware of the dignity of her position and the professional image she projects.

To apply for admission into this area of nursing you might plan to visit some of the industrial concerns that employ health service personnel. Make yourself known to the nurses employed there; once they are aware of your interest they may offer information that will aid you to think further about this as a possible career area. Daily newspapers, employment bureaus, or the professional counseling and placement services of your state nurses' association may have information that is helpful. In some instances information about the job and application papers are available through the personnel manager of a specific industrial plant.

The salary offered for these positions depends upon the industry to which you apply and the scale of payment established for nurses' services in the area. Salary usually increases with experience and advanced levels of responsibility. Policies governing employment, sick leave, vacations, and other fringe benefits may offer additional incentives.

A few admonitions are offered for your guidance as a prospective occupational health nurse:

1. It is not so much what job you do in industry that counts but rather the potential you possess for continuing growth and development as a valued worker.
2. Standing orders for administration of care to patients are a protection to both employee and the nurse. Nurses in occupational health assignments should have orders from the medical administrator as a guide for administration of nursing care.
3. Records of illnesses and injuries should be complete in every detail and expressed in simple, succinct language. Such records may become legal documents and a primary resource in the event they are needed in industrial claims.
4. Professional secrecy is of greatest importance. The nurse must exercise prudence in discussing matters both with employees and with management.
5. Knowledge of community facilities, particularly the agencies to which the employee or his family may be referred for health and medical services, is very important.
6. The nurse can play a vital part in the production efficiency of an industry if she knows and carries out those activities for which she is accountable. By efficient use of her skills and her knowledge in the

implementation of preventive and therapeutic programs, she aids in the return of the employee to his work following illness and in increasing his effectiveness on the job.

NURSING IN FEDERAL AGENCIES

UNITED STATES PUBLIC HEALTH SERVICE

Registered nurses interested in beginning positions with the United States Public Health Service may apply to the Division of Nursing for appointments either as a member of the commissioned corps or under the civil service system. In the former instance one's preparation for nursing must include a baccalaureate degree; graduates of diploma and associate degree programs may qualify as applicants by passing required civil service examinations.

Nursing service assignments include work in the various hospitals operated by the Service, the Indian Health Services, or the clinical center of the National Institutes of Health in Bethesda, Maryland. In every area there are opportunities for growth and professional development through clinical nursing, teaching, or research. Continued affiliation with the Division of Nursing may also provide opportunities in consultation and administration to qualified personnel.

Current and detailed information about openings in the Division of Nursing, United States Public Health Service may be obtained by writing to the Office of the Surgeon General, Chief Nurse Officer, United States Public Health Ser-

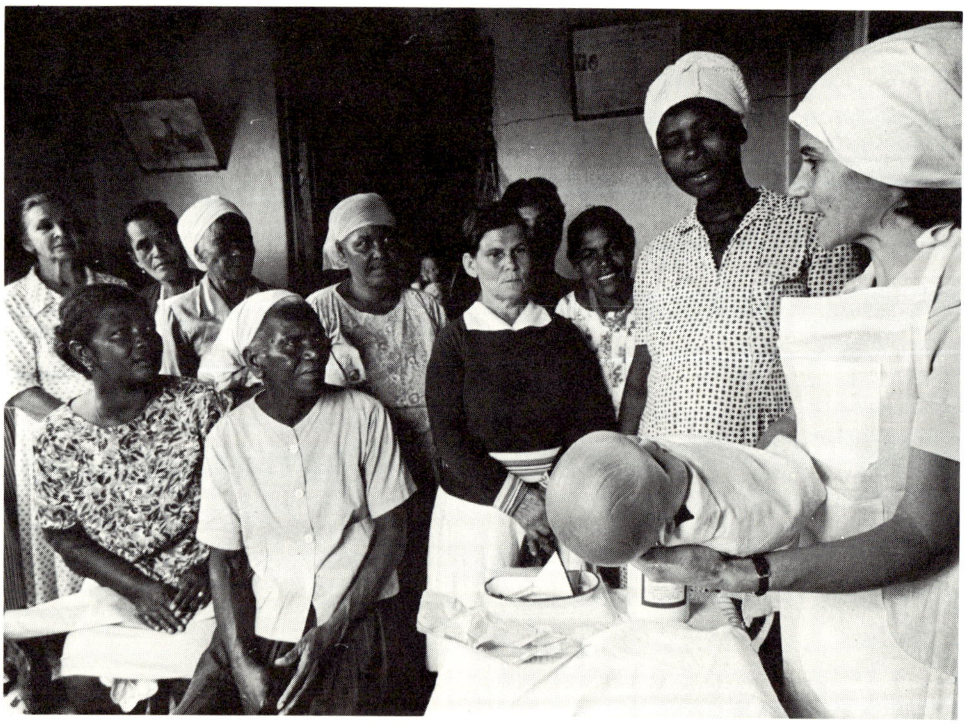

One of the 2,500,000 nurses in the world today reaching out to millions in the rural areas of Brazil—teaching infant care to interested onlookers. (Courtesy World Health Organization; from World Health publication.)

vice, U.S. Department of Health, Education and Welfare, 5600 Fishers Lane, Rockville, Md. 20852.

VETERANS ADMINISTRATION

Nursing service appointments in Veterans Administration hospitals are open to graduates of registered nurse and practical/vocational nurse programs. Hospitals and clinic services are provided for both men and women veterans of the military services. Except for maternity care, most of these hospitals provide facilities in all clinical areas. Some hospitals are exclusively for patients with respiratory conditions or with neuropsychiatric diagnoses.

Nurses serving in this branch of government nursing are eligible for advancement to a higher grade in their work classification with accumulation of work experience and/or educational preparation. Salary increments are based upon merit, and transfer from one hospital to another does not reduce the nurse's salary level or otherwise affect benefits gained through seniority. There are many opportunities for professional growth and education available to nurses working in VA hospitals. Information about the VA hospital system and its nursing services, together with application blanks and the addresses of the nearest area office and hospital facility in your region, may be obtained by writing to the Veterans Administration Headquarters, Nursing Service, Washington, D. C. 20420.

NURSING UNDER MILITARY AUSPICES

Nursing in the military includes service in the Army Nurse Corps, the Air Force Nurse Corps, and the Navy Nurse Corps. Military nurses have responsibilities as nurses and as

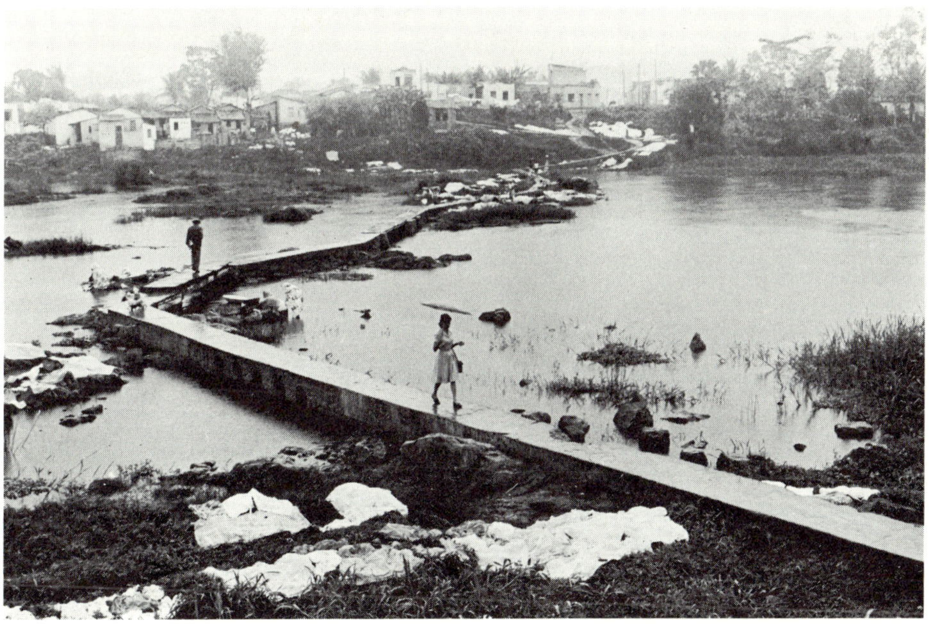

Part of a highly technical staff, this nurse climbs the slippery muddy slope of a hill in Brazil to do her job. Note the housing, sanitation, and laundry facilities amidst which she nurses. (Courtesy World Health Organization; from World Health publication.)

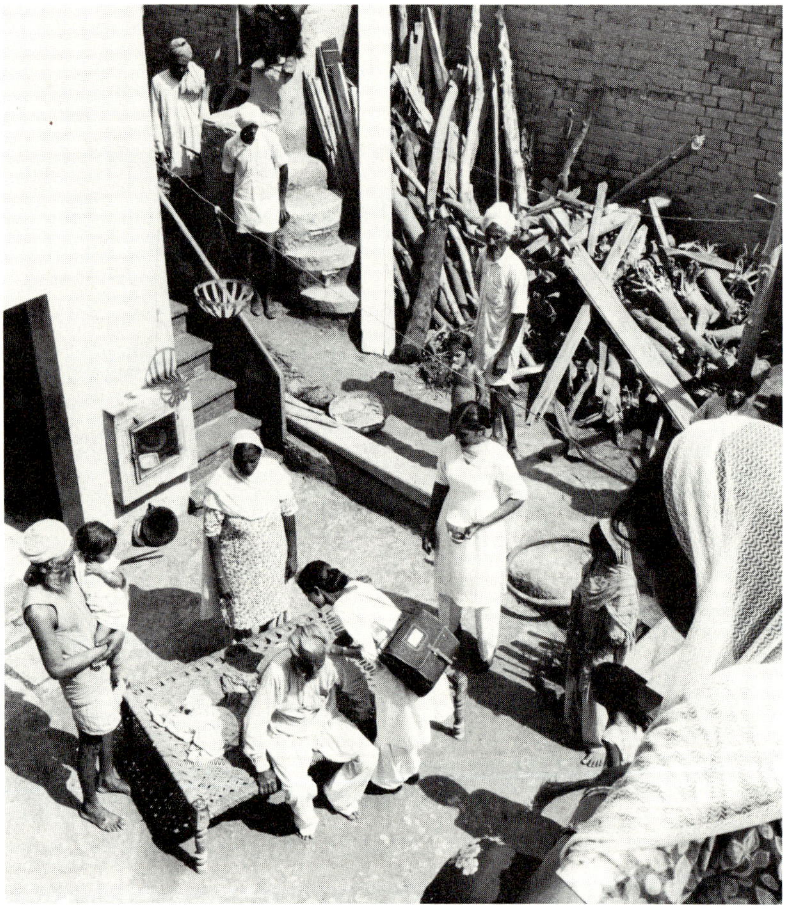

This nurse with advanced education in midwifery and public health nursing serves the people on the streets of India from her post in a primary health center. (Courtesy World Health Organization; from World Health publication.)

officers. They must be adaptable, able to meet challenges rapidly, exactly, and safely. They must utilize mature nursing judgment.

Since the beginning of the Air Force Nurse Corps in 1949, the number of nurses trained in flight nursing has mounted. With space medicine receiving more and more attention, space nursing may be selected as an area of specialization by qualified Air Force Nurses. Nurses serving in the Air Force Corps must be well oriented to the present as well as the future, for they will use knowledge of hospital nursing in peace time and disaster nursing during war emergencies. There are many nursing skills to be developed in even newer forms of air travel.

The Army offers opportunities for the professional nurse to obtain education at a civilian university. The Registered Nurse Student Pro-

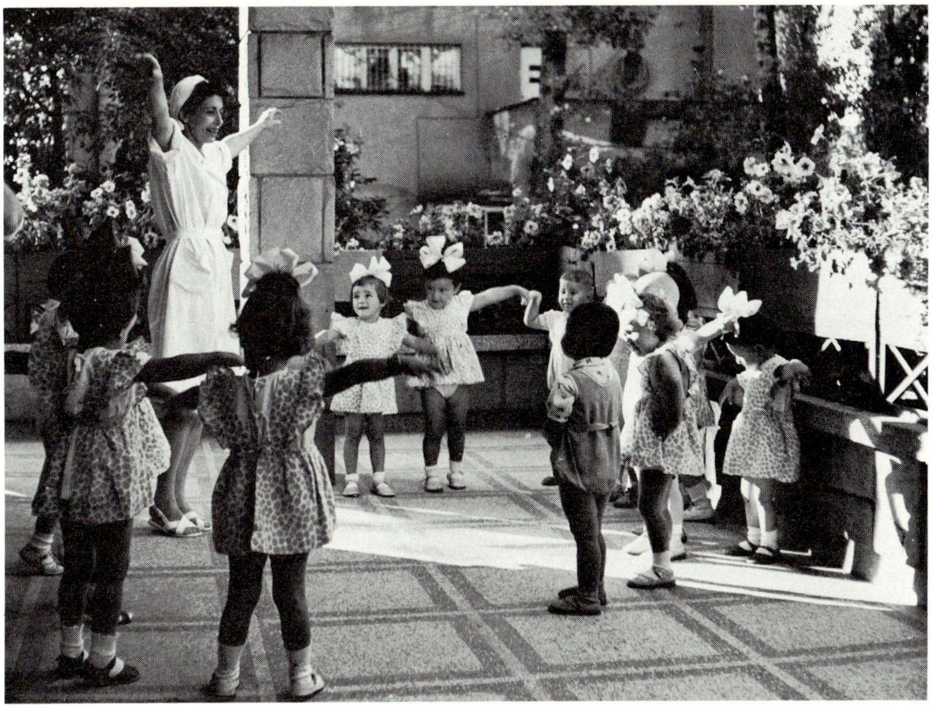

In Bulgaria this nurse is educating the children so that they may grow as healthy young citizens to whom the world may look with pride. (Courtesy World Health Organization; from World Health publication.)

gram is for those nurses currently enrolled in colleges or universities who are studying toward a bachelor's or master's degree. The selected candidates are commissioned and permitted to attend school on a full-time basis. They must be able to complete their education within one calendar year. They receive monthly pay plus allowances, and upon graduation they fulfill a two-year period of service.

The Navy also extends financial assistance to student nurses by accepting Nurse Corps Candidates. It allows qualified senior student nurses from fully approved basic collegiate schools of nursing to join the Navy while continuing their education. Tuition and salary are provided, and the nurse is commissioned as an ensign for the last six months. She is obligated to serve with the Navy for a minimum of two years.*

There are requirements that must be met for nursing for the federal government. The following requirements are maintained for all positions. The applicant must:

1. Be a graduate of a school of nursing which offers a basic curriculum of not less than 27 months (this stipulation automatically exempts graduates of associate degree programs)

*Eligible senior student nurses may apply to the Navy Nurse Corps Candidate Program by writing to the Director of Nurse Corps, Bureau of Medicine and Surgery, Navy Department, Washington, D. C. 20390.

2. Be an American citizen or have declared your intention to become one
3. Have active nurse registration in at least one state for commission (however, applications may be made prior to graduation in all services)
4. Be in good health (you must be able to pass rigid physical and mental examinations)
5. Have good character references, which assure high personal, professional, and moral qualifications
6. Be 21 years of age (the ceiling on age will vary and can be determined for the specific fields)
7. Have no dependents under 18 years of age although applicants may be married (there may be exceptions made for the various fields)

At the present time only graduates of baccalaureate and hospital diploma programs qualify for commissioned officer rank. However, qualifications for service in the military nursing services have been revised in the past. For example, one revision made it possible to grant commissioned officer rank to male nurses, so it is possible that those requirements presently in force may be changed. Registered nurses who look to the military services as an area in which they can make a contribution as members of the nursing profession should be certain that they have current information concerning qualifications for entrance as they plan their future. Information is available from the following sources:

Office of the Surgeon General
United States Army (Nurse Corps)
Washington, D. C. 20314

Bureau of Medicine and Surgery
Nursing Division
Department of the Navy
Washington, D. C. 20390

Office of Surgeon General
United States Air Force (Nurse Corps)
Washington, D. C. 20330

Those who become members of the military nurse corps have opportunities to serve in hospitals, clinics, and special patient care facilities, which are similar to assignments in civilian hospitals, and there is the additional appeal of work assignments in foreign lands. In addition, nurses in military services are afforded opportunities for advancement in areas of administration, teaching, research and clinical specialization.

As officers comparable in rank to officers in other branches of military service, nurse corps members are entitled to similar rights and privileges; they are also subject to any limitations imposed by military regulations. There are many opportunities for professional development and personal growth during a tour of duty and, after twenty years, the nurse is eligible for retirement as an officer with corresponding rights and privileges.

Commissioned rank for the nurse who enters the Armed Forces after the completion of her basic course and state registration now stands as follows:

1. Army Nurse Corps—*second lieutenant*
2. Navy Nurse Corps—*ensign*
3. Air Force Nurse Corps—*second or first lieutenant*

The advantages of nursing with the Armed Forces are numerous and can be found in the pamphlets provided by each service. Among them are the following:

1. Opportunities to travel
2. Generous personnel policies, including retirement provisions after twenty years of service and good insurance programs
3. Recreation facilities
4. The finest hospital equipment and techniques
5. Chances for promotion on merit
6. Uniform dress that is accorded public recognition
7. The same privileges as other commissioned officers
8. Veteran's benefits upon return to civilian life

The disadvantages seem minor in comparison with the list of advantages offered, however, there are a few that can be listed:

1. The nurse must agree to remain in a military service for a definite period of

time (usually two years in the United States or three years for foreign duties).

2. The military training and way of life may not coincide with your professional desires.
3. The "rushing and waiting" routines may not fit your temperament.
4. The deep understanding of human nature and the strength of will power required of military personnel may be beyond your expectations.

For professional opportunities and future security it is hard to match service in the Armed Forces. If you are interested, investigate the field of your choice in greater detail. Read the pamphlets and references listed in the bibliography and talk with those in the services.

NURSING UNDER AUSPICES OF OTHER AGENCIES

Nursing, because it is a socially oriented profession, becomes involved with the problems that affect men's health and well being. Therefore, it is natural for nurses to become interested in and involved with health problems the world over. Nurses who wish to use their knowledge and skills for the service of people throughout the world may wish to consider opportunities for working with such agencies as the World Health Organization (WHO), administered by the United Nations, or the Agency for International Development (AID) and the Peace Corps, both of which are administered by the United States Government.

Nurses who serve in these agencies usually work with nursing personnel of the host country as planners and coordinators of nursing projects. When possible, they leave the planning situation and transfer these directing functions to the nurses of the country with whom they have been working. This work offers a chance to share professional skills and experiences with others, as they share their cultural heritage, their way of looking at the world, and their needs and abilities with you. Meeting and accepting other cultures, standards, and the ways of life is an enormously enlightening and rewarding experience should you choose to join any one of these organizations. If you are interested in nursing assignments of this nature, information about the requirements for application are available from these sources:

World Health Organization
Chief Nursing Officer
Avenue Appia
Geneva, Switzerland

Agency for International Development
Department of State
Medical Division for Foreign Programs
Washington, D. C. 20520

Peace Corps
Nursing Advisor
Medical Program Office
806 Connecticut Ave., N.W.
Washington, D. C. 20525

A LOOK TO THE FUTURE

BELONGING TO YOUR PROFESSIONAL ORGANIZATION

Every nurse who looks to the future with thoughts about opportunities for professional growth should think about the advantages of becoming a member of the appropriate professional association. As a student you are likely to have some experience as a member of a student nurses' association (see Chapter 11) during your basic program. The professional organizations open to you as a graduate licensed nurse will probably be discussed in detail in your classes in professional trends and developments so that you become familiar with their basic philosophy and purposes (see Chapter 25).

Graduates of accredited nursing programs who have earned a state license to practice owe it to themselves to apply for membership in the official nursing association that represents their level of preparation. Nurses, as do members of every other profession, need to recognize and appreciate the advantages, the privileges, the obligations, and the prestige afforded them through affiliation with their official association.

Members of a nursing organization have a voice and a vote in deciding matters pertaining to general policy, legislation, socioeconomic issues, and in the establishment and maintenance of standards that affect their future and that of their profession.

CONTINUING WITH YOUR EDUCATIONAL PREPARATION

If you are thinking about proceeding toward higher goals of achievement in your profession you should start considering the necessity for advanced education for any career in nursing in the future. You may find yourself in a position where you need financial aid either to complete current educational requirements or to plan for future educational programs. Your counselor, your teachers, and other faculty members can inform your about sources of financial assistance from local organizations and service clubs. Check into the possibility of scholarship assistance through state nursing organizations and state departments of health as well as with federal loan funds available through the Office of Health, Education and Welfare. The National League for Nursing can give you information concerning your particular request and perhaps a comprehensive list of possible sources of funds for educational assistance. You should also check monthly issues of the *American Journal of Nursing* and *Nursing Outlook* for information about the availability of grants-in-aid or scholarships and the possibility of new opportunities of education through the establishment of new funds for loans and grants to students who qualify for them.

NURSES EDUCATIONAL FUNDS, INC.*

Nurses Educational Funds, Inc. (NEF) was established by voluntary contributions from individual nurses and their organizations. Gifts from interested citizens and other sources are occasionally received by NEF, and these funds are administered to provide financial aid to nurses who wish to study. NEF is an independent corporation, functioning under the auspices of the national nursing organizations. It grants scholarships, fellowships, and loans to nurses who are interested in professional advancement in nursing. Qualified nurses may enroll in the accredited nursing program of their choice.

The numbers of scholarships and their amounts offered on an annual basis by NEF are determined by the money available and the nature of the applications. Loans are available for a stipulated period for full-time study in a program accredited by the National League for Nursing,* with repayment of the principal at a stated rate of interest. Applicants who desire consideration are advised to write directly to the Nurses Educational Funds, Inc., 10 Columbus Circle, New York, N. Y. 10019, before February 1, preceding the fall in which college entrance is desired. The Executive Committee reviews applications, selects the applicants, and notifies them of their eligibility for assistance in March.

At present approximately fifteen scholarships are awarded annually. The scholarships range from $1,000 to $1,500 each.

If you should decide to avail yourself of one of these educational funds to advance your educational preparation in nursing, there are three steps for eligibility that will need to be considered:

1. Education and experience. All of the financial grants under NEF require that the applicant be a graduate from a state-approved nursing program and that she have state licensure; four of these grants require, in addition, a B.S. degree; all require evidence of eligibility for admission to a college or university, and a minimum of one year's satisfactory experience as a practicing nurse is usually expected.
2. Plan for study. Three of the fellowships require a declared major in a specific subject, the others do not. The length of full-time study for each of the NEF grants is an academic year as defined by the university where student plans to enroll.

*Committee on Careers, National League for Nursing, 10 Columbus Circle, New York, N. Y. 10019. Complete and updated lists and applications may be obtained on request.

*Both baccalaureate programs and master's programs accredited by the NLN are published biannually in the February and June issues of *Nursing Outlook*.

3. Professional identification. All scholarships require two identifications: official evidence of state registration as a nurse and current membership in the American Nurses' Association.

Do not be disappointed if you do not receive acceptance on your first try. The competition for funds and scholarships is great, so it would be prudent to have some alternative plans to reach your anticipated goals.

You are reminded to research the possibilities for financial assistance and to write to the national nursing headquarters for detailed information. You know your interests and your scholastic standing. You know whether or not you are capable of competing with those seeking degrees on the bachelor, or master's, and eventually on the doctorate level. If you are determined to add to your basic education, financial help may be more accessible than you realize.

BIBLIOGRAPHY

ANA First Position Paper on Education for Nursing, American Journal of Nursing **65**:106-111, Dec. 1965.

American Nurses' Association: ANA Position Paper on Nursing Education, ANA in Review **14**:3, (Winter, 1967).

Baccalaureate Council reviews role of physicians' assistant, National League for Nursing News **18**:6, May-June 1970.

Bergen, H. J. A., and Zagormil, D.: Teaching nursing process to beginning students, Nursing Outlook **16**:38-41, July 1968.

Berry, E. J.: Hope docks in Guinea, American Journal of Nursing **66**:2238-2242, Oct. 1966.

Brown, E. L.: Nursing reconsidered, a study of change. Part I, Philadelphia, 1970, J. B. Lippincott Co.

Brune, P., and Shanahan, M.: Teaching Peace Corps volunteers, American Journal of Nursing **65**:96-99, Apr. 1965.

Bulbulyan, A., Davidites, R. M., and Williams, F.: Nurses in a community mental health center, American Journal of Nursing **69**:328-331, Feb. 1969.

Careers for nurses in the federal health programs service, Pub. No. 1922, Washington, D. C., 1969, U. S. Department of Health, Education and Welfare.

Careers in nursing, RN, Feb. 1969, pp. 37-100.

Caudland, L.: The home care administrator, Nursing Outlook **16**:30-34, Jan. 1968.

Cherescavich, G. D.: R. N.—a blurring image? American Nurses' Association Clinical Conference, 1969.

Clemons, B.: Operating room nursing's humane frontier, Association of Operating Room Nurses Journal **12**:54-56, Aug. 1970.

Coakley, J. M., and Parker, J. M.: Education of nurses for school nursing, American Journal of Nursing **65**:84-87, Nov. 1965.

Coffey, K. J.: Nurses and the Peace Corps, American Journal of Nursing **62**:50-52, July 1962.

Colman, M. E.: In service in nursing homes, Nursing Outlook **16**:43-45, Feb. 1968.

Donnelly, A.: The extended care facility as a clinical laboratory, Nursing Outlook **16**:32-35, Feb. 1968.

Douglass, L. M., and Bevis, E. O.: Team leadership in action; principles and application to staff nursing situations, St. Louis, 1970, The C. V. Mosby Co.

Erickson, R.: Visiting wide neighborhoods, Nursing Outlook **14**:34-37, Oct. 1969.

Farrisey, R. M.: Clinic nursing in transition, American Journal of Nursing **67**:305-309, Feb. 1967.

Germain, L. D.: Needed: changes in hospitals to utilize the new practitioner in nursing, Journal of Nursing Education **8**:25, Aug. 1969.

Goldfarb, A. T.: Responsibilities to our aged, American Journal of Nursing **64**:78-82, Nov. 1964.

Goostray, S.: Memoirs: half a century in nursing, Boston, 1969, Nursing Archive, Boston University Mugar Memorial Library.

Guinee, K. K.: The professional nurse, Toronto, 1970, The Macmillan Co.

Harty, M. B.: Trends in nursing education, American Journal of Nursing **68**:1039-1043, Apr. 1968.

Heidgerken, L. E.: Preference for a teaching or clinical nursing practice career, Nursing Research **19**:292-295, July-Aug. 1970.

Henderson, V.: Nature of nursing, American Journal of Nursing **64**:62-65, Aug. 1964.

Heneman, H. C.: Collective bargaining: major instrument for change, American Journal of Nursing **65**:1039-1043, May 1965.

Jacot, M.: Pioneer nurse, World Health **22**:25-29, Sept.-Oct. 1969.

Jackson, H. A.: The psychiatric nurse as a mental health consultant in a general hospital, Nursing Clinics of North America **4**:527-540, Sept. 1969.

Kain, C. M.: Nursing and the Agency for International Development, Nursing Outlook **11**:902-904, Dec. 1963.

Kelly, N. K.: The lure of the hills, Frontier Nursing Service Quarterly Bulletin **45**:17-25, Summer, 1969.

Kelly, Sister M. St. Dominic: In Hong Kong with the Maryknoll Sisters, Nursing Outlook **14**:54-56, Dec. 1966.

Killam, L.: The nursing director as the group facilitator, American Journal of Nursing **70**:1686-1690, Aug. 1970.

Kramer, M.: The new graduate speaks, American Journal of Nursing **66**:2420-2424, Nov. 1966.

Kreuter, F. R.: What is good nursing care? Nursing Outlook **5**:302-304, May 1957.

Levine, E.: Nurse manpower—yesterday, today and tomorrow, American Journal of Nursing **69**:290-296, Feb. 1969.

Mahoney, A. B., and Conlon, A. Y.: Bargaining rights for nurses, American Journal of Nursing **66**:544-548, Mar. 1966.

Maxwell, R. M.: Missionary nursing, Nursing Outlook **11**:895, Dec. 1963.

McGrath, M. E.: Teaching students to teach, Nursing Outlook **15**:69-71, Sept. 1967.

Millard, R.: Liberal and professional nursing education, Nursing Outlook **15**:69-71, Sept. 1967.

Mussallem, H. K.: The changing role of the nurse, American Journal of Nursing **69**:514-517, Mar. 1969.

National League for Nursing: Nursing service without walls, New York, 1963, The League.

Nursing careers among the American Indians, Washington, D. C., 1970, U. S. Department of Health, Education and Welfare.

O'Brien, M. E.: Widening horizons in occupational nursing, International Nursing Review **15**:280, Mar. 1968.

Pellegrino, E. D.: Rationale for education in the university, American Journal of Nursing **68**:1006-1010, May 1968.

Plaisted, L. M.: The clinical specialist in rehabilitation nursing, American Journal of Nursing **69**:562-564, Mar. 1969.

Reese, E. M.: Public health nursing and comprehensive health care, Nursing Outlook **16**:48-53, Jan. 1968.

Richards, J. F.: Integrating a clinical specialist into a hospital nursing service, Nursing Outlook **17**:23, Mar. 1969.

Rutherford, R.: What bothers staff nurses, American Journal of Nursing **67**:315-318, Feb. 1967.

Schmitt, M. H.: Role conflict in nursing, American Journal of Nursing **68**:2348-2350, Nov. 1968.

Schulman, D. P., and Schulman, S.: The nurse as a catalyst, American Journal of Nursing **68**:1890-1894, Sept. 1968.

Stobo, E.: Trends in the preparation and qualifications of the school nurse, American Journal of Public Health **59**:669-673, Apr. 1969.

Uhl, G.: The Division of Nursing USPHS, American Journal of Nursing **65**:82-85, July 1965.

Vaillot, Sister Madeline Clemence: Commitment to nursing, Philadelphia, 1962, J. B. Lippincott Co.

Walker, M.: Today's occupational health nurse, Nursing Outlook **13**:62-65, Nov. 1965.

Whitaker, J. G.: The nurse as a professional person, Nursing Outlook **9**:217-219, Apr. 1961.

Willcox, A. F.: The new professional's practical aspects of the use of new careerists in public service agencies, Mental Hygiene **54**:347-355, July 1970.

COMPLETE WORK SHEET ON PP. 353 TO 356

CHAPTER 25

The official nursing organizations

Both the American Nurses' Association and the National League for Nursing had their origins prior to 1900 (see Chapter 3). However, the revolutions in nursing following World War II brought changes in the numerous organizations that were in existence.

In 1944 a joint committee was formed by the six national nursing organizations then functioning: the American Nurses' Association, the National League of Nursing Education, the National Association of Colored Graduate Nurses, the National Organization of Public Health Nursing, the American Association of Industrial Nurses, and the Association of Collegiate Schools of Nursing. The joint committee was known as The Promoting Committee for the Study of the Structure of National Professional Organizations. This committee was to investigate the organization, administration, functions, and needs of nursing organizations. The study, known as the Structure Study, was directed by Raymond Rich Associates. It was financed by individual nurses, various groups of nurses, and the nursing organizations. The Rich Report offered a beginning for reorganization planning. In 1946 this study was terminated, but studies were continued by the American Nurses' Association and the boards of directors of the six national nursing organizations. The Structure Study originally recommended the unification of all nursing organizations into one group called the American Nursing Organization. Since such a move was not accepted by all of the joint committee on nursing, these groups combined in 1949 to form a Joint Committee on the Structure of National Nursing Organizations for further investigation of the proposals made by the Rich Report.

Each of the six nursing organizations had representation. Their common interests included patient welfare, the provision of nursing care, and the dissemination of health education. However, only two of the organizations, the National League of Nursing Education and the National Organization of Public Health Nursing, admitted lay members. Much work was done by the joint committee on a national level. State and local studies were made to offer individual nurses the opportunity to help in making vital decisions. Publicity was widely circulated in the *American Journal of Nursing* and state magazines concerning the proposed plan for and against one organization. The one-organization plan gave way to the two-organization plan, which seemed to have more advantages. The joint committee believed that unification would better serve the individual members of the profession and more readily meet the changes in society.

In June 1952, at the biennial convention in Atlantic City, the two-organization plan was accepted. The American Nurses' Association continued to function in the interest of *nurses*; a new national nursing organization, known as the National League for Nursing, was formed in the interest of *nursing education and service.*

After the two-organization plan had been in

*Addresses for all of the organizations discussed in this chapter are given in Appendix A, pp. 273 to 274.

effect for six years, a resolution was adopted at the 1958 ANA Convention in Atlantic City that the Board of Directors of this organization invite the NLN Board of Directors to cooperate in appointing a committee to study a one-organization plan for nurses and nursing. Among the resolutions proposed at NLN Convention in 1959 were (1) that these two national nursing organizations merge and (2) that one national nursing magazine be maintained. However, nursing leaders believed that such a proposal would need further consideration, both for the profession's welfare and for the welfare of individual nurses.

AMERICAN NURSES' ASSOCIATION (ANA)

History. The American Nurses' Association is the national professional organization. Only registered nurses are eligible for membership. Formed in 1896 as the Nurses Associated Alumnae of the United States and Canada, its constitution and bylaws were adopted at Manhattan Beach, New York in 1897. In 1901 the bylaws and constitution of the Nurses Associated Alumnae of the United States were incorporated in the state of New York. The Canadian Nurses formed their own association. The name was officially changed to the American Nurses' Association (ANA) in 1911, the name it still bears.

This association was the second to be organized on a national level in the interest of nurses and nursing. The first was the American Society of Superintendents of Training Schools for Nurses formed in 1893. This group became the National League of Nursing Education in 1912 and now exists as the National League for Nursing (NLN). Both the ANA and NLN were approved as nursing's organizations in June 1952, as a result of the Structure Study.

Membership. From the small group of associated alumnae meeting in 1896, total membership in the American Nurses' Association has grown to approximately 204,000 registered nurses. Members are drawn from a federation of fifty-five nurses' associations in fifty states, the District of Columbia, Guam, Puerto Rico, the Panama Canal Zone, and the United States Virgin Islands. There are 862 district nurses' associations.

Fees for annual dues are billed by, and paid to, the national office of ANA. The amount of membership dues retained nationally is established by the House of Delegates at biennial convention. The amount remitted to district and state associations varies for each district and state and is determined by these respective memberships. Registered nurses in good standing interested in any area of nursing practice are eligible for membership. For those nurses who do not anticipate employment during any calendar year, an associate membership is available. The associate member cannot vote, serve as a delegate to convention, or hold an office or chairmanship, but she can otherwise participate and benefit from all organization activities. Because of the limitations placed on an associate membership, dues are proportionately lower. Individual memberships are also available to qualified nurses who reside in a foreign country or territory.

Purposes. The ANA, which is comprised entirely of registered nurses, speaks authoritatively for its membership. ANA seeks to maintain high standards of nursing practice, to promote opportunities for professional advancement, and to improve the economic security and welfare of all registered nurses. Many programs are offered on the national, state, and local levels to implement the avowed purposes of the ANA.

As an ANA member, you are privileged to join one or two of the divisions on nursing practice. There are five divisions, which include community health, geriatric nursing, maternal and child health, medical-surgical nursing, and psychiatric and mental health nursing. Each division attempts to meet the needs of society and of the nurses employed in its area of service. Through active participation, you will receive the benefit of current concepts of research, the interpretation of this research, and guidance as to its implementation through reprints, institutes and workshops, and interaction with other members of your interest group.

Programs. To implement the purposes of the

Text continued on p. 258.

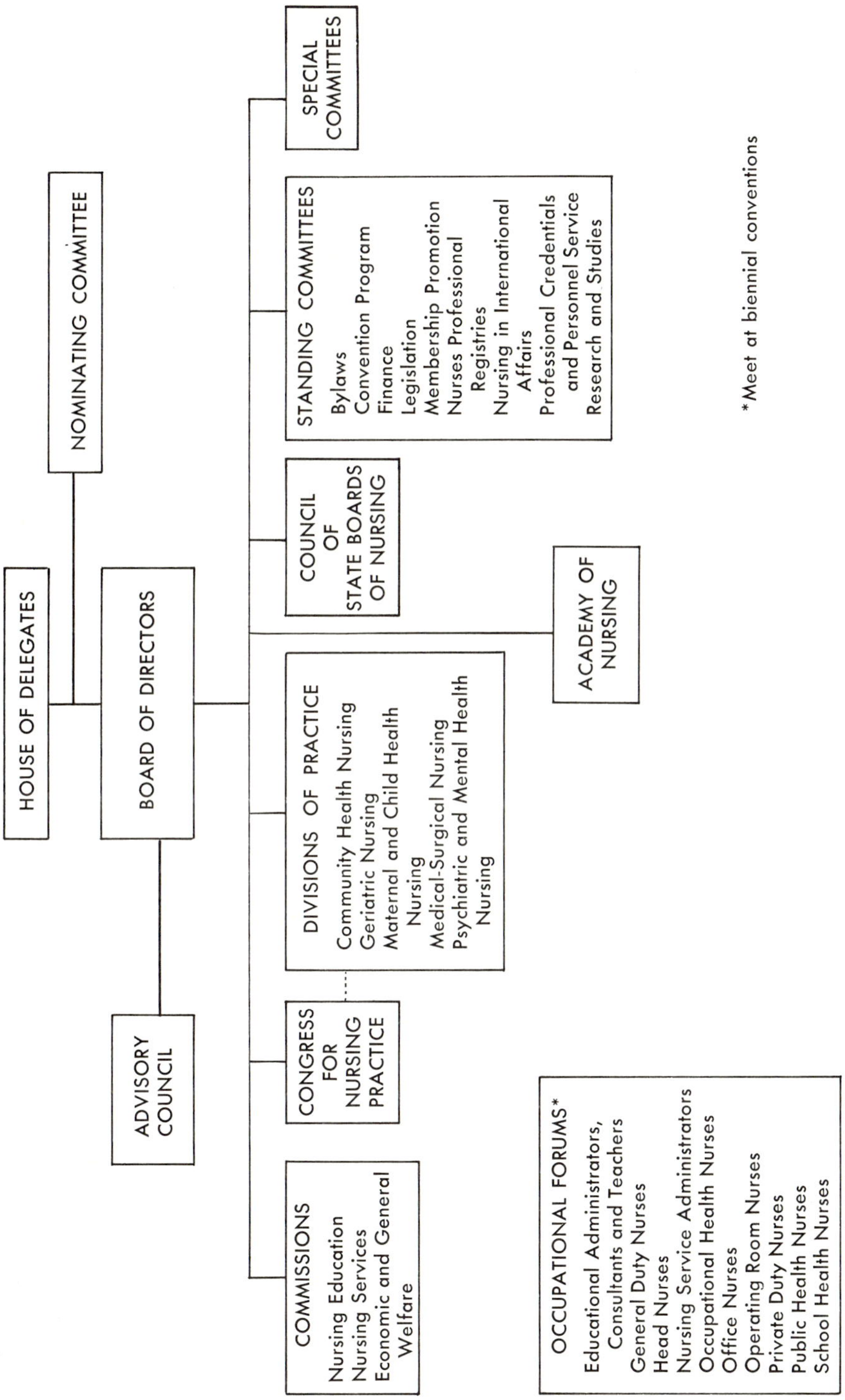

AMERICAN NURSES' ASSOCIATION ORGANIZATION CRART.

this is ANA

75th Anniversary 1896-1971

DATA ON AMERICAN NURSES' ASSOCIATION

What It Is

The national professional organization of registered nurses in 54 constituent state and territorial associations in the 50 states, District of Columbia, Guam, Puerto Rico and Virgin Islands. State nurses associations, in turn, have a total of 869 district associations.

History

Founded in 1896 as the Nurses Associated Alumnae of the United States and Canada. Became the American Nurses' Association in 1911.

Purposes

To foster high standards of nursing practice, to promote the professional and educational advancement of nurses and the welfare of nurses to the end that all people may have better nursing care.

Membership

Registered nurses in all areas of nursing practice are eligible.

Biennial Conventions

Held in even-numbered years in differing sites across the country to provide discussion and information of clinical and general interest to all nurses. Regular meetings of the House of Delegates, ANA's top policy making body, composed of delegates from all constituent associations.

Divisions on Practice

Members may affiliate with one or two of the five divisions on practice: community health, geriatric, maternal and child health, medical-surgical, psychiatric and mental health nursing. The divisions establish standards for nursing practice, provide for recognition of professional achievement, conduct clinical conferences and scientific sessions, stimulate research, and disseminate information to improve nursing practice.

Programs and Activities

Nursing Practice—ANA works continually to improve the quality of nursing care available to the public. The professional association defines the general aspects of professional practice; promotes adherence to ethical standards through a Code for Nurses; and advises on legal aspects of practice.

There are five divisions on nursing practice, each responsible for advancing the standards, knowledge and skills in one of these areas: community health nursing, geriatric nursing, maternal and child health nursing, medical-surgical nursing, psychiatric and mental health nursing.

An executive committee of expert practitioners in each division gives assistance to nurses interested in that area of practice through dissemination of current information relevant to practice, and by conducting various educational conferences. Each executive committee has appointed a standards committee to develop and implement written standards for practice in its area of concern and a certification board to develop and implement recognition of excellence in practice through the process of certification.

A Congress for Nursing Practice establishes the scope of nursing practice, evaluates relevant scientific and educational developments, encourages research, recommends action concerning federal and state legislation related to nursing practice, provides guidance to state committees or councils on practice regarding ethical, legal and professional aspects of practice, coordinates the work of the ANA divisions on practice. The Congress is composed of the chairman of each ANA division on nursing practice and four members who are appointed by the ANA board.

Academy of Nursing—The Association plans to establish an Academy of Nursing for the advancement of knowledge, education and nursing practice. Fellows will be selected for an outstanding contribution to nursing.

Nursing Education—Fundamental to the activities of ANA is the Association's position on nursing education which states that education for nursing practice should take place in the general educational system.

A prime ANA task is the implementation of the education position. To accomplish the orderly transition of nursing education into educational institutions, the Association has issued several major statements calling for community planning for nursing education throughout the United States.

ANA works to set standards and policies for nursing education. Activities of the ANA Commission on Nursing Education include the evaluation of relevant scientific and educational developments, changes in health needs and practice as they apply to nursing education; the encouraging and stimulating of research in all areas of nursing education and formulating policy and recommending action concerning federal and state legislation in the field of education.

Through the ANA-NLN Nursing Careers Program qualified people are recruited into nursing education programs. Particular emphasis is given to the career development of the registered nurse.

The Council of State Boards of Nursing, which includes one representative from each State Board of Nursing, establishes policies for the development and use of the State Board Test Pool Examination for nurse candidates in all states. State Boards are authorized by state law to license nurse practitioners.

The Council also recommends methods and procedures to encourage reasonable uniformity in state board standards and practice to facilitate interstate licensure. Another Council activity includes developing materials for use by boards in the approving of basic nursing education programs.

Through national annual meetings and education conferences ANA provides Council members with information on national trends and changes in nursing education, nursing practice and nursing services.

Nursing Services—ANA works to improve the quality of nursing services in all settings.

The ANA Commission on Nursing Services works to develop standards and guides, and to assist in other ways to bring about improvements in the organization and management of nursing services. The Commissioners are responsible for evaluating scientific and educational developments, changes in health needs and practices and their implications for nursing services, changes in health needs and care and estimating requirements for nursing manpower and resources. It formulates and recommends policy related to federal and state legislation where it affects the organized nursing services.

ANA maintains liaison with allied health groups such as the American Hospital Association, the American Society of Hospital Pharmacists, and the National Federation of Licensed Practical Nurses.

Plans for essential nursing services in the event of natural or man-made disaster have been developed by the ANA Committee on Emergency Health Preparedness and National Defense. This committee has developed criteria and guidelines for utilization of registered nurses in the event of disaster and has enumerated nursing functions that should be expanded during national emergency.

Continued.

Economic and General Welfare–This program is based on the principle that nurses have the right as well as the duty to participate in determining their salaries and conditions of employment. The program is carried out on local, district, state and national levels. The aim is to assure that (1) nurses receive fair compensation and benefits for their professional services, (2) employment conditions are conducive to providing high quality nursing care and (3) the number of qualified nurses necessary to meet the nation's health care needs is recruited and retained. To this end ANA advises and assists the constituent state nurses associations (SNA's) which in turn act as the representatives of nurses in all employment settings.

The ANA Commission on Economic and General Welfare formulates policies of the economic security program and has a program which provides direct assistance to SNA's on projects related to organizing and representing nurses. Commission responsibilities include developing and implementing general economic standards and an economic education program; formulating policy and recommending action related to federal and state economic security legislation interests; and studying and evaluating the economics of health care as well as the economics of nursing.

Government Relations ANA studies and interprets trends in government and promotes legislation relating to nurses, nursing and health. ANA assists state nurses' associations in promoting nursing practice acts that adequately protect the profession and the public from unqualified practitioners and offers consultation on other state legislative measures affecting nurses. ANA speaks for nurses in promoting federal health, education, civil rights and other social legislation that affects the health and well-being of the public, and facilitates communications between the respective programs of the Association and appropriate government agencies.

Intergroup Relations–Since the need for nursing services is universal, ANA works for full integration of all qualified nurses into the profession. Membership and full participation in the Association is open to all registered nurses. ANA, through its Divisions, Commissions, and committees at the national level and through state and district associations, promotes equal opportunities in education, employment and advancement in nursing and supports and assists in the implementation of civil rights legislation so that all people have access to health care.

International–The American Nurses' Association is the United States representative in the International Council of Nurses, participating with 74 counterpart national nurses' associations in programs to improve nursing practice and to meet health care needs. ANA supports the United Nations and its specialized agencies. It works cooperatively with State Boards of Nursing, state nurses' associations, and U.S. government departments in maintaining and interpreting nursing standards as they relate to alien nurses entering the United States. The ANA serves as a central source of nursing information for inquiries from overseas and for Americans seeking information about nursing abroad.

ANA Professional Credentials and Personnel Service–Provides professional record service for members, and encourages and supports counseling and placement activity by state nurses' associations. A cumulative record of the nurse's professional education and experience, including references from previous employers, is compiled and updated as needed throughout the nurse's professional career. A summary of the record, called a professional biography, is sent to employers on request by the nurse. Information about employment opportunities is available from state nurses' associations.

Public Relations–Information about ANA programs, activities and goals is disseminated to nurses, the public, allied professional and health groups, the government and its special agencies through the public relations department for the purpose of education and interpretation, and to win understanding and support for ANA programs.

Research and Statistics—ANA studies are made relating to the program interests and needs of the Association. Current and comprehensive manpower and economic data are compiled and analyzed. Information about ANA and its membership, informational support to all ANA departments and programs, and information to nurses and the public is disseminated through *Facts About Nursing* and other reports.

The ANA Commission on Nursing Research encourages and stimulates research in all areas of nursing. Its responsibilities include participating in the establishment of standards of nursing research; recommending priorities for the profession's research concerns; assisting organizational units in identifying research needs to expand nursing knowledge; assisting constituents in developing nursing research programs; developing and disseminating research-related documents; assisting in the dissemination of nursing research findings; conducting nursing research workshops; developing and maintaining liaison with appropriate groups, such as the American Nurses Foundation.

Advisory Council

ANA's Board of Directors and two representatives of each constituency, meet three times a year to discuss new developments, proposals for changes in policy, and suggestions for ways to strengthen and advance the Association's activities. This meeting is called by the Board of Directors or a majority of the constituents.

Research Foundation

ANA sponsors the American Nurses' Foundation which was established in 1955 and which has as its objectives conducting and promoting scientific nursing research in patient care, providing financial support for research, providing interdisciplinary research experience, disseminating and promoting dissemination of research findings, and conducting experimental investigation in methods of implementing research results.

Student Association

The American Nurses' Association maintains close relationship with the National Student Nurses' Association as the preprofessional organization for nursing students. NSNA is a separate legal corporation.

There is an ANA-NSNA Committee on Common Interests and Goals and similar committees are being established in a number of states. Through this liaison committee and through board-to-board contacts, augmented by close working relationships of the headquarters staffs of the two organizations, registered nurses and nursing students work together.

Official Publications

American Journal of Nursing, published by the American Journal of Nursing Co., an ANA wholly owned subsidiary. *Facts About Nursing,* annual statistical sourcebook of latest data and information on nurses and nursing. *ANA in Action,* the membership publication which provides information on Association and nursing activities.

National Officers

President, Hildegard E. Peplau, Ed.D., Madison, New Jersey; *First vice-president,* Mrs. Evelyn Cohelan, Ed.D., Washington, D.C.; *Second vice-president,* Jessie M. Scott, McLean, Virginia; *Third vice-president,* Virginia M. Paulson, Minneapolis, Minnesota; *Secretary,* Josephine A. Brandt, Moline, Illinois; *Treasurer,* Rosamond C. Gabrielson, Phoenix, Arizona.

Headquarters

Maintains national offices at 10 Columbus Circle, New York, New York, 10019. For further information write to: Eileen M. Jacobi, Ed.D., Executive Director or Mrs. Anne. R. Warner, Public Relations Director.

American Nurses' Association
10 Columbus Circle, New York, N.Y. 10019

American Nurses' Association as stated in its bylaws, many programs are conducted.

Government relations program. Government relations programs are promoted on federal, state, and district levels. The association speaks for nursing when pending legislation concerns general health and welfare programs or reflects directly on the nurse practitioner. An advisory staff and office for the purpose of monitoring proposed legislation is maintained at the New York headquarters* and in Washington, D. C.,† so that the association may assist any of its constituencies.

Research and statistics program. The research and statistics program conducts surveys of available nurse resources, collects data concerning American Nurses' Association membership, and conducts research relative to the advisability and application of association programs. Publication of *Facts About Nursing,* and other reports of research studies are also a part of this program.

Public relations program. The public relations program interprets ANA and its activities to nurses, allied professional and health groups, the government and its special agencies, and the public. It provides an education and information service for the nursing profession.

Organization services program. This group strives for improved intergroup relationships and correlates activities of interest and importance on national, state, and district levels. The group is comprised of staff members assigned to special interest areas, and members serve in an advisory capacity at all levels.

The Professional Credentials and Placement Service (PC and PS) serves graduate registered nurses who are members of ANA. This program maintains a cumulative record of the educational achievement and professional experience (and references) of nurses and offers assistance to nurses in choosing positions so that there will be maximum nurse-employer satisfactions.

Nursing education program. The ANA Commission on Nursing Education assists in establishing educational standards for the preparation of nurse practitioners. This program attempts to correlate the education of the nurse to the health needs of the nation.

State boards of nursing. A committee of state boards of nursing is composed of one representative from each jurisdiction. It meets annually and considers problems and makes recommendations in regard to optimum standards relating to licensure, education, and Nurse Practice Acts.

Nursing practice program. The Congress on Nursing Practice, the five Divisions of Nursing Practice (Community Health, Geriatric, Maternal and Child Health, Medical-Surgical, and Psychiatric and Mental Health Nursing), and other related programs all strive to implement the ANA Code for Nurses. This implementation of the code assures quality nursing care, that is safely and ethically administered. Through this program it is hoped ANA will establish an Academy of Nursing with Fellows selected for an outstanding contribution to nursing as designated by the Nursing Practice divisions.

Economic and general welfare program. The ANA Commission on Economic and General Welfare is responsible for implementing the American Nurses' Association's economic security program. This program is based on the premise that nurses have the right to a voice in establishing the conditions under which they will work. The economic security program is established to promote and protect the economic status of nurses. The American Nurses' Association supports legislation related to the economic welfare of all people including nurses, and the state nurses' associations implement the economic welfare programs of the national organization by representing nurses and negotiating with local employers.

International program. The ANA supports international relationships in nursing and is an active member of the International Council of Nurses. It implements the program for exchange of nurses between the United States and other countries for educational and service training. The ANA has been designated as an official sponsor of the United States State Department Exchange-Visitor Program and is responsible for

*10 Columbus Circle, New York, N. Y. 10019.

†1030 Fifteenth Street, N. W., Washington, D. C. 20005.

determining the qualifications of nurses coming to the United States and for assisting them in adjusting to employment conditions. As a national association of nurses the ANA is also instrumental in securing the type of education and experience that will be profitable to the foreign nurse and will benefit the nursing profession in her own country. This program challenges the interests of nurses in their fellowman and enhances international fellowship among nurses. The ANA supports the United Nations and the World Health Organization in their various activities.

As a registered nurse you may join:

The American Nurses' Association (ANA)
1—Membership is attained through district or state associations, or, in special cases, by direct application to the national office.
2—Dues are determined according to organizational needs. They will be established to include district, state, national, and international dues.

↓

Your State Association of ANA
1—Membership is in the state where you are employed. It will provide programs of individual interests in nursing.
2—Dues will be itemized with the national billing and forwarded by national to your state.

↓

Your District Association of ANA
1—Membership is in the district where you are employed. It will provide programs of individual interests in nursing.
2—Dues will be itemized with the national billing and forwarded to your district.

The International Council of Nurses
1—Membership is automatically attained by national membership from nations retaining such membership.
2—Dues are determined on a per capita basis according to membership of a national association. They are forwarded by the treasurer of ANA.

The nursing organizations offering membership to every registered nurse through ANA.

Special points for consideration. The first president of the ANA was Isabel Hampton Robb. The current presidents are voted on at the biennial conventions by the membership through representation in the House of Delegates, the highest authority in the association. Hildegard E. Peplau, R.N., Ed.D., is the current president and Eileen M. Jacobi, R.N., Ed.D., is Executive Director. The name of the president may be obtained from the Directory of the *American Journal of Nursing,* which supplies information concerning national, federal, and state organizations.

Meetings are held on a biennial basis in the larger cities of the United States that can accommodate the number of nurses who attend.

The Coordinating Council is composed of officers and board members of the ANA and the NLN. This council coordinates areas of mutual concern to both organizations. The National Student Nurses' Association functions as an independent organization under the auspices of this council. The official publication of ANA is the *American Journal of Nursing.*

THE INTERNATIONAL COUNCIL OF NURSES (ICN)

All members of the American Nurses' Association are also members of the International Council of Nurses. The International Council of Nurses is a federation of fifty-nine national associations of nurses. The purpose, as stated by the Council, is "to attain high standards of Nursing Service and Nursing Education, to develop Nursing as a Profession and to safeguard the Social and Economic Welfare of Nurses in their own countries."*

As a member of ICN, you have the opportunity to contribute to international understanding and cooperation.

*International Council of Nurses, London, England, 1962, The Council.

History. The International Council of Nurses is the oldest international association of professional women. It was organized in 1899 by an English nurse, Mrs. Bedford-Fenwick, who was assisted on a provisional committee by nursing leaders from several countries. Mrs. Bedford-Fenwick became the first president of ICN, and the constitution was adopted in 1900. The first meeting of the Council was held in Buffalo, New York, in 1901.

Membership. Originally nurses were admitted as individual members, but by 1904 there were three countries that had national organizations sufficiently organized for affiliation with the ICN as charter members: England, Germany, and the United States.

The ICN offers its members many activities of interest to nurses. Members can attend international congresses and conferences, and they have the opportunity to visit other countries for study, employment, or observation. These exchanges are sponsored by the Exchange of Privileges Programme of the ICN. Members of the ANA can also receive information, advice, and assistance from the ICN Information Centre.

ICN publications serve to keep the nurse informed about new developments in nursing and nursing education in all parts of the world.

Special points for consideration. The headquarters for the International Council of Nurses is located in Geneva, Switzerland.

The official publication of the ICN is *The International Nursing Review,* which is an illustrated bimonthly journal. Articles on nursing and allied subjects are published in English, German, and Spanish. The *Review* is available in more than one-hundred countries.

An International Congress is held every four

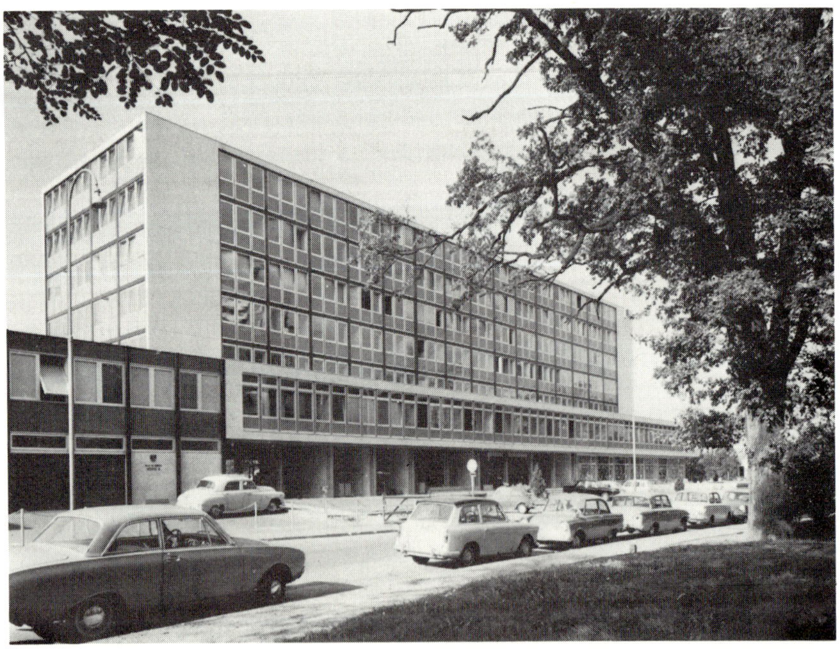

HEADQUARTERS OF INTERNATIONAL COUNCIL OF NURSES
(ICN photograph)

years. Occasionally interim conferences are held to discuss professional problems. The city chosen for a Congress is decided according to invitations received from member associations and is voted on by the ICN Grand Council. The country in which the Congress is held is responsible for some of the arrangements for the Congress. The 1965 Congress was held in Frankfurt Main, Federal Republic of Germany, and the 1969 Congress met in Montreal, Canada. The 1973 Quadrennial is scheduled to be held in Mexico City. Margrethe Kruse of Denmark was elected president at the 1969 Congress with Dorothy A. Cornelius of the United States as first vice president, Alice Girard of Canada as second vice president, and Ruth Elster of Germany as third vice president.

Adele Herwitz of the United States was appointed as the executive director of the International Council of Nurses in 1970. She had served as acting director of the ICN for six months prior to her appointment.

The following is a summary of the international functions of the ICN:

1. ICN is on the Consultative Register of the Economic and Social Council. All members of the ICN therefore have direct contact with the United Nations and its specialized agencies.
2. The ICN is officially connected with the World Health Organization (WHO).
3. The ICN acts in a consultive capacity for nongovernmental organizations. A list of such consultive agencies is maintained by the International Labor Organization.
4. The International Council of Nurses is a member of the International Hospital Federation and the World Federation for Mental Health.
5. The ICN works in cooperation with the International Committee of the Red Cross, League of Red Cross Societies, World Medical Association, International Confederation of Midwives, United Nations Educational Scientific and Cultural Organization, United Nations International Children's Emergency Fund, and Union of International Associations.

Committee activities and dissemination of professional information are a part of ICN. The members of the functioning committees are nominated by the member national nurses' associations and are elected by the Board of Directors for the subsequent quadrennial period. Reports of the activities of the committees and other professional information are distributed to the membership from headquarters. Research in nursing is promoted and conducted by the headquarters staff.

The Florence Nightingale International Foundation (FNIF) was established as an educational trust in 1934. Its purpose was, and is, to be a living memorial to Florence Nightingale.

During World War II the activities of the foundation were necessarily diminished. Reorganization in 1949 resulted in its establishment as the Educational Division of the International Council of Nurses.

In 1957 it was decided that the FNIF should come more closely within the administrative framework of the ICN, and a division called the Florence Nightingale Education Division was established. Its purpose is to undertake the current educational work of the organization previously carried on by the FNIF.

An Exchange of Privileges Programme has been provided through the ICN. This program, which offers individual nurses the opportunity to study and work in other countries, has contributed to the improvement of standards and the understanding of nursing internationally. The ANA International Unit implements the international exchange of nurses in this country. Through the Exchange of Privileges Programme, nurses may obtain assistance from their national organization to study or work in other countries for a temporary period. Prospective exchange visitors should request information from ICN headquarters or the national ANA headquarters concerning salary and employment, student or tourist visa privileges, and work-study experiences which have been made available to nurses who seek exchange.

ICN services for student nurses include the facilities of its information center. The center promotes the national student nurses associations and gives advice concerning their establishment and development. Contact among national student nurses associations and among individual student nurses throughout the world is encouraged. Student nurses are permitted to attend ICN Quadrennial Congresses. By being a member of a national organization, you share in the privileges of the activities of this international organization. You will learn of international relationships and nursing needs and may aspire to becoming an active member in the years to come.

THE NATIONAL LEAGUE FOR NURSING (NLN)

History. In 1893 the first national organization for nurses was formed during the Chicago World's Fair under the title of The American Society of Superintendents of Training Schools for Nurses. This society admitted members from America and Canada. In 1907 the Canadian nurses withdrew, and in 1912 the name of the organization was changed to the National League of Nursing Education. This organization functioned effectively until it was concluded that greater efficiency could be obtained by revamping the organization plan for American nurses. In June 1952, the National League of Nursing Education gave way to the new organization, the National League for Nursing. This organization speaks for members on matters related to nursing service and nursing education. It cooperates with other national organizations and federal agencies for improvement of the health and welfare of the American people.

Having studied in detail the organization of the American Nurses' Association, consider the details of the membership organization chart of the NLN, which is presented on p. 263.

Membership. Both individual and agency memberships are available in the National League for Nursing.

Individual membership is open to anyone interested in nursing—both nurses and laymen. Agencies offering health care services or involved in the preparation or education of health care personnel are eligible for agency membership.

Under the new structure there are forty-five state constituent leagues for nursing, one metropolitan constituent league (Cleveland), and another in the District of Columbia. The presidents of these constituent leagues, plus the chairmen of the two division coordinating committees, make up the Assembly of Constituent Leagues for Nursing. This assembly helps to implement the program of the NLN. Interest groups in local areas work with constituent leagues to further the work of the organization.

In addition to membership in a constituent league, membership is also organized into two divisions and seven councils. The two divisions are the Division of Individual Members and the Division of Agency Members. The Division of Individual Members has one council, the Community Planning for Nursing, to which all individual members belong. Agency members select the council in their area of interest: Associate Degree Programs, Baccalaureate and Higher Degree Programs, Diploma Programs, Hospital and Related Institutional Nursing Services, Practical Nursing Programs, and Public Health Nursing Services. Each council elects its own leadership.

Purposes. The National League for Nursing fosters the development and improvement of nursing education and of nursing service.

Programs. Specific services related to nursing education include the NLN's Evaluation Service, which offers achievement tests to schools of nursing and examinations for use in the selection, guidance, and placement of students in basic professional, graduate nurse, and practical nurse programs. The Service also offers licensing examinations for use by state boards of nursing.

The NLN accrediting program nationally accredits schools of nursing and the NLN Committee on Careers conducts a national nursing recruitment program, which is co-sponsored by the ANA, the American Hospital Association, and the American Medical Association. This committee further sponsors the approximately 4,000 Future Nurse Clubs, which are organized in high schools throughout the country.

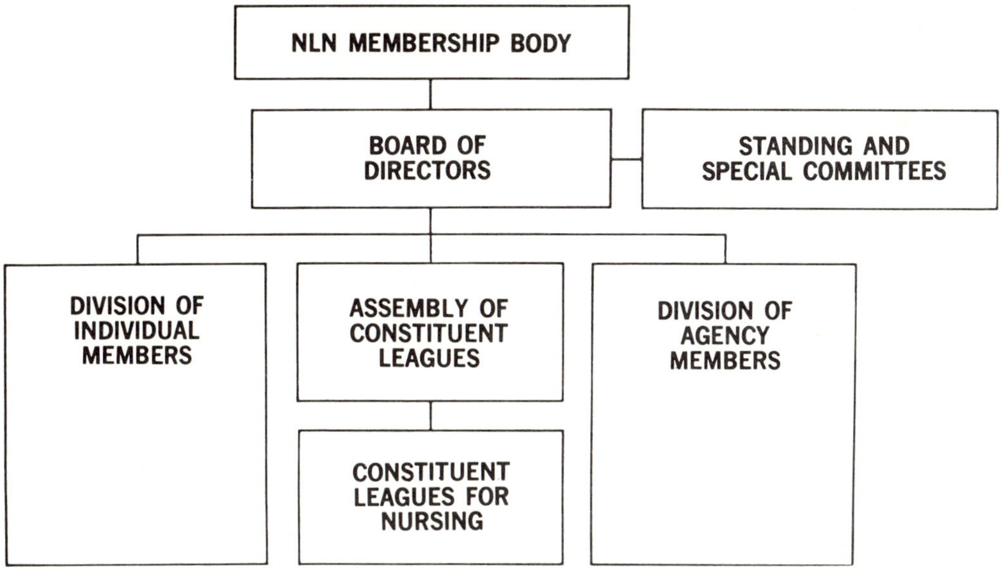

NATIONAL LEAGUE FOR NURSING

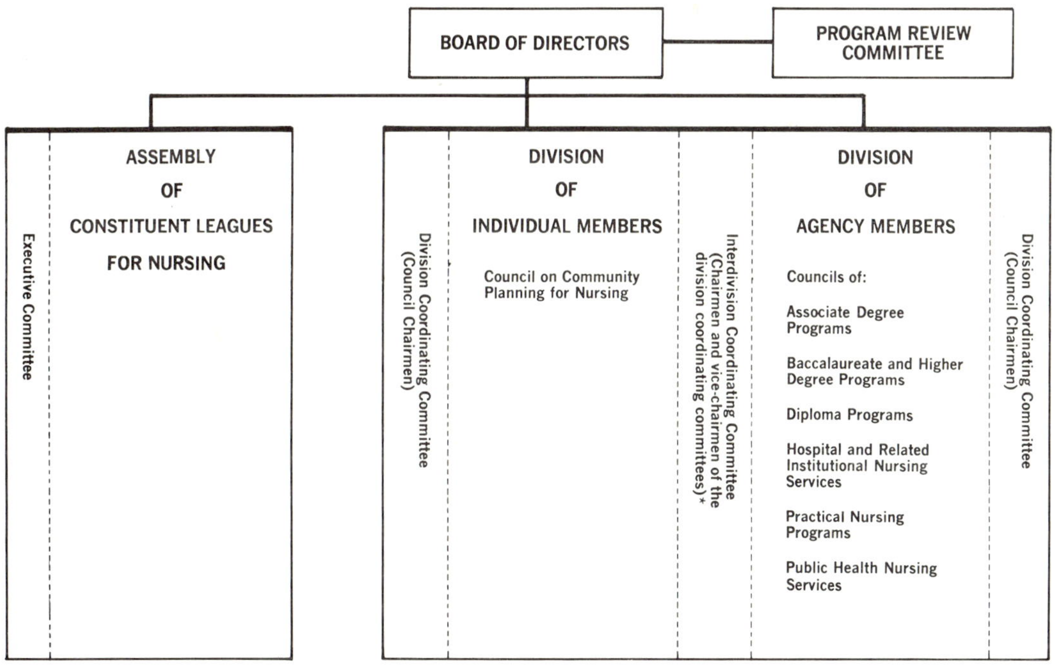

* Also the chairman and vice chairman of the Assembly of Constituent Leagues for Nursing by vote of the NLN Board of Directors, January 1968.

2

NATIONAL LEAGUE FOR NURSING ORGANIZATION CHARTS.

Services of the NLN to improve nursing service include encouraging and assisting action groups and constituent leagues to develop programs to meet the changing nursing needs of society. The NLN also assists nursing staffs in hospitals and extended care facilities in the utilization of new techniques of patient care. Other services include motivating and preparing qualified leadership personnel for nursing education and nuring service and establishing and maintaining high standards of education in the facilities preparing nurses.

NATIONAL ASSOCIATION FOR PRACTICAL NURSE EDUCATION AND SERVICE (NAPNES)

History. A small group of professional nurses involved in practical nurse education organized the Association of Practical Nurse Schools in 1941. Their purpose was to improve and to standardize the education and preparation of the practical nurse. The Association of Practical Nurse Schools became the National Association for Practical Nurse Education in 1942. The addition of "and Service" to its name in 1959 identified the purposes of this association in preparing qualified licensed practical nurses to meet the needs of the consumer of their services.

Membership. NAPNES welcomes both individual and group membership. Individual membership is open to all nurses, both licensed practical and registered, as well as to faculty and students of schools of practical nursing. Eligible for individual membership, also, is anyone interested in practical nursing. This includes all health service personnel (professional and nonprofessional), consumers of nursing service, and vocational and general education personnel. Health agencies, health facilities, alumnae associations of schools of practical nursing, and practical nurse associations may become group (or agency) members.

Organization. The Board of Directors is the governing body of the National Association for Practical Nurse Education and Service. Serving on the board are representatives from hospital administration, medicine, nursing, and vocational and general education.

Purposes and programs. NAPNES serves as the accrediting agency for practical nurse education programs, provides consultation service to upgrade all existing and new schools, offers continuing education programs for educators and practical nurses, attempts to meet the needs of licensed practical nurses through workshops and conventions, and publishes a list of schools of practical nursing accredited and approved by its organization.

The official publication of NAPNES is *The Journal of Practical Nursing.*

NATIONAL FEDERATION OF LICENSED PRACTICAL NURSES (NFLPN)

History. The National Federation of Licensed Practical Nurses (NFLPN) is the organization of licensed practical or vocational nurses. Organized in 1949 and incorporated in the State of New York, NFLPN serves as the national voice of all licensed practical or vocal nurses. It is a federation of constituencies (state associations), which include divisional associations and members-at-large.

Membership. Membership is open only to licensed practical (vocational) nurses. A member may either join through the state association or directly through the national office.

Purposes. The purposes of the NFLPN all emanate from three primary goals. These are (1) to improve the quality of nursing administered by practical nurses, (2) to ensure the economic and general welfare of all licensed practical (vocational) nurses, and (3) to help the licensed practical nurse meet the health needs of the American people.

Organization. Through representation in the House of Delegates, each NFLPN member assists in developing policies and programs of the organization. The House of Delegates consists of elected representatives from each state constituency. These representatives elect the Executive Board, which includes officers and board members. The Executive Board transacts all business of the association requiring specific action between conventions.

The official publication of NFLPN is the

American Journal of Practical Nursing which is published bimonthly.

RELATED NURSING ORGANIZATIONS

AMERICAN ASSOCIATION OF NURSE ANESTHETISTS (AANA)

History. The American Association of Nurse Anesthetists was founded in 1931 by a group of forty nurse anesthetists. They were the first nurses specialists to organize. One of the prime concerns of the AANA was the development of a national examination for nurse anesthetist and a program for the inspection and evaluation of schools of anesthesia. From 1933 to 1940, in cooperation with the American Hospital Association, the AANA educational committees investigated ways of implementing both goals. A survey of schools of anesthesia was undertaken in 1941, but was discontinued with the outbreak of World War II.

On May 19, 1949, the American Hospital Association endorsed the accreditation plan of the AANA. The Council on Professional Practice of AHA assisted in an advisory capacity and in 1960 new minimum requirements for approved schools were adopted. Upon completion of an approved eighteen-month course, nurses take a qualifying examination, which prepares them to become Certified Registered Nurse Anesthetists (CRNA).

Purposes. The purposes of this organization are to develop educational standards for nurse anesthetists, to improve the skill of the nurse as she administers to patient welfare as a member of the surgical team, and to acquaint both health professionals and those outside the profession with the role of the nurse anesthetists. It publishes a journal and pamphlets to keep members informed about new developments in anesthesiology, educational programs, and the various activities of local associations.

The official magazine of this organization is the *Journal of the American Association of Nurse Anesthetists,* which is published bimonthly. A *News Bulletin* is published bimonthly for members of the association. AANA headquarters are maintained in Chicago.

THE AMERICAN ASSOCIATION OF INDUSTRIAL NURSES (AAIN)

History. The American Association of Industrial Nurses was organized in 1942 as an association for professional nurses employed in industry. The organization was incorporated in 1944. Types of membership offered are active, associate, and patron. Besides the national organization there are also state and local units. At the time of the Structure Study this organization was one of the six national nursing organizations. When the two-organization plan (ANA and NLN) was accepted in June 1952, the American Association of Industrial Nurses retained its identity as a separate organization, with headquarters in New York.

Purposes. The purposes of AAIN are similar to the purposes of other nursing organizations. They include maintaining the honor and character of the nursing profession and improving community health through improved nursing service to workers. AAIN also seeks to promote and develop standards for industrial nurses and for industrial nursing services. The organization provides a forum for discussion of problems relating to industrial nursing, and seeks to stimulate industrial nurse participation in all levels of nursing activities.

The official publication of AAIN is *Occupational Health Nursing* (formerly the *American Association of Industrial Nurses' Journal*) which is published monthly. It provides reports, articles, and announcements related to industrial nursing, information on educational opportunities, and the activities of various industrial nursing associations. Other literature and pamphlets are prepared by AAIN. Those who are interested in the standards established for nurses engaged in occupational health may request them from the national headquarters office.

ASSOCIATION OF OPERATING ROOM NURSES (AORN)

History. The Association of Operating Room Nurses was the outgrowth of interest among nurses in this specialty over a period of years. It was organized into a national association in

1957, and local organizations function in many states, including Alaska and Hawaii. The national headquarters office is maintained in Englewood, Colorado.

Purposes. AORN strives to develop the specialty of operating room nursing by an exchange of ideas and possible solution of problems that are specific to this clinical area, to improve service to patients in the operating room, and to bring about more effective interpersonal relationships between operating room nurses and those in other professional areas.

An annual congress is held each year for AORN nurses, and other members of the surgery team may participate in this congress.

AORN Journal is the official publication and is published bimonthly. This journal offers articles of interest to nurses in the operating room and contains reports and announcements concerning institutes, opportunities, and trends.

AMERICAN NURSES' FOUNDATION, INC. (ANF)

In 1955 the American Nurses' Association established the American Nurses' Foundation, Inc. to advance research and to study all phases of nursing. At the onset the foundation received contributions from interested individuals and groups. By 1960 the needs for research continued to mount, and the Foundation requested aid from state and district nurses' associations. Individuals, nursing organizations, and individuals and groups from allied professions who were sympathetic with the nursing project were encouraged to contribute to this drive. As a member of the American Nurses' Association, you will continue to support this foundation through your dues. Donations are also received from business, industry, and other sources that wish to promote nursing. The ANF sponsors research projects, plans and coordinates research activities, and evaluates and distributes research findings.

The office of ANF is maintained with the national nursing organizations in New York. Information concerning the activities of this organization and applications for grants may be obtained from this office. The ANF makes research grants available to universities, colleges, hospitals, and nonprofit organizations who apply and meet specific requirements. It also cooperates in channeling research data pertaining to nursing, in stimulating interest in projects, and in providing services that will guide those persons developing programs promoting educational opportunities such as workshops, conferences, and publications of value to nurses.

THE AMERICAN NATIONAL RED CROSS

History. The Red Cross organization originated from the interest of Henri Dunant, a Swiss banker, who observed the need for volunteers to care for the wounded at the Battle of Solferino in 1859. He stimulated interest in his idea and obtained the cooperation of others. Meetings were held and representatives from various countries were invited to participate in the development of a worthy cause. By 1864 it was decided that a permanent society should be formed for the purpose of assisting in the care of the wounded during times of war. The International Red Cross Treaty was written and signed at this time in Geneva, Switzerland. However, the United States did not join until years later, since it was engaged in the Civil War at that time. The wounded of the Civil War were being cared for by the United States Sanitary Commission, a group similar to the Red Cross; thus there seemed to be no need to join the International Red Cross Society.

The American National Red Cross as we know it today was developed through the efforts of Clara Barton. She became the first president when it was formed in 1881. The developments therafter make interesting history. It carried out numerous relief operations during wars and during peacetime emergencies such as earthquakes, floods, and fires.

In 1909 the nursing service division of the American National Red Cross was organized; Jane Delano was the first national director. Registered nurses have contributed to local and national needs since that time. They have also served on an international basis during the world wars by volunteering their services with the nursing service division of the American Red Cross. Red Cross nurses participated further in one of the federal government services as the Army or Navy Nurse Corps.

Purposes of the Red Cross Nursing Service. The Red Cross Nursing Service is dedicated to maintaining a nationwide program that will extend ordinary community nursing and health resources during emergencies. Emergency services and instructional programs include the following:

1. Training and assigning nurses and coordinating emergency nursing services with hospitals and other health organizations during natural disasters
2. Providing instruction in:
   a. care of the sick and injured
   b. mother and child care
   c. family care
3. Instructing laymen to function as nursing assistants during emergencies
4. Conducting discussion groups on the maintenance of health of senior citizens
5. Training volunteer nurse's aides to assist in hospitals and health agencies, during disasters, and in the Red Cross Blood Program
6. Providing professional nursing service in Red Cross blood centers and other community health programs
7. Maintaining a reserve of qualified volunteer nurses, who have had Red Cross training and experiences, to:
   a. serve during disasters, including epidemics
   b. teach volunteer nurse's aide and home nursing courses
8. Assisting in planning study programs for nursing scholarship students and study visitors from other countries

The headquarters of the Red Cross Nursing Service are maintained in Washington, D. C. For the address, the name of the directors of various programs, and the area offices, refer to the Official Directory in a recent issue of *The American Journal of Nursing*. Information is also available from your area office or from your local chapter.

Membership. During World Wars I and II, the Red Cross Nursing Service acted as a reserve of the Army and the Navy Nurse Corps. Since 1947 it has cooperated with these corps, but enrollment has been secured by the individual corps rather than through the Red Cross.

Application for membership as a Red Cross Nurse may be made through the local chapters. There are approximately 3,600 chapters throughout the nation.

Papers must be filled out and high qualifications met, including registration, personal and professional good standing, good health, and a willing spirit. You may request membership for volunteer duties, for paid services, and for occasional or full-time employment. Payment for services is made on a basis similar to that of an Army or Navy nurse, but only when a member is engaged in active duties.

As a Red Cross nurse you do not pay dues, but once you have been accepted as a member, you retain membership unless you withdraw by returning your appointment card and badge or your membership is annulled for some definite reason.

There is a fee for those who desire to become members of the Red Cross Society. Anyone may become a member by making the annual payment. However, joining this organization is not to be confused with *Red Cross Nursing Service* membership.

Advantages of being a Red Cross nurse are:

1. It makes you a part of an organization that was founded and is maintained for humanitarian purposes.
2. It offers you opportunities to serve your fellow men in unusual places and in dire need. This can be a most gratifying and worthwhile experience, especially if you have been engaged in routine nursing duties.
3. It offers opportunities to teach or to share your nursing knowledge with others, even though you may be inactive in nursing and can devote only a limited amount of

time to committee participation, home nursing, or community welfare.

4. It extends to you the privilege of allying yourself with an organization that is closely associated with other federal nursing services, and you can therefore hope for special consideration should you desire to enter one of these services.

BIBLIOGRAPHY

A.N.A.—help in economic programs reaches nurses in fifteen states, American Journal of Nursing **70**:11, Jan. 1970.

Belote, M.: Nurses are making it happen, American Journal of Nursing **67**:284-289, Feb. 1967.

Bridges, D. C.: The growth and development of a profession, Canadian Nurse **65**:32-35, June 1969.

Bridges, D. C.: A history of the International Council of Nurses, 1899-1964, Philadelphia, 1967, J. B. Lippincott Co.

Foundation reviews activities of 1969, Nursing Research Report **4**:7, Dec. 1969.

Geister, J. M.: One organization—why? Occupational Health **18**:14-15, Mar. 1970.

Haynes, I.: N.L.N. at ten, Nursing Outlook **10**:372-377, June 1962.

I.C.N.—how did nursing students view it? Imprint **16**:9, Nov. 1969.

Lewis, E. P.: The Fairview story, American Journal of Nursing **66**:64-70, Jan. 1966.

Monteiro,—: Involvement is the key to a revitalized league, Nursing Outlook **17**:20-26, Feb. 1969.

NAPNES 29th Annual Convention, Practical Nurse **20**: 32-40, 1970.

National League for Nursing Convention, Nursing Outlook **17**:42-61, June 1969.

Nurses, nursing, and the A.N.A., American Journal of Nursing **70**:808-815, Apr. 1970.

Nurses in peace, RN **33**:38-44, Feb. 1970.

Nurses in war, RN **33**:48-56, Feb. 1970.

Of spirit, for strength, American Journal of Nursing **69**: 1649-1650, Aug. 1969.

Peplau, H.: A.N.A.'s new executive director states her views, American Journal of Nursing **70**:84-88, Jan. 1970.

Quinn, Sheila: I.C.N.—the immediate past, the urgent present and focus on the future, International Nursing Review **16**:241-246, Mar. 1969.

Society in crisis. Report of ANA Biennial Convention, Nursing Outlook **18**:44-49, June 1970.

The International Council of Nurses 14th Quadrennial Congress, Nursing Outlook **17**:36-41, Aug. 1969.

The world of nursing meets in Montreal for the Fourteenth Quadrennial Congress of the International Council of Nurses, American Journal of Nursing **69**: 1684-1689, Aug. 1969.

Walsh, M. E.: N.L.N. faces the seventies, Nursing Outlook **18**:327, Mar. 1970.

What means to what ends? American Journal of Nursing **69**:1433, July 1969.

Pamphlets

Many ANA and NLN pamphlets are available on request.

Check the monthly journals and state publications for current lists. American Red Cross pamphlets can be obtained from your local Red Cross Chapter. International Council of Nurses pamphlets are obtained from the office in Geneva, Switzerland.

COMPLETE WORK SHEET ON PP. 357 TO 360

CHAPTER 26

American Nurses' Association position paper

IMPACT OF POSITION PAPER

The publication of the American Nurses' Association's first *Position Paper on Education for Nursing* (December 1965)* created a controversy among those responsible for administering health care. Although some believed it to be the solution to all of nursing's problems, a large percentage of the American Nurses' Association membership thought it was degrading—an insult to the quality of their educational preparation. The position paper roused many silent members from their apathy into a more vocal role. Much of the clamor that arose was the result of emotional reactions. Letters and articles appeared defending or rejecting the position paper in every publication dealing with nursing or allied health professions. These were often expressions of the individual's fear of change of status as a nurse practitioner. Although the status quo is comfortable and secure nursing is a dynamic profession and as such it must be prepared for the inevitable changes required in order to meet the health needs of the American people. What is true of nursing as a whole is equally true of each individual nurse.

Standard setting for any professional group is the privilege and the reponsibility of members of that profession; therefore, nurses must determine the best method of preparing nurse practitioners. The American Nurses' Association adopted the recommendations of its Committee on Current and Long-Term Goals in 1960, which stated that the American Nurses' Association should "continue to work toward baccalaureate education as the basic education for nursing practice." In 1963, the American Nurses' Association Board of Directors authorized its Committee on Education to prepare a position paper as a guideline to facilitate this goal. The position paper was prepared after this committee carefully studied social trends as they reflect on health care needs, reviewed nursing practice, both present and future, and evaluated the individual needs of nurse practitioners. This study, review, and evaluation of the nurse's role took cognizance of the current focus on American education, the changing pattern of health care, and the shortage of qualified nursing personnel. The fact that a position paper is a statement of beliefs and identified goals of the involved group was lost sight of in the controversy that followed the publication of this paper. These expressed goals are attained only through the activities of involved people by a slow and orderly process.

CURRENT FOCUS ON EDUCATION

Traditionally, nursing education took place in a hospital school where the student gave service in exchange for her education. It has been ten to fifteen years since this exchange system was abolished. As the result of knowledgable educators' awareness of nursing's complexity and

*American Journal of Nursing **65**:106-111, Dec. 1965.

their desire to maintain high standards required for NLN accreditation, nursing programs in hospitals (diploma) schools became increasingly education-oriented rather than service-oriented. Each student's hospital clinical laboratory experience was carefully selected and directed by instructors to correlate with current classroom theory. To enhance the student's ability to meet society's needs additional courses such as psychology, sociology, and English were added to school curriculum. Why then did the American Nurses' Association Committee on Education believe that nursing education should "take place in institutions within the general system of education"? Three social forces are effectively helping to accomplish this shift to a totally educational environment. They are:

1. *The high cost of maintaining a diploma school.* Qualified faculty, education and nursing facilities, a well equipped library, science laboratory, and nursing laboratory (hospital) are all expensive to maintain. Although the student pays tuition, this amount is only a small part of the overall cost. The rest of the cost is absorbed through federal funding to schools and through patient fees. Since colleges and universities are maintained by society through various channels, this additional strain on patient fees is a form of double taxation.

2. *College oriented society.* One of the aspirations of most immigrants to the United States was education for their children, not possible in many other countries. Today a large percentage of American youth is able to achieve this goal. They expect and choose to enter college and it is predicted that this trend will continue. The percentage of high school graduates entering nursing education in preference to going to college is decreasing.

3. *The complexity of nursing practice.* Scientists continue to make discoveries, technologists continue to develop new therapeutic devices, and social forces are increasingly placing nursing in the community setting. Since this places more and more pressure on the nurse practitioner, the basic preparation of the nurse must add depth and breadth, including experience in a variety of nursing agencies in the community. To enrich the diploma program in order to meet these stated needs would create an even greater financial burden and the additional pressure of looking for more qualified faculty.

Placing nursing education in a junior or senior college as an established major and utilizing the available faculty of the college would reduce the cost to student and community. It has also been suggested by many, and tried by some, to establish a health care curriculum available in colleges and universities, reducing overall cost and placing greater stress on the health team concept and the need for interaction.

Let no one lose his perspective. Remember the statement made earlier in this chapter that a position paper is meant as a guideline, not an accomplished fact, and that stated goals are only attained through a slow and orderly process. Neither the position paper nor this chapter intends to belittle any registered nurse graduating from an accredited school of nursing. It is wise to keep in mind that Nurse Practice Acts require nurses to keep current in order to meet society's needs. Remember, too, that other professions prepare their practitioners in a college environment. Why not nursing? The demands on the individual nurse require utilization of mature judgment, sound reasoning, and the application of knowledge and skills.

The American Nurses' Association Committee on Education, after careful evaluation of the focus on education and the needs of nursing service, recommended that nursing should prepare two types of nurse practitioners—professional and technical. They believe, as do many nursing leaders, that the professional nurse should have a baccalaureate degree in nursing and that the technical nurse should be prepared with an associate degree education. Since December 1965, many diploma schools have closed and many associate degree programs in nursing have been established. The trend is here. Even though many nurses object strenuously to being called "technical," a nurse's conduct should always be professional regardless of the level of preparation received. She is a part of the profession of nursing.

CHANGING PATTERN OF HEALTH CARE

Reflected in the pattern of health care in 1963 (and in the 1970s) were the increased life-span, the changing birth rate, the hospitals for the acutely ill, the nursing homes and extended care facilities for the chronically ill, and the needs of the geriatric patient. Not to be excluded in a study of a community's nursing needs is the prevalence of emotional illness at all age levels, so much a part of today's society. Since science and technology have played a major role in altering the approach to, and the methods of, patient therapy, this too is a factor. Nursing education strives to prepare the nurse to administer quality patient care, and nursing service is constantly striving to improve the patient care administered. It was believed by the American Nurses' Association Committee on Education that nursing should utilize all community facilities of health care in order to prepare a nurse that would meet the needs of her community. Placing the basic preparation for the nurse in other than one hospital helps to facilitate this goal.

The current patterns of health care administration requires the two suggested types of nursing education. The professional nurse whose basic education was derived from a baccalaureate program can assume leadership roles after experience and orientation and can continue her education by becoming an educator, administrator, nurse clinician, supervisor, or head nurse. The technical nurse is needed to give quality patient care, seeking guidance when needed, and to assume responsibility for direct patient care. The technical nurse can continue an educational program, if desired, in order to advance her position.

SHORTAGE OF QUALIFIED NURSING PERSONNEL

Following the depression in the 1930s there was a shortage of nurses. From 1963 to 1965, when the American Nurses' Association Committee on Education prepared the position paper, this shortage had become more critical. The supply (number graduating and actively employed) cannot keep up with the demand (population explosion and longer life-span). Many new career opportunities were opening up for the college bound and for those headed for a technical school. Other professions offered a life of scholarship, service, satisfaction of achievement, social prestige, and material reward. Accessibility of universities and colleges have worked a hardship on otherwise aspiring nursing leaders. Obtaining an advanced degree in a major other than nursing has also played a part in depleting the numbers of qualified personnel.

In the summary report of the National Commission for the Study of Nursing and Nursing Education, published in the February 1970, issue of *The American Journal of Nursing*, the question is raised as to whether there is really a nursing shortage or just poor utilization of the available nurses. However, there is a shortage of prepared nurse educators, of prepared nurse clinicians, of prepared public health nurses, and of nurses at the bedside in nursing homes, extended care facilities, and hospitals. This shortage is more acutely felt in the areas away from the large, metropolitan medical centers, yet these patients are entitled to the kind of care administered by qualified and well-prepared nurses.

CONCLUSIONS

The American Nurses' Association's first *Position Paper on Education for Nursing* is six years old. Some of the original impact has gone. The changes as foreseen by this farsighted committee are occurring. Established baccalaureate programs are revising their curricula, new baccalaureate programs are opening, an ever-increasing number of junior and community colleges are developing nursing programs, and many diploma schools of nursing are closing. But, accredited and excellent diploma schools of nursing will continue to produce graduates qualified to pass state board examinations, to become registered, and to render excellent nursing service. The trend, however, is for graduates of both diploma and associate degree programs to continue seeking educational advancement following graduation from their basic program. It may be that this advanced education will be a requirement of the future.

BIBLIOGRAPHY

American Nurses' Association's first position paper on education for nursing, American Journal of Nursing **65**: 106-111, Dec. 1965.

Christman, L. O., and Jelinek, R. C.: Old patterns waste half the nursing hours, The Modern Hospital **108**:79, Jan. 1967.

Dineen, M. A.: Current trends in collegiate nursing education, Nursing Outlook **17**:22-26, Aug. 1969.

National Commission for the Study of Nursing and Nursing Education, American Journal of Nursing **70**:279-294, Feb. 1970.

Toward quality in nursing, Report of the Surgeon General's Consultant Group on Nursing (Pub. no. 992), Washington, D. C., 1963, U. S. Public Health Service Government Printing Office.

U. S. National Advisory Commission on Health Manpower: Report, vol. 1, Washington, D. C., 1966, Government Printing Office.

COMPLETE WORK SHEET ON P. 361

APPENDIX A

Organizations and their addresses

American Association of Cardiovascular Nurses
2000 Church Street
Nashville, Tennessee 37203

American Association of Industrial Nurses
79 Madison Avenue
New York, New York 10016

American Association of Junior Colleges
1785 Massachusetts Avenue, N.W.
Washington, D. C. 20006

American Association of Medical Social Workers
1860 Broadway
New York, New York 10023

American Association of Nurse Anesthetists
111 East Wacker Drive
Chicago, Illinois 60611

American Cancer Society
219 East 42nd Street
New York, New York 10019

American College of Nurse Midwives
50 East 92nd Street
New York, New York 10028

American Dietetic Association
620 North Michigan Avenue
Chicago, Illinois 60611

American Heart Association
44 East 23rd Street
New York, New York 10010

American Hospital Association
840 North Lake Shore Drive
Chicago, Illinois 60611

American Medical Association
535 North Dearborn Street
Chicago, Illinois 60610

American Nurses' Association
10 Columbus Circle
New York, New York 10019

American Nurses' Foundation
10 Columbus Circle
New York, New York 10019

American Occupational Therapy Association
250 West 57th Street
New York, New York 10019

American Physical Therapy Association
1790 Broadway
New York, New York 10019

American Psychological Association
1333 Sixteenth Street, N.W.
Washington, D. C. 20006

American Public Health Association
1790 Broadway
New York, New York 10019

American Red Cross Nursing Programs
17th and D Streets, N.W.
Washington, D. C. 20006

American Society of Medical Technologists
Hermann Professional Building
Houston, Texas 77025

Association of Operating Room Nurses
8085 East Prentice
Englewood, Colorado 80110

Catholic Hospital Association
1438 South Grand Boulevard
St. Louis, Missouri 63104

Conference of Catholic Schools of Nursing
1438 South Grand Boulevard
St. Louis, Missouri 63104

Christian World Mission
Missionary Nursing
475 Riverside Drive, Room 1466
New York, New York 10027

International Council of Nurses
Box 42
1211 Geneva 20, Switzerland

Medical Library Association, Inc.
Executive Office
919 North Michigan Avenue
Chicago, Illinois 60611

National Association for Practical Nurse Education and Service
1465 Broadway
New York, New York 10036

National Federation of Licensed Practical Nurses
250 West 57th Street, Room 323-25
New York, New York 10019

National Foundation for Poliomyelitis
800 Second Avenue
New York, New York 10017

National Health Council
1790 Broadway
New York, New York 10019

National League for Nursing
10 Columbus Circle
New York, New York 10019

National Rehabilitation Association
1025 Vermont Avenue, N.W.
Washington, D. C. 20005

National Research Council
2101 Constitution Avenue, N.W.
Washington, D. C. 20007

Nurses Christian Fellowship
620 North Carroll Street
Madison, Wisconsin

Nurses Educational Funds
10 Columbus Circle
New York, New York 10019

Office of Education
Department of Health, Education and Welfare
Bureau of Adult Vocational and Library Programs
Washington, D. C. 20202

Pan American Health Organization
Pan American Sanitary Bureau
525 23rd Street, N.W.
Washington, D. C. 20037

The American Society of X-ray Technicians
16 Fourteenth Street
Fond du Lac, Wisconsin

United States Civil Service Commission
Federal Job Information Center
1900 E Street, N.W.
Washington, D. C. 20415

United States Department of Health, Education and Welfare
The Surgeon General, Public Health Service
5600 Fishers Lane
Rockville, Maryland 20852

World Federation of Neurosurgical Nurses
250 East Superior Street
Chicago, Illinois 60611

World Health Organization, Personnel Section
Avenue Appia
Geneva, Switzerland

APPENDIX B

Parliamentary procedures

Just as moral and social codes have been established for the welfare of an individual's self-government and character development, so a code has been provided for group government. An organization will progress in a more orderly manner if this code is put into practice by the individual participants of the group. Thus, parliamentary usage is of value to the student nurse of today.

Following is a brief description of the history, definition, purpose, principles, and method of using parliamentary procedure.

Parliamentary procedure was first used in England by the British Parliament. Since that time it has undergone transformation and has been planned as a systematic procedure to serve any group of people.

Parliamentary procedure (or law) is the accepted system of rules for conducting business, preserving order, and governing debate in deliberative or legislative groups.

The purpose may vary, but it is primarily the fair and orderly accomplishment of the business before the group. The rules are usually definite and, if followed, will achieve orderly and desired results.

By using the principles of parliamentary procedure, a group can transact business in an orderly manner, thereby promoting cooperation and harmony. Considerations included are the following:

1. Every significant point presented deserves full and free discussion.
2. Motions follow a definite order or precedence.
3. Each member should understand at all times the question before the group and what its effect will be.
4. Only one question can be considered by the group at a time.

Equality and fairness are to be provided for all members regarding rights, privileges, and obligations. Considerations included are the following:

1. Officers should be elected in a democratic manner for the interests of the group.
2. The chairman or president must serve impartially for the welfare of the group.

The group is ruled by the majority, and the rights of the minority are to be protected.

Method of using parliamentary procedure

The method herein described is simplified for the general use of student nurses. Details may be supplied by reference to a text which has been written by a recognized authority.*

Constitution and bylaws of an organization. Every member has definite rights according to the constitution and bylaws of the organization. Among these are to receive notices, to attend and participate fully in meetings, to exercise rights for enforcing rules of the organization, and to hold office. The rights may be changed, and members may be suspended or expelled for reasons stated in the organization rules. In case of the latter, the member must be notified. She is then entitled to a hearing before a prescribed group.

*Robert's rules of order or Sturgis' standard code of parliamentary procedure.

Meetings. A brief description of meetings follows:

Suggestions for conducting meetings

Although each member contributes to the success of a meeting, the following suggestions will be helpful to the presiding officer:

1. Before the meeting, determine what reports and communications are to be given in order that they may be presented in a businesslike manner.
2. Begin the meeting promptly.
3. Keep the meeting moving. Do not let it "run down."
4. Pay recognition and tribute to those doing outstanding work.
5. Close the meeting with a final challenge, provocative thought, or inspirational statement. Adjourn always by motion and vote.

Types of meetings

In general, a meeting is an assembly of the members of an organization for a definite period of time. At this time the will of the group is made known, and each individual member protects her interests by attending. Meetings may be classed as:

Regular. This type is described in the constitution and bylaws of the organization with respect to the day and time.

Special. This type is called by an authorized person (usually the president or a number of persons as designated in the bylaws).

Adjourned. This meeting is an continuation of a regular or special meeting. Any information which was discussed at the original meeting can be continued at this time.

Quorum for a meeting

A quorum is the number of members necessary to hold a meeting. This number is usually stated in the constitution and bylaws of the organization. It refers to the number of members in good standing, and not to the total membership. For a committee meeting it usually refers to the majority.

Order of business (agenda)

This is usually established in the bylaws of the organization and can be changed only by a two-thirds vote of the membership. The president or chairman ordinarily acts as the presiding officer and proceeds to conduct the meeting in the following order:

1. *Call to order.* This is an announcement and may be followed by an invocation.

2. *Reading of the minutes of the previous meeting.* This is requested from the secretary and may be followed by roll call.

3. *Report of the treasurer.* This is requested from the treasurer.

4. *Reports of boards and standing committees.* These are requested from the chairman of each committee.

5. *Reports of special committees.* These are requested from the chairman of each committee.

6. *Unfinished business.* This is presented to the group.

7. *New business.* This may be presented, or it may be brought up by a member of the group. (Elections at annual meetings are included here.)

8. *Announcements.* These are requested from the members and then offered by the presiding officer.

9. *Adjournment.* This is done by a motion made and seconded by members. The announcement is then made by the presiding officer.

Courtesies followed during a meeting

The presiding officer of a meeting may be called a speaker, a chairman, or a president and is addressed as Madam Speaker, Chairman, or President (or Mr. Speaker, Chairman, or President).

The presiding officer speaks of herself as "The Chair" and should never say "I" when presiding. She may not make, second, nor discuss a motion while occupying the chair. If she wishes to do so, she should call upon the vice-president to preside.

A member waits for a speaker to yield the floor before rising to ask recognition.

A member who has the floor should not be interrupted unnecessarily.

A motion should be discussed before the entire assembly, not whispered in small groups.

The officers on a platform (and members of the group) should avoid conversation or moving about while a person is speaking or while a program is in progress.

If it is necessary to move about while business is being carried on, passing between the presiding officer and a member who has the floor should be avoided.

All remarks made from the floor should be addressed to the presiding officer, not directly to another member.

Technique of offering and voting on a motion

A motion is a statement of a proposal or question which is presented in a formal manner for the consideration of the group. The steps are as follows:

1. *A member obtains the floor.* She rises, addresses the presiding officer, and waits for recognition. (She gives her name in a large group in which the members are not readily known to one another.)

2. *The member is recognized by the presiding officer.* This may be given by repeating the member's name, by other verbal recognition, or by a nod of the head.

3. *The motion is proposed.* The member who has the floor states, "I move that ________________" or "Resolved that ________________." A clear statement is given (verbally or in writing) and the member is seated.

4. *The motion is seconded.* This is offered by another member who remains seated and states, "I second the motion." This second is required for all routine motions. If none is offered, the motion is lost.

5. *The presiding officer states the motion.* She does this by saying, "It has been moved and seconded that ________________."

6. *The presiding officer opens the pending question to debate.* She can do this by saying, "Is there any discussion?" "Are there any remarks?" or "What is your pleasure?"

7. *The presiding officer puts the question to a vote.* Following the discussion of the pending question, the presiding officer inquires, "Are you ready for the question?" If the group is ready, a member (or members) will reply, "Question."

The most usual method of voting is the viva voce or "voting by voice." Thus, the presiding officer says, "All those in favor, please indicate by saying 'aye,'" and waits for the response. Then, "All those opposed indicate by saying 'no.'" The motion is accepted or lost according to the strength of the replies.

8. *The presiding officer declares the vote.* The presiding officer states, "The question ________________ has been carried," or "lost" as indicated by the votes.

Classification of motions

Space does not permit the discussion of motions in detail; however, some of those used most frequently are listed according to precedence.

1. *Privileged motions*
   a. *Adjourn.*
   b. *Recess.* A speaker may not be interrupted in order to present these two motions. They must be seconded, and they must have a majority vote.
   c. *Question of privilege.* This is to obtain an immediate action upon a matter which concerns the conveniences, comforts, or rights of the organization as a whole or any individual member. Example: "to have the speaker talk louder." It is presented by a member who rises (need not wait for recognition) and interrupts the speaker. This motion needs no second since it is a request and needs no vote.

2. *Subsidiary motions.* These all require a second, cannot interrupt a speaker, and need a majority vote to be carried (unless otherwise indicated).
   a. *Postpone temporarily* (lay on the table)—has the purpose of suspending consideration
   b. *Vote immediately*—has the purpose of preventing discussion and requires a two-thirds vote because it limits the privilege of debate
   c. *Postpone definitely*—has the purpose of

allowing a lapse of time to consider the question outside the meeting

d. *Refer to committee*—has the purpose of permitting further investigation or action (the motion should state the type of committee, name the chairman or members, and give instructions to be followed)

e. *Amend*—has the purpose of changing or modifying the motion being considered

f. *Postpone indefinitely*—has the purpose of suppressing the question without permitting it to come to a vote (this is the same as the complete rejection of a motion)

3. *Main motions.* These, on the whole, cannot interrupt the speaker, require a second, and need a majority vote. They are the following:

a. *General or original*—used to introduce new business

b. *Specific or incidental*—used during the action of the meeting, such as:

(1) *Reconsider*—can interrupt speaker, has the purpose of taking up a matter again as if it had never been voted on before

(2) *Rescind*—has the purpose of nullifying a motion previously passed (this will delete the original motion from the record)

(3) *Resume consideration*—take from table; has the purpose of taking a motion from the table to be considered at this time

4. *Incidental motions.* These, on the whole, can interrupt the speaker, do not require a second (not true motions), and need no vote.

a. *Appeal*—has the purpose of checking on the decision of the presiding officer (this requires a second and a majority vote of the group)

b. *Point of order*—has the purpose of checking a point of parliamentary law which is being used during the course of the meeting

c. *Withdraw a motion*—has the purpose implied; cannot interrupt the speaker

d. *Object to consideration*—has the purpose of avoiding a discussion which seems inadvisable at the time (it requires a two-thirds vote)

e. *Division of a question*—has the purpose of separating a motion into distinct parts (the chairman decides on this and then presents it)

f. *Division of assembly*—has the purpose of clarifying a voice vote by having the members rise in order that opinions can be checked

Technique of amending a motion

A motion may be amended in order that the original motion will express more satisfactorily the opinion of the group. This amendment will require a second and a vote. The proposed amendment may be further amended, but only two amendments are permitted before the original motion can be voted upon.

1. *Form for amendment.* This is stated, "I move to amend the motion by__________."

2. *Methods for amendment*

a. By striking out a certain word or words

b. By inserting or adding a certain word or words

c. By substituting

d. By dividing the question

Technique of making a resolution

A resolution is a long motion, or one of special importance, which is usually required to be in writing.

1. *Form for resolution.* This is stated, "Resolved that ____________." It requires a second and a group vote.

2. *Reasons for resolution.* These may be indicated and should be given before the resolution by using "Whereas." Example: "Whereas, _____ _____. Resolved that ______."

Voting at a meeting

This is the method by which the will of the individual members and of the group as a whole is made known. Various methods of voting are the following:

1. *Viva voce* (see *Technique of offering and voting on a motion*)

2. *Silent assent* is demonstrated when the presiding officer says, "The minutes stand approved as read."

3. *Division of the group* is demonstrated by a show of hands or a standing vote (the count may be made by the presiding officer or the secretary)

4. *Ballot* is a written vote (the votes are counted by designated tellers appointed by the presiding officer; the teller named first is the chairman, unless otherwise stated, and is responsible for checking the number of ballots cast and the number needed for the vote; candidates may not act as tellers; a written report of an election must be signed by all tellers)

Ballots are preserved until a motion is made to destroy them. Tie votes are lost votes since there is no majority. However, the presiding officer may vote to break a tie. Regardless of the method used in voting, the presiding officer makes the announcement of the vote. She first states whether the motion is carried or lost, and then she restates the substance of the motion.

Minutes of a meeting

These should include the following information:

1. Name of the organization
2. Kind of meeting held
3. Place, date, and hour (unless always the same)
4. Name of the presiding officer
5. The presence or absence of officers and the names of substitutes
6. The approximate number of members present
7. The disposition of the minutes of the previous meeting
8. The business transacted including reports (details need not be written), motions carried or lost, and resolutions adopted (written out in full)
9. Vote taken by ballot, stating number for and against a motion
10. Communications received
11. Manner and time of adjournment
12. Signature of the secretary (also the president in some instances)

Officers of an organization

Being an officer of an organization implies certain general responsibilities to that office. In the first place the acceptance or nomination and election is an ethical pledge of the candidate's confidence in her ability to serve and of her willingness to perform the duties of the office. Second, absences from meetings, without reasonable excuse, or neglect of responsibilities may require the forfeiting of an office by resignation. Thus some suggested abilities and duties of the officers of an organization are given here to increase the understanding of these responsibilities.

President

(Presiding officer, chairman, speaker, or moderator)

Abilities. The president, or presiding officer, should be chosen because of the qualifications which she is believed to possess.

1. Ability to lead (this implies an understanding and an appreciation of human nature, the importance of the group, and the necessity of individual consideration)

2. Ability to preside (this implies a knowledge of parliamentary procedure and an ability to carry out the will of the majority)

3. Ability to show a genuine interest in the suggestions and discussions of the group and its individuals

4. Ability to cooperate with the other officers, committees, and members in activities

5. Ability to be an example of right spirit and policy of the organization

6. Ability to remain impartial and to keep the business of an organization moving ahead

Duties. These will be given in the constitution and bylaws of an organization but usually include the following:

1. To act as the official representative of the group

2. To assume the major responsibility of the organization

3. To preside at all regular or special meetings

4. To arrange special meetings in accord-

ance with the convenience of the board and members

5. To sign all acts or orders necessary to carry out the will of the group

6. To call the meetings to order at the appointed time and to follow the established procedure of the meeting

7. To control the meeting by following parliamentary procedure, including:

(a) To stand when addressing the group or a member and to be seated only during the longer speeches

(b) To announce the business which should come before the group in its proper order

(c) To keep the group in order, recognizing those who wish to speak

(d) To acquaint the group with all questions, motions, and results of voting

8. To vote in case of a tie when authorized to do so.

9. To act as an ex officio member on all committees, as directed by the bylaws

10. To determine whether or not the officers are functioning efficiently and cooperatively

11. To give credit where it is due, that is, to officers, committees, and members

First vice-president

Abilities. The vice-president should have abilities which are similar to those of the president and should have the potentialities of a president.

Duties. The duties of the first vice-president include the following:

1. To perform the duties of the president in the absence of that officer, and, in the event of a vacancy in the office of president, to become president for the unexpired term

2. To cooperate with the president

3. To maintain an interest in the plans of the group and assume a responsibility in carrying out the plans

4. To fulfill the duties specified by the bylaws

5. The first and subsequent vice-presidents usually assist the president and may direct some of the committees or other duties specified by the bylaws

Secretary

Abilities. The secretary should have the ability to understand records and the routine business of the group and the personal ability of being orderly, responsible, and painstaking.

Duties. The duties include the following:

1. To take notes during a meeting in a rough form (No comments are to become a part of a permanent record; the notes are to be transferred later into accurate minutes of the proceedings of the meeting)

2. To handle the various correspondence that may be required for the transaction of the business of the group

3. To issue all calls for meetings under the direction of the president

4. To prepare a roll call of members and call it when necessary

5. To call the meeting to order in the absence of the presiding officers

6. To report on and obtain information from previous meetings when requested by the officers or members

7. To preserve all records, reports, and papers of the group

8. To assist the presiding officer by preparing before each meeting an order of business, list of unfinished business, list of committees which are to report, and list of announcements

9. To provide the chairman of each committee with a list of the members of her committee and with information concerning committee functions

10. To read all reports and papers at the request of the presiding officer at a meeting

11. To bring to each meeting a copy of the constitution and bylaws, the standing rules, and a list of members of all committees

12. To notify all officers, committees, and delegates of their appointments

13. To keep copies of all reports, correspondence issued and received, bulletins, programs, and privileges extended to the group

14. To be responsible for the correct form and details, good penmanship, and typing in all reports and correspondence

15. To sign all records, including the minutes of meetings, and, together with the president, all orders on the treasurer

NOTE—The position of secretary may be one of three offices:

Recording secretary, who primarily takes the minutes of meetings; *corresponding secretary,* who takes care of the correspondence, including the sending of notices; or *executive secretary,* who directs her abilities toward the administration of an organization by assisting officers and committees (she is usually given financial remuneration for her services)

Treasurer

Abilities. The treasurer must have the following abilities:

1. Ability to handle money in an accurate manner
2. Knowledge of bookkeeping and ability to retain meticulous records of all money received and paid out
3. Ability to maintain honesty and financial integrity in the dealings with the group
4. Ability to develop an understanding of the economic transactions in bank accounts and checking accounts

Duties. Her duties include:

1. Keeping a record in permanent form of all money received and paid out
2. Giving receipts for all money received
3. Paying out money only upon orders properly signed by the presiding officer and the secretary
4. Assuming the responsibility for placing the group's funds in a bank and for keeping an accurate record of the source of all money
5. Keeping a record of money paid out and giving a summary of finances at each meeting, if called for by the presiding officer, and a complete report at least annually
6. Supplying records to support or clarify the report, including accounts, checks, bills, and other notes
7. Preparing records for an annual audit by an auditing committee or one appointed for this purpose (this is a protection to the group and to the treasurer; such a report must be voted on for acceptance)
8. Signing all checks with the president or executive secretary
9. Acting upon a resolution made by the group (when retiring from office) to send an official notice to the bank and provide for new signatures

The parliamentarian

Abilities. The parliamentarian must have:

1. Knowledge of the details of parliamentary procedures
2. Ability to think clearly and quickly
3. Ability to make corrections in an unoffending, tactful manner

Duties. Duties including the following:

1. To assist the presiding officer by giving her information as needed (this is in the position of giving advice, but the presiding officer may take or disregard this advice)
2. To assist in maintaining the method of conducting the meeting under parliamentary procedure and to direct points of dispute

Committees

A brief description of the role of committees is presented.

Purposes

The main purpose of a committee is to take a discussion into a smaller group which can devote more time and consideration to it. These groups do much of the work (by deliberation or action) and report back to the organization. The members of a committee assume the responsibility of fulfilling certain duties. They prepare the members for teamwork and leadership. Their decisions are usually accepted by the organization.

Kinds of committees

Standing committee. This is one formed for a definite period of time, usually over the year following the appointment. It carries out matters which are permanently connected with the organization.

Special committee. This is one formed for a specific task, and as soon as this task is completed the committee no longer functions; for example, a committee for a Christmas program.

Membership on a committee

Each *member* (particularly the chairman) should be carefully chosen and should:

1. Accept the membership before the appointment is made
2. Possess a knowledge of, or interest in, the committee itself
3. Attend the meetings and assume some responsibilities
4. Work with others harmoniously
5. Know the duties expected of a member of a committee

The *chairman* of a committee is usually a leader and maintains a specific interest. If the presiding officer of an organization appoints the whole committee, the first named may be the chairman. The presiding officer may appoint only the chairman, who in turn appoints the other members of the committee.

Ex officio members are usually persons who hold definite offices. These members act as informers or coordinators to other related groups. They are expected to help, not hinder, the progress of a committee. When an ex officio member leaves an office, she ceases to be a member of a committee.

Information for committees

Information should include such matters as the original motion referred to the committee with all information previously discussed by the group; the name of the chairman and all members; directions for the deliberation or action to be taken by the committee; and the date when the report is to be given to the organization.

Duties of the committee

Duties are usually specified by the presiding officer or by the constitution. The chairman is to familiarize each member of the committee with the purpose and the relationship of the report to the organization. The chairman is also responsible for seeing that the members attend the meetings and work together for the cause.

The members usually act on motions in an informal manner, but all work of the committee should be definite with a record kept by a secretary (or designated member).

Committee reports

A definite form may be used, but it is to be remembered that the committee only summarizes a report and makes recommendations concerning the original motion. If the recommendations are lengthy, the committee may rewrite the amendments and recommend that the new proposal be submitted for the original. A plan for a report is as follows:

1. The statement of the question given to the committee
2. Method used by the committee for investigation
3. Information obtained in a summary form
4. Conclusions
5. Recommendations

The report should be brief and clearly stated in the third person. Credit is given to those who contributed in a special manner. All resolutions should be submitted separately. It is then signed by the chairman and all members who approve the recommendations.

The report is presented to the organization by the chairman or a designated member who recommends its acceptance upon the completion of the presentation.

APPENDIX C

Social etiquette: guides for use in correspondence

SPECIAL CORRESPONDENCE

The thank you letter. A thank you letter is written:

1. After spending a week-end with friends
2. To acknowledge Christmas or other gifts, regardless of how small
3. For a courtesy shown by another person

The letter should be written while the occasion is still in the minds of all concerned. You should write to the giver of a gift or your hostess a few friendly lines expressing gratitude in your own personal way.

March 4, 1971

Dear Mary,

After a grand weekend with you and your family, I am having a little difficulty in resuming my studies and duties. However, the memory of the good meals, the theater party, and your hospitality will be recalled for many days to come.

It was wonderful to spend the days with you, and I thank you a million times for remembering me in your plans.

Lovingly,
Ann

Invitations

Informal invitations

1. *Written* invitations are preferred, for they give the recipient time to accept or decline. However, they may be "face to face" or by telephone.

2. A *reply* is always indicated immediately. R.S.V.P., meaning "Reply, if you please," is often stated on the invitation when it is necessary to have a reply for definite plans.

3. The *acceptance* (like the reply to decline) should be written in an informal manner. This carries with it an obligation to appear after one has once accepted the invitation.

Formal invitations

1. The *form* used may be:
   a. Written in longhand
   b. Engraved on the first page of white or ivory stationery (it should contain no abbreviations)

Mr. and Mrs. Weare Flyinghigh
request the pleasure of
Miss Youare Invited's
company at a dance
Sunday, the tenth of October
at ten o'clock
Maumee Country Club

2. The *envelopes* (as for graduation invitations) should include:
   a. *Inside* envelope:
      (1) The tissue over the engraving on the invitation or announcement is left in place.

(2) The inside envelope is left unsealed.
(3) Names are written on this envelope including the Christian name:
"Mr. and Mrs. Pride"
(4) When younger members of the family are to be included, do not write "and family," but add the Christian names, such as:
"Mr. and Mrs. Pride
Sarah and John"
(5) Another adult member in the family should receive a separate invitation with the name "Miss Pride" on the inside envelope.
(6) If two sisters or two brothers are to receive an invitation, they would be addressed as "The Misses Pride" or "The Messrs. Pride," respectively.
(7) After the names have been written on the inside envelope (in blue or black ink), it is placed in the outer envelope with the names facing the flap.

b. *Outside* envelope:
(1) The complete names of the recipients are written on the outside envelope.
(2) Abbreviations of titles, cities, and states are not used.
(3) The outer envelope is sealed.
(4) The return address may be written on the flap if desired.

3. The *reply* should follow the form and type of phrasing used in the invitation.

a. *Acceptance:*

Miss Youare Invited
accepts with pleasure
the kind invitation of
Mr. and Mrs. Weare Flyinghigh
to a dance
Sunday, the tenth of October

b. *Refusal:* This follows the same plan as illustrated for "acceptance," except that the line
"Accepts with pleasure"
is replaced with two lines:
"Regrets that a previous engagement
prevents her from accepting."

NOTE: You need not give a reason for regrets, but it is more courteous to do so.

Wedding invitations

1. *Engraved* invitations are used only when the wedding in formal.

2. The *form* used:

a. For a *church* wedding:

Mr. and Mrs. John Henry Parent
request the honor of your presence
at the marriage of their daughter
Only
to
Mr. Fine Husband
Tuesday, the fourth of October
at ten o'clock
The Trinity Cathedral
Columbus, Ohio

b. For a *home* wedding:
The same form is used as above except:
(1) House address is substituted for the Church.
(2) R.S.V.P. is placed in the lower left corner.
(3) The *tissue* paper may or may not be removed according to the bride's preference.

3. *Envelopes.* There are always two used. The inner one is unsealed and bears only the name of the person (or persons) to whom the invitation is sent. Avoid the use of "and family"—include all names. This one is inserted in the outer envelope with the writing toward the back of the outer envelope.

4. Response to a wedding invitation:

a. An invitation to a church wedding does not require an answer.

b. A reply is required to an invitation to a reception or a breakfast.
c. A reply is required to a home wedding.

Miss Ima Invited
accepts with pleasure
(or regrets that she is unable to accept)
Mr. and Mrs. John Henry Parent's
kind invitation for
Tuesday, the fourth of October
at ten o'clock

VISITING CARDS (NAME CARDS)

These are convenient and sometimes necessary. They are usually on white Bristol board. The sizes will vary according to the user; 2 by 3 inches is correct for an unmarried woman.

1. *Name used:*
   a. The full name with Miss, Mr., or Mrs. to be printed or engraved
   b. The use of initials not correct
2. *When used:*
   a. Enclosed with gifts
   b. Left when calling
   c. Used with invitations or as invitations
3. *How used:*
   a. In altered form when used with invitations
   b. Informal:
      (1) To convey a message (in this instance the name becomes the signature, and the Miss, Mr., or Mrs. is crossed out)
      (2) To serve as an invitation to picnics, teas, or parties
4. *Response* to visiting card invitations:
   a. Regardless of how the response is made, it is a "must."
   b. You may make your reply by phone, especially if R.S.V.P. has been used.
   c. It is considered more courteous to give a reason for refusing an invitation, but this is not a "must."

TITLES AND THEIR USE IN CORRESPONDENCE

Personal titles

1. A *man* who has no other title uses "Mr." preceding his name in the United States.

2. An *unmarried woman* uses the title "*Miss*." If one is in doubt concerning a woman's title, it is correct to use "Miss" rather than "Mrs."

3. A *married woman* uses her own first name and signs as "Mary Smith." However, if she wishes to include her title, it consists of her husband's name preceded by "Mrs." Example: Mary Smith (Mrs. Robert Smith).

4. A *widow* uses her first name in writing, such as "Mary Smith." However, she continues to be addressed by her husband's title as "Mrs. Robert Smith." It is not correct, according to some authorities, for her to be addressed as "Mrs. Mary Smith."

5. A *divorced woman* may have her maiden name restored to her and will be called "Miss Mary Hughes." Or, she may legally retain her husband's last name, such as "Mrs. Hughes Smith," but not his complete title as "Mrs. Robert Smith."

6. A *professional married woman* may continue to retain her maiden name for professional or other reasons. In addressing this woman, you would follow her personal preference.

Professional titles

1. *Physician or dentist:*
   a. A doctor of medicine or dentistry, in this country, is addressed by his professional title "Doctor" which may be abbreviated: "Dr. John Jones."
   b. When addressing the doctor and his wife, use "Dr. and Mrs. John Jones."
2. *Wife of a professional man:*
   a. The wife of a professional person uses the title of "Mrs." The same is true for a minister's wife.
   b. As in professional usage, the minister and his wife are addressed as "Reverend and Mrs. James North."
3. *Academic titles:*
   a. Men in academic fields are most com-

The personage	*Envelope title*	*Salutation title*
Clergy of Non-Catholic Churches		
Anglican Bishop	The Lord Bishop of ______	My Lord Bishop: (formal)
Episcopal Bishop	To the Right Reverend ______ ______ Bishop of Boston	My dear Bishop ______:
Methodist Bishop	The Reverend Bishop ______	Dear Bishop______:
Other Protestant Clergymen	The Reverend ______ or The Rev. Dr. ______ ______ (if entitled to a degree)	My dear Mr. ______: or Dear Doctor ______:
Jewish Rabbi	Rabbi ______ ______ or The Reverend ______ ______	My dear Mr. ______: Dear Rabbi:
Clergy of the Roman Catholic Church		
The Pope	His Holiness Pope ______ ______ or His Holiness the Pope	Your Holiness: or Most Holy Father:
Cardinal	His Eminence Cardinal ______	Your Eminence:
Archbishop	His Excellency, The Archbishop of ______ or The Most Reverend Archbishop of ______	Your Excellency: or Most Reverend Archbishop: or Dear Archbishop ______, (*informal*)
Bishop	His Excellency, Bishop of ______ or The Most Reverend Bishop ______	Your Excellency: or Dear Bishop ______, (*informal*)
Monsignor:		
Papal Household	The Very Reverend Monsignor ______	My dear Monsignor:
Domestic Prelate	The Right Reverend Monsignor ______	My dear Monsignor:
Priest	The Reverend John Doe, O.P. or The Reverend Father Doe	My dear Reverend Father: or My dear Father Doe: or Dear Father,
Members of religious institutions (Initials of the order may be used following the name)		
Superior of a Sisterhood	Reverend Mother ______ or Reverend Mother Superior	My dear Reverend Mother: or Dear Reverend Mother,
Member of a Sisterhood	Sister Joan Mary, C.P.P.S.	My dear Sister Joan Mary: or Dear Sister Joan Mary,
Superior of a Brotherhood	Reverend Brother ______, S.J.	My dear Rev. Brother: or Dear Brother,
Member of a Brotherhood	Brother ______, C.S.C.	Dear Brother ______,

monly addressed by their titles, such as President, Professor, Doctor, or Dean.

b. A man who is both a professor and a doctor, except of medicine, is usually addressed as "Professor." When a professional title is used to precede the name, the degree does not follow—thus "Doctor John Jones" (without M.D. or Ph.D. following).

c. "Professor" is the correct title for all who hold positions as professors, whether they are professors, assistant professors, or associate professors. In writing they are always addressed as "Professor." If the degree is to be indicated, then the title is omitted–thus "John Jones, Ph.D."

d. A college instructor, tutor, or teacher who has no doctor's degree is addressed as Mr., Miss, or Mrs. according to the individual. No degree below the doctorate (such as B.A. or M.A.) is used in titles when one is corresponding.

4. An *attorney* is usually addressed as:

"John Smith, Attorney"
or
"Mr. John Smith
Attorney-at-law"

Titles for clergy and government officials in the United States

The titles of "Reverend" and "Honorable" are used in many instances. In each the title indicates respect and should be followed by two names: "The Honorable John Smith," not "The Honorable Smith."

1. *Reverend* may be used with other academic titles and abbreviations for academic degrees to denote respect:

a. "The Reverend John Adams" (abbreviated "Rev.")
b. "The Rev. President John Adams"
c. "The Rev. Professor John Adams"
d. "The Rev. John Adams, D.D."

2. Honorable may be used in addressing the following: ex-presidents, governors, cabinet officers, senators, congressmen, American ambassadors, American ministers, the secretary to the president, assistant secretaries of the executive departments, judges (not of the Supreme Court), heads of the independent boards of commissioners, and mayors of cities.

Titles for officials in Washington are fixed by established usage. The highest are addressed in social correspondence by their titles rather than by their names. Refer to a reliable text or person of authority for detailed information in addressing government officials and military personnel.

Notations concerning the use of titles for Army and Navy personnel are as follows:

1. In each instance the rank and last name is used on the envelope.
2. In the salutation you use the rank and name only for those who have the rank above a captain. Otherwise, the title of "Mr." is used with the name.
3. In the case of a general or admiral, where there are varying degrees of rank, you use only the saluation of "My dear General ________" rather than "My dear Major General."
4. Medical officers who have the rank of captain or above are addressed by their titles. Those who are lieutenants are addressed as "Doctor."
5. Chaplains are addressed as "Chaplain" regardless of their grade.
6. Noncommissioned officers are addressed by their titles on the envelope and in the salutation as "My dear Mr. ________."

The complimentary close in general may follow the correct usage of "Very truly yours" (more formal), "Sincerely yours" or "Respectfully yours" (more informal forms).

Index

A

Ability, 83
Academic policies and scholarship requirements for nursing school, 117-122
essential, interpretation of, 112-122
Academic problems, value of counseling for, 130
Acceptance of others, importance of in interpersonal relations, 135
Accompanying patient in public, 190
Accomplishments to present, personal, 188
Administering patient care, 189-190
Administrative positions in hospital nursing services, 234-235
Admission, requirements for
in collegiate nursing programs, 52-53
in community college nursing programs, 54-55
in hospital nursing programs, 50
in practical nursing programs, 57
Agencies, outside, for private duty nurses, 236
Agency for International Development, nursing opportunities with, 247
Agenda, 276
Air Force Nurse Corps, 244
Alexian Brothers in history of nursing, 8
Ambition, 70
American Association of Industrial Nurses, 251, 265
history of, 265
purpose of, 265
American Association of Industrial Nurses' Journal, 265
American Association of Nurse Anesthetists, 265
history of, 265
purposes of, 265
American Journal of Nursing, 207, 235, 236, 248, 251, 271
Directory of, 259
American Journal of Practical Nursing, 265
American Medical Association code of ethics, 101-102
American National Red Cross, 266-268
history of, 266-267
membership in, 267-268
purposes of, 267
American Nurses' Association, 31, 36, 251, 252-259
code of ethics of, 101
Commission on Economic and General Welfare, 258
Commission on Nursing Education, 258
Committee on Education, 269-272
history of, 252
membership in, 252
National Student Nurses' Association Committee on Common Interests and Goals, 125-126
occupational health nursing defined by, 241
organization chart of, 253
position paper of, 269-272
changing pattern of health care in, 271
current focus on education in, 269-270
impact of, 269
shortage of qualified nursing personnel in, 271
position of in two-organization plan, 251
programs of, 252, 258-259
economic and general welfare program, 258
government relations program, 258
international program, 258-259
nursing education program, 258
nursing practice program, 258
organization services program, 258
public relations program, 258
research and statistics program, 258
state boards of nursing, 258
Public Health Nurses' Section of, 238
purposes of, 252
role of in founding of National Student Nurses' Association, 123
and social security for nurses, 202-203
special points for consideration, 259
American Nurses' Foundation, Inc., 266

American Red Cross Nursing Service
in World War I, 35
in World War II, 38-40
American reforms in nursing, 15
American Society of Superintendents of Training Schools for Nurses, 31, 252, 262
Analysis, occupational, 188
Anointing the sick in Roman Catholicism, 184-185
Application for job, 217-222
forms for, 221-222
letter for, writing of, 218-220
personal interview in, 220-221
Application form for nursing school, 113-114
Apprentice nursing, 2, 8-16
Civil War, 15-16
in the Crusades, 8-10
definition of, 8
impact of social revolutions on, 10-14
in New World, 14-16
Pre-Civil War, 15
Reformation and, 11-12
Aptitude tests in selection of students for nursing school, 116
Area of nursing practice, selection of, 188-189
Armistice period, nursing in, 35-36
Army, nursing opportunities with, 144-145
Army Nurse Corps in World War I, 35
Army School of Nursing, 35
Assault and battery, 176
Assistant director of hospital nursing service, 235
Associate degree programs for nurses, 53-55
Associated Alumnae, 31
Association of Collegiate Schools of Nursing, 251
Association of Operating Room Nurses, 265-266
history of, 265-266
purposes of, 266
Association of Operating Room Nurses Journal, 266
Association of Practical Nurse Schools, 264
Atomic energy, effect of on nursing, 43
Attendance, importance of, 118
Attitudes
development and evaluation of, 82-83
effect of on communication, 146-147
Augustinians, 9
Authority
flow of in hospital, 138
recognition of, 66

B

Babylonia, ancient, regulation of medical practice in, 3
Baccalaureate program for nurses, 51-53
Baptism
in Protestant churches, 185
in Roman Catholicism, 184
Barton, Clara, 266
Beguines, 9
Bellevue system of nurse education, establishment of, 29
Benedictines, 9
Boards of nursing, state, 173, 258
Bolton Nurse Training Law, 38-39
Bonds, government savings, 200-201
Books, role of in personal development, 206
Budgeting, 192-196
Bylaws and constitutions of an organization, 275

C

Caduceus, medical, origin of, 5
Cap, nurse's, 29-30
significance of, 81-82
Care
administration of, liability for, 180
extended, post-hospital, coverage of under Medicare Hospital Insurance, 212
home health, post-hospital, coverage of under Medicare Hospital Insurance, 212
of patient, administering, 189-190
Career in nursing
opportunities for pursuing, 233-250
"second thoughts" about, 61-63
Cathrine of Siena, Saint, 10
Cavell, Edith, 33-34
Certified Registered Nurse Anesthetists, 265
Character, attributes and importance of, 63-65
Character references, use of in selection of students for nursing school, 114-115
Charge accounts, 199-200
Charity, 64-65
organized, rise of, 11
Child Health Act of 1967, 213
Christian philosophy, transition to from pagan philosophy, 5-7
Christianity, precepts of, 184
City taxes, 202
Civil Rights Act of 1964, 213
Civil War, nursing during, 15-16
Clarification, use of questions for, 158-159
Clarke, Alice, 40
Cleanliness, 81
Clergy, titles of, 287
Clergyman, role of in nursing school counseling program, 130
Clinical areas, special, nursing in, preparation for, 235
Clinical Nursing Specialist, 206
Clinical psychologist, role of in nursing school counseling program, 130
Clinical situation
counseling in, 130-131
interpersonal relations in, 136-138
Clothing, budgeting for, 197
Collegiate nursing program, 51-53
Commitment to nursing, 88
Common law, 172

Communication, 142-154
  definition of, 143
  effect of attitudes and prejudices on, 146-147
  factors to remember in, 145-154
  lines of
    in hospitals, 138
    student's, 139-140
  listening in, importance of, 153-154
  in nursing, importance of, 142
  person-to-person, 143-145
  privileged, 177
  process of, 144-145
  purpose of, 145-146
  right time for, 146
  skills and techniques in, 155-164
    direction giving, 161-162
    information gathering, 155-159
    information giving, 159-161
    report giving, 162-164
  use of feedback in, 147-148
  verbal and nonverbal, 142-143
Communicative purpose, 145-146
Communion
  in Protestant churches, 185
  in Roman Catholicism, 184
Community college for education of nurses, 53-55
Community Mental Health Centers Act of 1963, 213
Community Mental Health Centers Staffing Act of 1965, 213
Companionship capacity, assisting patient in, 190-191
Computers, effect of on nursing, 43-44
Conduct, professional, in public, 190-191
Congress on Nursing Practice of American Nurses' Association, 258
Connotative meaning of words, 149-150
Consent, patient's, 177-178
Constitutions and bylaws of an organization, 275
Contemporary nursing, 2, 42-46; *see also* Nursing, contemporary
Context, meaning of words from, 150
Continuing care unit, modern, 74
Continuing education, 209-210
Conversation, impression created by, 86-87
Cooperation, importance of to nursing, 109-111
Correspondence
  special guides for, 283-287
  titles in, 285-287
Counseling
  in the clinical situation, 130-131
  in nursing program, role of, 128-133
  program for participants in, 129-130
  reasons for seeking, 130-131
Counseling relationship, 131-133
Counselor, role of in nursing school counseling program, 129
Credit ratings, 199-200
Credit union membership, 201
Crimea, Florence Nightingale in, 26-27
Crimes relating to nurses, 175-177
Crusades, nursing in, 8-10
Cultured person, meaning of, 205-206
Curriculum, design of
  in collegiate nursing programs, 53
  in community college nursing program, 55
  in hospital nursing program, 50-51
  in practical nursing programs, 57

D

Debts, budgeting for, 197-198
Dedication, pledges of, 103-104
Delano, Jane, 266
Denotative meaning of words, 149
Depression, great, nursing in, 36-37
Development, personal
  opportunities for in nursing care team, 170
  role of books in, 206
Diagnosis, agents for, effect of on nursing, 44
Diploma program for nurses, 50-51
Diploma school, high cost of maintaining, effect of on educational orientation in nursing preparation, 270
Directions, giving of, skills and techniques involved in, 161-162
Director of hospital nursing services, 235
Discretion, 69
Disposition, 83
Dress, 81-82
Drug Abuse Control Amendments, 179
Drug abuse and the nurse, 178-180
Drugs
  administration of, liability for, 180
  dangerous, control of, 179-180
Dunant, Henri, 266
Duties
  to patient, 189-190
  to physician, 190
  to profession, 189
Dying patient, spiritual needs of, 185-186

E

Economic and general welfare program of American Nurses' Association, 258
Economic security, building for, 192-204
Economics, personal, 192-204
Educated nursing, 2, 25-41
  in the Armistice period, 35-36
  foundations of, 25-28
  in the great depression, 36-37
  in the Spanish-American War, 31-32
  in the twentieth century, 32-40

Educated nursing—cont'd
in the United States, 28-32
in World War I, 33-35
Education
continuing, 209-210, 248
current focus on in American Nurses' Association position paper, 269-270
in-service, 209
for nurses
collegiate school (baccalaureate program), 51-53
community or junior college (associate degree program), 53-55
early twentieth century, 32
foundations of, 25-28
hospital school (diploma program), 50-51
Nightingale system of, 25-28
opportunities in, 237-238
practical/vocational nursing program, 56-58
preservice programs, 47-58
standards for, setting of, 32-33
types of programs, 48-58
in the United States, cornerstone of, 28-32
Educational grants and loans for nursing students, 198-199, 213-214, 248-249
Educational records, official transcripts of, use of in selection of students for nursing school, 114
Educational setting, interpersonal relations in, 138-140
Entrance requirements for nursing schools, reasons for, 112-113
Ethics
code of
American Medical Association, 101-102
American Nurses' Association, 101
functions of, 103
International Council of Nurses, 102-103
medical, 101-102
nurses', 101
and etiquette, differences between, 100
nature of, 99-100
for nursing, 99-104
professional, 100-103
functions of, 103
Etiquette
and ethics, differences between, 100
social, guides for use in correspondence, 283-287
Examination, physical, use of in selection of students for nursing school, 115-116
Exchange of Privileges Programme, 260, 261
Extended care, post-hospital, coverage of under Medicare Hospital Insurance, 212
Extreme Unction in Roman Catholicism, 184-185

F

Facts About Nursing, 208, 258
Facts, study of in problem-solving, 95-96
Far East, nursing in, 4
Federal agencies, nursing in, 242-247
requirements for, 245-246
Federal income taxes, 202
Feedback
clarification of, 148
in communication, use of, 147-148
provisions for in giving directions, 162
Finances
for hospital nursing program, 50
personal, management of, 192-204
Florence Nightingale Education Division, 261
Florence Nightingale International Foundation, 261
Followership
importance of, 98
and leadership, 110-111
Food, budgeting for, 196-197
Fortitude, 65
French leave, 223
Friendships, new, forming of, 61

G

Goodrich, Annie W., 35
Government officials of the United States, titles of, 287
Government relations program of American Nurses' Association, 258
Government savings bonds, 200-201
Grade point average, derivation of, 120-122
Grading system in nursing school, 118-120
Grants and loans, educational, for nursing, 198-199, 213-214, 248-249
Greece, ancient, nursing in, 4-5
Gretter, Lystra E., 104
Grief and mourning, stages of, 186
Group living
adjustment to, 59-60
respecting rights of others in, 85-86
Growth, personal, opportunities for on nursing care team, 170

H

Harrison Narcotic Act, 179
Head nurse, 234-235
Health
maintenance of, 91-92
and medical services, coverage of under Medicare Medical Insurance, 213
public; *see* Public health
spiritual, basic considerations for, 182-187
Health Amendments Act of 1956, 213
Health care
changing pattern of, in American Nurses' Association position paper, 271
prepaid, effect of on nursing, 45
Health center environment, new, assisting patient in, 190

Health legislation, 211-213
Health Manpower Act of 1968, 214
Health record, use of in selection of students for nursing school, 115-116
Health team, 166
Hebrews, hygienic regulations of, 4
Hippocrates as father of medicine, 5, 17
History
of American Association of Industrial Nurses, 265
of American Association of Nurse Anesthetists, 265
of American National Red Cross, 266-267
of American Nurses' Association, 252
of associate degree program, 53-54
of Association of Operating Room Nurses, 265-266
of collegiate nursing programs, 51-52
of International Council of Nurses, 260
of National Association for Practical Nurse Education and Service, 264
of National Federation of Licensed Practical Nurses, 264
of National League for Nursing, 262
of National Student Nurses' Association, 123-124
of nursing, 1-7
of practical nursing programs, 56-57
Home health visits, coverage of under Medicare Medical Insurance, 213
Honesty
attributes and importance of, 65-67
evidences of, 66-67
Honor, 65
Hospital
administration team of, 165
functions and organization of, 136-138
interpersonal relations in, 136-138
lines of communication in, 138
medieval, 18
new, assisting patient in, 190
Hospital Insurance under Medicare, 212
Hospital nursing, 233-234
Hospital nursing services
administrative position in, 234-235
assistant director of, 235
director of, 235
supervisor of, 235
Hospital school for education of nurses, 50-51
Hospitalization, coverage of under Medicare Hospital Insurance, 212
Hotel, care for patient in, 190
Housemother, role of in nursing school counseling program, 130
Housing, budgeting for, 196
Humor, sense of, 68, 92-93

I

Immigration Law of 1965, 213
Imprisonment, false, 176-177
Industry, nursing in, 240-242
Information
gathering of
skills and techniques involved in, 155-159
use of questions for, 158
giving of, skills and techniques involved in, 159-161
In-service education, 209
Installment buying, 199-200
Institutes on nursing skills, 209
Institution of Kaiserswerth as first school of nursing, 13-14
Insurance, budgeting for, 201-202
Integrity, 65
Intelligence, 92
Intensive care unit, modern, 74
International Council of Nurses, 258-262
code of ethics of, 102-103
history of, 260
international functions of, 261
membership in, 260
purposes of, 259
special points for consideration, 260-262
International Nursing Review, 207, 260
International Pledge, 103-104
International program of American Nurses' Association, 258-259
International Red Cross Treaty, 266
Interpersonal relations, 134-141
in clinical situation, 136-138
in educational setting, 138-140
importance of in public health nursing, 239
between individuals, 140-141
meaning of, 134
satisfactory, characteristics of, 134-136
Interview, personal
in job application, 220-221
in selection of students for nursing school, 116-117
Intuitive nursing, 2-7
in ancient Greece, 4-5
definition of, 2
in Far East, 4
in Near East, 3-4
Investments, 201
Invitations, 283-285
formal, 283-284
informal, 283
wedding, 284-285

J

Jacobi, Eileen M., 259
Jargon, medical, 151
Jewish patient, religious consolation for, 183-184
Job
application for, 217-222
personal interview in, 220-221

Job—cont'd
  application form for, 221-222
  dismissal from, 223
  first, 215-224
    importance of, 216-217
  handling yourself on, 222
  resignation from, 222-224
  right, finding of, 217-218
  selection of, 215-217
Johns Hopkins Hospital School of Nursing, 30
Joint Committee on the Structure of National Nursing Organizations, 251
Journal of the American Association of Nurse Anesthetists, 265
Journal of Nursing Education, 208
Journal of Practical Nursing, 264
Journal of Psychiatric Nursing and Mental Health Services, 208
Journals and periodicals, professional, 206-209
Judgment, attributes and importance of, 68-69
Junior college for education of nurses, 53-55
Justice, 64

K

Kaiserswerth, Institution of, as first school of nursing, 13-14
"Kashruth," 183-184
Knight of Malta in battle dress and in hospital confines, 9
Knights of St. John of Jerusalem, 8
Knights of St. Lazarus, 8

L

Language; *see also* Words
  and meaning, 148-149
  use of in communication, 148-151
Last Rites in Roman Catholicism, 184-185
Laura D. Smith scholarship, 126
Laws
  common, 172
  licensing, for nurses, 172-173
  mandatory, 173
  permissive, 172-173
  purpose of, 172
  statutory, 172
Leadership
  and followership, 110-111
  qualifications for, 97-98
Learning
  continuation of throughout career, 105
  and working as student in nursing program, 85-98
Legal accountability of nurses, 172-177
Legal aspects of nursing functions, 174-175
Legal aspects of nursing practice, 172-181
Legal status of nurses, 172-174
Legislation
  health, 211-213
  nursing, 44-45, 213-214
Leone, Lucille Petry, 39
Letter
  of inquiry and application, writing of, 218-220
  thank you, 283
Liability
  for administration of care, 180
  for administration of drugs, 180
  of nurses, off-duty, 175
  for supervision, 180-181
Licensing laws for nurses, 172-173
Licensure of nurses, 172-174
  annual renewal of, 173
  denial, revocation, and suspension of, 173-174
  by endorsement, 173
  by examination, 173
  process of, 173
  by waiver, 173
Life
  philosophy of, relationship of to view of nursing, 87-88
  symmetrical, building of, 87-88
Limitations and strengths, recognition of, 188-189
Listening, importance of to communication, 153-154
Lister, Joseph, 19
Loans
  budgeting for, 197-198
  and grants, educational, for nursing, 198-199, 213-214, 248-249
Loyalty, attributes and importance of, 67

M

Maas, Clara Louise, 31
Malpractice, 176
Mance, Jeanne, 14-15
Manpower Development Training Act of 1962, 213
Meaning
  and language, 148-149
  of words
    connotative, 149-150
    from context, 150
    denotative, 149
Medical caduceus, origin of, 5
Medical ethics, principles of, 101-102
Medical and health services, coverage of under Medicare Medical Insurance, 213
Medical Insurance under Medicare, 213
Medical jargon, 151
Medicare, 212-213
  effect of on nursing, 45
Medicine, space, effect of on nursing, 44
Medieval hospitals, 18

Meetings, 276-279
conducting, 276
courtesies followed during, 276-277
minutes of, 279
motions in, 277-278; *see also* Motions
order of business in, 276
types of, 276
voting in, 278-279
Membership
in American National Red Cross, 267-268
in American Nurses' Association, 252
in International Council of Nurses, 260
in National Association for Practical Nurse Education and Service, 264
in National Federation of Licensed Practical Nurses, 264
in National League for Nursing, 262
in National Student Nurses' Association, 124-125
Men in nursing during the Crusades, 8
Military auspices, nursing under, 243-247
Mind, peace of, 92
Minority groups, involvement of nursing with, 45
Moderation, attributes and importance of, 71-72
Motions
amending, technique of, 278
classification of, 277-278
incidental, 278
main, 278
offering and voting on, 277
privileged, 277
subsidiary, 277-278
Motivation, attributes and importance of, 70
Mourning and grief, stages of, 186

N

Name cards, 285
Narcotics, control of, 179-180
National Association of Colored Graduate Nurses, 251
National Association for Practical Nurse Education and Service, 264
history of, 264
membership in, 264
purposes and programs of, 264
National Commission for the Study of Nursing and Nursing Education, 271
National Conference of Professional Students, 126
National Defense Medical Center in Taipei, Taiwan, 126-127
National Federation of Licensed Practical Nurses, 264-265
history of, 264
membership in, 264
organization of, 264-265
purposes of, 264
National League for Nursing, 252, 262-264
Committee on Careers, 262
National League for Nursing—cont'd
history of, 262
information on educational preparation for teaching, 238
membership in, 262
organization chart, 263
position of in two-organization plan, 251
programs of, 262-264
purposes of, 262
role of in founding of National Student Nurses' Association, 123
National League of Nursing Education, 31, 32, 36, 251, 252, 262
standard curriculum for nursing education set by, 32
National League for Nursing Evaluation Service, 262
National Organization of Public Health Nursing, 36, 251
National Student Nurses' Association, 123-127
activities of, 125-127
committees of, 125
history of, 123-124
membership in, 124-125
official emblem of, 124
organization of, 125
purpose of, 125
Navy, nursing opportunities with, 245
Near East, nursing in, 3-4
Negligence, definition and proof of, 176
New World, nursing in, 14-16
Nightingale, Florence
nursing activities in the Crimea, 26-27
nursing school established by, 27-28
preparation for nursing, 26
system of nursing education established by, 25-28
Nightingale Pledge, 103-104
Nonverbal and verbal communication, 142-143
Nurse Practice Acts, 172-175, 180, 270
Nurse-instructors, role of in nursing school counseling program, 129-130
Nurse-patient relationship, 140
Nurse Training Act of 1964, 214
Nurses
code of ethics for, 101
contemporary, evolution of, 2
costumes of
American nurse during Spanish-American War (1898), 22
Catholic order of Canonesses (1242), 20
in court of Henry VIII of England (1540), 20
early uniform (1880), 22
"Flapper age" (1925), 23
through history, 20-24; *see also* Uniforms, nurse's
modern habit of religious order, 24
modern uniform, 24
volunteer nurse at Battle of Gettysburg (1863), 21
crimes and torts relating to, 175-177
drug abuse and, 178-180
education of; *see* Education for nurses
first historical mention of, 4

Nurses—cont'd
functioning of, legal aspects of, 174-175
graduate, first job of, 215-224
head, 234-235
legal accountability of, 172-177
legal status of, 172-174
licensing laws for, 172-173
licensure of, 172-174
annual renewal of, 173
denial, revocation, and suspension of, 173-174
by endorsement, 173
by examination, 173
process of, 173
by waiver, 173
male, during the Crusades, 8
off-duty liability of, 175
organizations of, addresses of, 273-274
Nurses Associated Alumnae of the United States and Canada, 252
Nurses Educational Funds, Inc., 248
Nursing
American reforms in, 15
apprentice, 2, 8-16; *see also* Apprentice nursing
"awakening" of, 30-31
career in
opportunities for pursuing, 233-250
"second thoughts" about, 61-63
commitment to, 88
communication in, importance of, 142
concepts of, 105-107
contemporary, 2, 42-46
effect of atomic energy on, 43
effect of computers on, 43-44
effect of diagnostic and therapeutic agents on, 44
effect of prepaid health care on, 45
effect of scientific and technical research on, 43-44
effect of space medicine on, 44
involvement with minority groups, 45
legislation affecting, 44-45
social forces affecting, 44-46
technologic efficiency affecting, 45-46
"dark period of," 11-12
definitions, 107-108
educated, 2, 25-41; *see also* Educated nursing
education for
career opportunities in, 237-238
grants and loans for, 198-199, 213-214, 248-249
effect of social reforms on, 12-14
ethics for, 99-104
in federal agencies, 242-247
requirements, 245-246
history of, 1-7
hospital, 233-234
importance of cooperation in, 109-111
interpretations of, 105-111
intuitive, 2-7; *see also* Intuitive nursing
under military auspices, 243-247
as an occupation, 105
Nursing—cont'd
occupational health, 240-242
office, 235-236
orders of, religious, rise of, 8-9
organizations of, official, 251-268
practice of
area of, selection of, 188-189
complexity of, effect of on educational orientation in nursing preparation, 270
legal aspects of, 172-181
private duty, 236-237
as a profession, 48, 105-106
profession of, official publications of, 206-208
program of
counseling in, role of, 128-133
first days in, 59-84
learning and working as student in, 85-98
public health, 238-242; *see also* Public health nursing
recruitment for by National Student Nurses' Association, 126
reformation and, 11-12
school, 240
schools of
academic policies and scholarship requirements of, 112-122
early development of, 47-48
entrance requirements for, reasons for, 112-113
Institution of Kaiserswerth as first, 13-14
student selection for, 113-117
in United States, 28-30
scope of, 107-109
in special clinical areas, preparation for, 235
specialization in, 32
staff, advantages and disadvantages of, 233-234
state boards of, 173, 258
view of, relationship of philosophy of life to, 87-88
Nursing care team, 166-170
evolution of, 166-167
leader of, 168-169
opportunities for personal growth and development in, 170
organization for service, 167-169
purpose of, 167
working in, 169-170
Nursing Council for National Defense, 38
Nursing education program of American Nurses' Association, 258
Nursing Forum, 208
Nursing legislation, 213-214
Nursing Outlook, 207, 235, 248
Nursing personnel, qualified, shortage of, in American Nurses' Association position paper, 271
Nursing practice program of American Nurses' Association, 258
Nursing Research, 207
Nursing saints, 9-10

Nursing service administration team, 165-166
Nursing services, hospital, administrative positions in, 234-235

O

Obedience, 66-67
  importance of to interpersonal relations, 87
Observation, importance of in nursing, 69
Occupation, nursing as, 105
Occupational analysis, 188
Occupational Health Nursing, 265
Occupational health nursing, 240-242
Office nursing, 235-236
Officers in organization, 279-281
Old-Age, Survivors, Disability, and Health Insurance Program of Social Security, 211-212
Opening Doors Wider in Nursing, 126
Operating expenses, budgeting for, 197
Opportunities
  in nursing education, 237-238
  for pursuing a career in nursing, 233-250
Organization services program of American Nurses' Association, 258
Organizations
  constitutions and bylaws of, 275
  nursing, addresses of, 273-274
  nursing, official, 251-268
  officers of, 279-281
Outpatient hospital diagnosis services, coverage of under Medicare Hospital Insurance, 212

P

Pagan philosophy, transition from to Christian philosophy, 5-7
Parliamentary procedures, 275-282
Patience, 68
Patient
  accompanying in public, 190
  duties to, 189-190
  dying, spiritual needs of, 185-186
  Jewish, religious consolation for, 183-184
  Protestant, religious consolation for, 185
  religious needs of, 182-187
  Roman Catholic, religious consolation for, 184-185
  traveling with, 190
Patient's consent, 177-178
Peace Corps, nursing opportunities with, 247
Peace of mind, 92
Penance in Roman Catholicism, 184
Peplau, Hildegard E., 259
Periodicals and journals, professional, 206-209
Perseverance, 70
Personal accomplishments to present, 188
Personal adjustment to nursing programs, 60-61
Personal development, role of books in, 206
Personal economics, 192-204
Personal growth and development, opportunities for on nursing care team, 170
Personal interview
  for job, 220-221
  in selection of students for nursing school, 116-117
Personal problems, value of counseling for, 131
Personal resources, proper use of, 91-93
Personal titles, 285
Personality, 72, 81-82
Perspectives in Psychiatric Nursing, 208
Philosophy
  of life, relationship to view of nursing, 87-88
  transition from pagan to Christian, 5-7
Physician
  duties to, 190
  role of in nursing school counseling program, 130
Physician's and surgeon's services, coverage of under Medicare Medical Insurance, 213
Pitch in speaking, 152
Pledges of dedication, 103-104
Poor Clares, 9, 10
Position; *see* Job
Position Paper on Education for Nursing, 269
Post-hospital extended care, coverage of under Medicare Hospital Insurance, 212
Post-hospital home health care, coverage of under Medicare Hospital Insurance, 212
Posture, 72
Practical nursing program, 56-58
Pre-Civil War nursing, 15
Pre-entrance tests in selection of students for nursing school, 116
Prejudices, effect of on communication, 146-147
Preservice nursing education programs, 47-58
Private duty nursing, 236-237
Privileged communication and the nurse, 177
Problem, identifying and defining, 94-95
Problem-solving, technique of, 93-96
Profession
  definition, 105
  duties to, 189
  nursing as, 48, 105-106
    ethics of, 100-103
Professional, definition, 106-107
Professional conduct in public, 190-191
Professional Credentials and Placement Service, 258
Professional journals and periodicals, 206-209
Professional organization, belonging to, 247-248
Professional practice, hallmarks of, 189-191
Professional registries for private duty nurses, local, 236
Professional and social responsibility, 205
Professional titles, 285-287
Promoting Committee for the Study of the Structure of National Professional Organizations, 251
Protestant, religious consolation for, 185
Prudence, 64

Psychologist, clinical, role of in nursing school counseling program, 130
Public, accompanying patient in, 190
Public Health Nursing, 207
Public health nursing, 238-242
  occupational health nursing, 240-242
  school nursing, 240
  after World War I, 35
Public Health Service, United States, nursing opportunities in, 242-243
Public relations program of American Nurses' Association, 258
Publications
  of nursing profession, official, 206-208
  professional, 206-209
Punctuality, importance of, 118

Q

Questions
  asking of, techniques for, 157-159
    to draw out information, 158
    to get another's thinking, 159
    to get clarification, 158-159
  importance of in information gathering, 156-159
  structured, use of, 156-157
  types of, 156-157
  unstructured, use of, 156-157

R

Rate of speaking, importance of to communication, 152
Recommendations, use of in selection of students for nursing school, 114-115
Records, 178
Recreation
  budgeting for, 197
  importance of, 88-89
Red Cross Nursing Service, purposes of, 167
Reformation and nursing, 11-12
Registered Nurse Student Program, 244-245
Registries, professional, for private duty nurses, local, 236
Relations, interpersonal, 133-141; *see also* Interpersonal relations
Reliability, attributes and importance of, 69-70
Religious consolation for patient, 183-185
Religious needs of patient, 182-187
Religious nursing orders, rise of, 8-9
Report
  delivery of, 163-164
  giving of
    organization of material for, 163
    skills and techniques involved in, 162-164
Research, scientific and technical, effect of on nursing, 43-44
Research and statistics program of American Nurses' Association, 258
Residence
  director of, role of in nursing school counseling program, 130
  in hospital nursing program, 50
Resignation from job, 222-224
Resolution, making of, technique of, 278
Resourcefulness, attributes and importance of, 70
Resources, personal, proper use of, 91-93
Respect for job, importance of in interpersonal relations, 135-136
Responsibility, social and professional, 205
Restraints, 176-177
Results, evaluation of in problem-solving, 96
Revolutions, social, impact of on nursing, 10-14
Rights of others, respect for, 85-86
RN, 208
Robb, Isabel Hampton, 30, 31, 259
Roman Catholic patient, religious consolation for, 184-185
Rubber gloves, origin of use of, 30

S

Saints, nursing, 9-10
Savings
  budgeting for, 200-201
  club or special fund for, 200
Savings accounts
  general, 200
  special, 200-201
Savings bonds, government, 200-201
Scholarship requirements and academic policies of nursing schools, 117-122
Scholastic achievement in nursing school, 118-122
School for Aerospace Nursing, 44
School nursing, 240
Schools of nursing in the United States, 28-30
Scientific research, effect of on nursing, 43-44
Security, sense of, 92
Self-acceptance, importance of in interpersonal relations, 134-135
Self-analysis in identification of strengths and limitations, 188-189
Self-awareness, importance of in interpersonal relations, 134
Self-evaluation, 63-72, 81-82
Self-restraint, attributes and importance of, 71-72
Sensitivity to others' needs, importance of in interpersonal relations, 135
Sick, anointing of in Roman Catholicism, 184-185
Slang, use of, 151
Social etiquette, guides for use in correspondence, 283-287
Social forces affecting nursing, 44-46
Social and professional responsibility, 205
Social reforms, effect of on nursing, 12-14
Social revolutions, impact of on apprentice nursing, 10-14

Social Security Amendments Act, 203
Social Security taxes, 202-203
Solutions, testing of in problem-solving, 96
Space medicine, effect of on nursing, 44
Spanish-American War, nursing in, 31-32
Speaking
  manner of, 151-153
  rate of, importance of to communication, 152
  voice pitch in, 152
  voice quality in, 152-153
  volume in, control of, 151-152
Specialization in nursing, 32
Speech, impression created by, 86
Spending, wise, 196
Spiritual health, basic considerations for, 182-187
Spiritual needs of patient, meeting, 182-185
Staff nursing, advantages and disadvantages of, 233-234
Standards for nursing education, setting of, 32-33
State boards of nursing, 173, 258
State taxes, 202
Statutory law, 172
Stewart, Isabel, 38
Stimson, Julia, 35
Strength and limitations, recognition of, 188-189
Student government activities, participation in, 96-98
Student-learner, role of, adjustment to, 60-61
Student selection for nursing schools, 113-117
Student War Nursing Reserve, 39
Study
  attitude for, development of, 89-91
  purpose of, 90
  techniques of, improvement of, 90-91
Supervision, liability for, 180-181
Supervisor of hospital nursing service, 235
Surgeon's and physician's services, coverage of under Medicare Medical Insurance, 213
Sympathy, 68

T

Tact, 69
Taiwan project of National Student Nurses' Association, 126-127
Taxes
  budgeting for, 202-203
  Federal income, 202
  Social Security, 202-203
  state and city, 202
Teaching in schools of nursing, 237-238
Teams
  health, 166
  hospital administration, 165
  nursing care, 166-170; *see also* Nursing care team
  nursing service administration, 165-166
  types of, 165-166
  working in, 165-171
Technical research, effect of on nursing, 43-44
Technologic efficiency, effect of on nursing, 45-46
Temperance, 65
Tertiaries of St. Dominic, 9, 10
Tertiaries of St. Francis, 9
Tests
  aptitude, in selection of students for nursing school, 116
  pre-entrance, in selection of students for nursing school, 116
Teutonic Knights, 8
Therapy, agents for, effect of on nursing, 44
Time
  for communication, choosing right, 146
  proper use of, 67, 91
Titles
  of clergy, 287
  in correspondence, 285-287
  of government officials in United States, 287
  personal, 285
  professional, 285-297
Tolerance, attributes and importance of, 67-68
Torts relating to nurses, 175-177
Transcripts of educational records, official, use of in selection of students for nursing school, 114
Traveling with patient, 190
Truthfulness, 65
Tucker, Pearl E., 44
Twentieth century, nursing in, 32-40

U

Understanding, 68
Uniform, nurse's, 81; *see also* Nurses, costumes of through history
  early (1880), 22
  "Flapper age" (1925), 23
  modern, 24
  origin of, 29-30
United States Cadet Nurse Corps, 39
United States Public Health Service, nursing opportunities in, 242-243
Unselfishness, 68
Ursulines, 9

V

Vacations, budgeting for, 197
Valuable papers and documents, care of, 203
Verbal and nonverbal communication, 142-143
Veterans Administration, nursing opportunities with, 243
Viaticum in Roman Catholicism, 184-185
Visiting cards, 285
Visiting Nurse Service of New York, 239

Vocational Education Act of 1963, 213
Vocational nursing program, 56-58
Voice quality in speaking, 152-153
Volume in speaking, control of, 151-152
Voting Rights Act of 1965, 213

W

Welfare program, general, of American Nurses' Association, 258
Wholesome Meat Act of 1967, 213
Wisdom, 68
Words; *see also* Language
  connotative meaning of, 149-150
  denotative meaning of, 149
  meaning of from context, 150
  usage of, 150-151
Working and learning as student in nursing program, 85-98
Workshops, 209
World Health, 208
World Health Organization (WHO), 42-43
  nursing opportunities with, 247
World War I, nursing in, 33-35
World War II, nursing in, 38-40

Work sheets

Work sheets pertaining to the material presented in the individual chapters of this edition follow. It is recommended that you avail yourself of opportunities to communicate your thoughts verbally and in writing, as the exercises provide, and to participate actively in discussions of various questions. You are also encouraged to formulate your own work sheets when they will be beneficial in expressing yourself in writing and then, if indicated, have others validate your contribution.

NAME ____________________

WORK SHEET

DATE ____________________

NURSING'S HISTORICAL FOUNDATIONS

1. Consider the unkempt, unwashed look of the penitent sinner who dedicated himself to a life without pleasures of the flesh, and the unkempt, unwashed, barefoot rebel of the 1970s. Is there any basis for comparison besides appearance?

2. Read Moloney, Sister Margaret Mary, "Some Impressions of Nursing and Nursing Education in the Middle East," Nursing Outlook 18:56-60, Aug. 1970. How does this nursing compare to that of the United States? Is there still superstition and a remnant of intuitive nursing prevalent in the U. S.?

WORK SHEET

NAME

DATE

THE PERIOD OF APPRENTICE NURSING

1. Social revolutions throughout the ages have had an influence on nursing development. For example, when people are imbued with a desire for power and personal ambition, normal feelings of understanding and sympathy are replaced with skepticism. To overcome guilt feelings, the affluent then dole out charity to those in blighted slum areas. Is charity the answer to the masses of people in slums?

2. Nursing care during the Crusades was given by military nursing orders such as the Knights of St. John of Jerusalem and the Teutonic Knights. Why was this nursing care more successfully given by men than by women?

3. The Renaissance (1200 A.D. to 1500 A.D.) was a period of renewed interest in art, science, literature, and music. Why did this time of exploration and growth in many of the arts and sciences not include a growth in nursing as well?

4. Louis Pasteur's "germ theory," Dr. Lister's theories on asepsis, and Dr. Semmelweiss' and Dr. Oliver Wendell Holmes' achievements in regard to puerperal fever all significantly affected later developments in medicine. What impact did the work of these great men have upon nursing? Defend your answer.

WORK SHEET

NAME

DATE

THE PERIOD OF "EDUCATED" NURSING

1. Miss Nightingale admitted two classes of students into her school. The regular probationer received one year of training followed by three years of supervised practice and was paid a stipend for service. The "lady probationer" paid fees for her program of a one year formal curriculum and two years of supervised practice, which prepared her as a leader. Compare the public image of the nurse who graduated from the early Nightingale School to the public image of the graduate nurse today.

2. Could a woman born into a less affluent family in Victorian England have accomplished the monumental tasks attributed to Florence Nightingale? Support your answer with special reference to the status of women of that period.

3. In the second half of the nineteenth century three wars were fought. Select the war which you feel had the greatest influence on nursing. Describe social conditions that the cessation of hostilities produced and state why nursing education either made strides forward or regressed as a result of these social conditions.

4. Nursing is still feeling the aftereffects of the depression of the 1930s. How do you feel that this effect is manifested? What measures would you suggest to prevent recurrence?

5. Compare the drive of the pioneer woman traveling in her Conestoga wagon across the wilderness to the drive of these pioneers in nursing.

   a. Lillian Wald

   b. Ethel G. Fenwick

   c. Mary Eliza Mahoney

   d. Pearl E. Tucker

WORK SHEET

NAME ______________________

DATE ______________________

THE PERIOD OF CONTEMPORARY NURSING

1. In early American schools of nursing doctors helped plan, direct, and teach much that was included in the student nurses' education. At that time the nurse functioned unquestioningly at the beck and call of the doctor. Compare or contrast the proposed new career for nurses as physician's assistant with this earlier relationship.

2. Involvement is the order of the day. What community involvement can you subscribe to in regard to:
   a. Air pollution

   b. Equal opportunity for employment

c. Equal opportunity for education

d. Equal opportunity for housing

e. Improved health care

Describe your selected issue, plan, implementation, evaluation.

NAME

WORK SHEET

DATE

PRESERVICE NURSING EDUCATION PROGRAMS

1. Why did you select the nursing program in which you are now enrolled?

2. What made you decide to become a nurse? Has what you have learned about nursing, so far, enhanced or fallen short of your expectations? Why?

3. As a student in the nursing program you should be interested in and know something about the historical background and achievement of your school of nursing. Write a short account of the history and development of your program.

4. As you are preparing for a career in nursing, what are some of the immediate goals you have set for yourself? What thought have you given to some long-range goals?

NAME ______________________

WORK SHEET

DATE ______________________

YOUR FIRST DAYS IN THE NURSING PROGRAM

1. Summarize what was included in your school's program of orientation.
   a. Indicate the various topics and/or experiences which you found most helpful.

   b. Suggest some additional problems of adjustment new students need help with that are not provided for in your orientation program.

2. What are some personal qualities you consider most essential for a nurse? List eight to ten of these qualities in order according to your opinion of their importance.

3. With reference to the habits of moral practice and attributes of character discussed in this chapter, *make a personal inventory for your own use* of the strengths you recognize in your own character and the weaknesses you must work on. From time to time make a special effort to review this inventory and gauge yourself on the progress you are making.

4. As human beings we must accept the attributes that Nature gave us. What is your interpretation of the statement: One is much more likely to make himself effective by emphasizing the good qualities he has in large measure than by undue effort to develop those in which he is weak.

NAME

WORK SHEET DATE

LEARNING AND WORKING AS A STUDENT IN NURSING

1. A hobby is something a person likes to do or study in his spare time. What does a hobby contribute to the mental health of a person? Make a list of your hobbies. Tell how you became interested in them and what they contribute to your life and enjoyment.

2. For a period of two weeks keep a detailed record of your study habits and routines and the amount of time you spend in study and preparation of assignments for each subject.
   a. Using the *problem-solving techniques* described in this chapter devise a daily schedule that will provide time for study and class preparations and other demands of daily living which must be met.

   b. Test the workability of your schedule for two to three weeks and make the adjustments indicated for a pattern to be consistently followed.

   c. Evaluate the effectiveness of your revised study pattern and schedule in terms of whether it:
      (1) Provides for a proportional amount of study time for difficult and easy subjects
      (2) Relieves the pressures and anxieties of meeting deadlines for written assignments
      (3) Results in improvements in class grades

3. Study the constitution and bylaws of your school's student government association and identify the:
   a. Official name of the group

   b. Purpose and functions of the association

   c. Qualifications for membership

   d. Officers: numbers and titles, individual duties, qualifications for serving, methods for selection and their duties

   e. Meetings of the association

   f. Executive board; duties

   g. Committees

   h. Techniques for amending bylaws

NAME ______________________

WORK SHEET

DATE ______________________

ETHICS FOR NURSING

1. Study the American Nurses' Association Code of Ethics and make a list of some specific ways you translate the provisions of this Code into practice in your daily nursing activities.

2. a. What is your understanding of what is meant by personal ethics and professional ethics?

   b. Give some examples of instances where one might be in conflict with the other.

3. Why is it considered unethical for a nurse to engage in or allow her name to be used in advertisements of commercial products?

WORK SHEET

NAME ______________________________

DATE ______________________________

SOME INTERPRETATIONS OF NURSING

1. A useful working definition must be one the nurse clearly understands, has examined critically, has found possible to approve, and one that provides direction in her service as a nurse. Profiting by a study of the definitions proposed by others, prepare a definition of nursing that is satisfactory to you.

2. Obtain a copy of the Nurse Practice Act of your state covering registered nurses and licensed practical/vocational nurses. Read and summarize the provisions for each pertaining to:
   a. Official definition as practitioners

   b. Scope and regulation of their practice

NAME ____________________

WORK SHEET

DATE ____________________

INTERPRETING ESSENTIAL ACADEMIC POLICIES AND REQUIREMENTS

1. To be successful any educational program must be a partnership between the school and the student. Each partner must be fully acquainted with the conditions governing the enterprise and the factors that control its continuance. In the catalogue of your school look up the conditions and requirements stipulated for your nursing program:

   a. Description of the kind of nurse the program wishes to graduate

   b. Entrance requirements

   c. Personal health requirements

   d. Program of study (description and sequence of courses)

   e. Grading system and standards of scholastic achievement (including conditions under which students may be placed on probation or be subject to dismissal because of poor standing)

   f. Requirements for graduation

2. As a student your success in the nursing program will be judged according to your scholastic achievements. This being the case, what is your personal feeling about "working for grades"?

WORK SHEET

NAME

DATE

THE NATIONAL STUDENT NURSES' ASSOCIATION

1. What is the name of the publication for your district, state, or national student nurse association?

Third district
Mo. State Student Nurses Association

If you were writing an article how would you present the problem(s) related to the following social and health situations in this publication?

a. Malnutrition in the United States

b. Health care for all citizens

c. Education for family living

What plan would you develop in order to get your group concerned and involved?

2. How are NSNA delegates selected for state conventions? for national conventions? What is the ratio of district membership to state membership delegates representing you at a national convention of National Student Nurses' Association?

3. a. Who is the current president of National Student Nurses' Association and what is the home school of this nursing student?

b. Who is the current president of your state association and what school of nursing does this student represent?

4. Identify the current NSNA purposes. How do they relate to the purposes of your local group?

NAME ____________________

WORK SHEET

DATE ____________________

THE ROLE OF COUNSELING IN NURSING PROGRAMS

1. A friend of yours asks you to describe in detail the counseling program and the facilities for guidance in your school of nursing. State, in outline, what information you will give her.

2. Think about two instances in your life when you needed counsel and guidance with problems. Indicate how you sought this assistance, acted on the guidance received, and benefited from the experience.

3. Distinguish between personal growth which results from dependence on 'Do this' or 'Don't do that' guidance, and that which is gained from choosing a plan of action and accepting the consequences of it.

4. Describe, briefly, your feelings about counseling and guidance.

NAME

WORK SHEET

DATE

INTERPERSONAL RELATIONS

1. An organization chart is only a series of boxes connected by lines unless it is *studied and understood* by the workers that make up the organization. The purpose of the hospital organization chart is to delineate the areas of responsibility and authority relationships that exist in the hospital. In other words, it tells us "who does what" and "who is responsible to whom." Many of the problems in hospital administration and management can be traced to two major causes: (1) individuals who make decisions on problems outside of their jurisdiction (area of authority and responsibility) and (2) "by-passing" (individuals going around instead of through the chain of supervision).

   For this exercise, study the organization chart of the hospital where you are receiving your clinical practice experience and note the various departments and services, the titles of positions, and the number of levels of control.

   a. Trace the line of authority that flows from the hospital administrator downward to the director of nursing service and through the nursing department organization to the unit where you are assigned for your clinical practice. Give the position title and the name of each person filling each position.

   b. Follow the channels of official communication from the nursing unit upward through the nursing department organization to the hospital administrator.

c. Suppose a problem arises on one of the nursing units involving a diet maid who frequently speaks to patients in a rough and abrupt manner. The handling of this problem falls under whose area of responsibility? Explain your answer.

d. Suppose the section supervisor decides to send a staff nurse from one nursing unit to help out on another unit that requires extra staffing because of the heavy work load. What procedure should the supervisor follow? Explain your answer.

e. Suppose you, the student, accidently threw away a urine specimen that was to be part of a 24-hour urine test. To whom should you report this mistake? Explain your answer.

2. Interpersonal relations, in all its aspects, has to do with the acceptance of others and a sensitivity to another's needs. With this in mind, draw up a "bill of rights" for patients. Set down what, in your opinion, every patient has a right to expect from the personnel who provide his nursing care.

3. As a team leader you will give orders to other members of the nursing care team and will be accountable for the way they perform their work.
   a. How does this change in status affect your relationship with the team members?

   b. What are some difficulties that might arise as a result of the way you perceive your role? As the result of the way team members perceive you?

   c. What should you do to prevent or minimize these difficulties?

4. Either as a student or as a graduate, a member of the nursing team will be responsible to the team leader, will work with others who hold similar positions, or will work with persons who have jobs subordinate to her own. These are three different roles. In working with others, interpersonal relationships involve the same qualities of personality whether you are working as a subordinate, a peer, or a person in a higher status. Explain how you see each of the following operating in each role:
   a. Courtesy

   b. Tact

   c. Cooperation

   d. Consistency

   e. Loyalty

   f. Honesty

NAME ____________________

WORK SHEET

DATE ____________________

COMMUNICATION

1. List ten important causes of communication failure.

2. A nursing educator is quoted as saying, "You may have more opportunities to improve your communication skills while a student in nursing than at any other time in your life." Enumerate the specific advantages and benefits she might have had in mind as you interpret her meaning.

3. Based on your answer in Question 2, how might you, or do you, use these opportunities to develop or to improve your own communication skills? Explain.

4. Listen to several casual conversations for trite expressions that are used over and over again by people, for example, "You know what?" "If you know what I mean," "So what?" "The darlingest." Then listen to yourself in your casual conversation and make a list of the overworked words or phrases in your own speech for which you should occasionally substitute others or eliminate altogether.

NAME ____________________

WORK SHEET

DATE ____________________

COMMUNICATION SKILLS AND TECHNIQUES

1. In what practical ways, if any, has the substance of this chapter been helpful to you and relevant to the tasks you perform daily? Explain.

2. Recall a communication situation in which you failed to tune in on the implicit message in another's question and tell what were the effects on both of you.

3. What is the pitfall in giving advice to someone else?

4. Anticipate some therapeutic procedure or diagnostic test one of your patients will receive and plan what you will tell the patient in order to prepare him for the test or procedure.

5. Assume that you have been assigned to admit a patient and to orient him to the nursing unit. It happens that he has never been a patient in a hospital until now.
   a. Describe what you would include in the orientation of this patient.

   b. What information would you give the patient's wife who is also present?

NAME ____________________

WORK SHEET

DATE ____________________

WORKING IN A TEAM

1. How do you interpret the following?
   a. Team nursing

   b. The nursing care team

2. Assuming that the hospital(s) where you are receiving your clinical practice experiences uses the nursing care team method for assigning patient care, outline in detail how the nursing care team functions.

3. As a student you may be given some supervised experience as a team leader. This will mean giving individual team members their assignments and making sure that the doctors' orders and nursing care of all patients for whom your team is responsible are carried out in a complete and satisfactory manner. How should you conduct yourself to get off to a good start in your relationships with your team members?

NAME

WORK SHEET

DATE

LEGAL ASPECTS OF NURSING PRACTICE

1. The American Nurses' Association Code for Nurses states that nurses use their "individual competence as a criterion in accepting delegated responsibilities and assigning nursing activities to others." In your local and state regulations affecting nursing practice what is the policy regarding a nurse performing:
   a. Closed chest cardiopulmonary resuscitation

   b. Intravenous infusion

   c. Blood transfusion

   d. Intravenous injection

2. In what ways could you bring about cause for litigation in the following?
   a. The application of leather restraints to the extremities of a difficult and belligerent patient?

   b. As an act of human kindness, the administration (without a physician's order) of a routine medication for relieving pain to a patient who seemed to be suffering extensively.

   c. The failure to check a patient's condition at a specific time because of concentration on other duties that seemed more essential.

WORK SHEET

NAME ______________________

DATE ______________________

BASIC CONSIDERATIONS FOR SPIRITUAL HEALTH

Consult a rabbi, Catholic priest, and a minister concerning the following questions. Compare the answers from each spiritual leader. Is there a great difference between their responses?

1. How do your ministrations as a clergyman spiritually differ in meeting the needs of the terminally ill patient and the patient who will recover?

2. Are you, as a nurse, free to proselyte your patient?

WORK SHEET

NAME ______________________

DATE ______________________

LOOKING AHEAD

1. Many active nurses are married, carrying both family and nursing responsibilities. Weigh the responsibility of the married nurse to self, family, and profession. Determine which comes first and whether there are lines of demarcation for:
   a. The man in nursing

   b. The woman in nursing

   What are the differences?

2. Look carefully at the objectives of your educational program in nursing. Determine from these the positions you would be qualified to assume upon passing your state board examination.

3. Many state nursing associations have identified the beginning positions that nurses would be qualified to assume upon graduation from their specific type of nursing education program. Does your state association have such identified positions available? If so, do these statements correspond to the stated objectives of your school of nursing?

NAME

WORK SHEET

DATE

BUILDING FOR ECONOMIC SECURITY

1. Make out a spending plan that suits your present situation. Devise your own budget with allocations to fit your own needs and preferences.
   a. Keep accurate record of all your expenditures for a period of one month, as described in this chapter.

   b. Analyze your spending record to see where your money goes. Determine where you spent more or were able to keep within the limits of or spent less than the budget allocations.

   c. Determine how your spending must be adjusted the following month in order to work within your spending plan.

2. What kind of documents and important papers would you place in a safety deposit box for safe-keeping? List some important papers that are best kept in a safe place at home so they are available for ready reference.

3. One way in which you build for your future financial security is by your payments in Social Security. A very important point to remember is that the individual has the responsibility for ascertaining that his earnings have been correctly recorded during his working years and that the individual must request the benefits to which he is entitled.
   a. Where would you obtain information about the benefits under the Social Security Act?

   b. How would you find out whether your employment is covered under Social Security?

c. What is the procedure if you change your name or lose your Social Security card?

d. What is the procedure for checking records to determine whether your earnings have been correctly reported?

WORK SHEET

NAME ______________________

DATE ______________________

KEEPING UP TO DATE

1. Evaluate the quotation from Alexander Pope's *Essay on Criticism* as to its application to you as a nurse practitioner and community member.

   A little learning is a dangerous thing;
   Drink deep, or taste not the Pierian spring;
   There shallow draughts intoxicate the brain,
   And drinking largely sobers us again.

2. You have elected to prepare to become a clinical nurse specialist. Identify your major area of interest. Then, after a careful review of the educational courses in colleges and universities offering this advanced clinical preparation, outline the educational plan and the nursing experiences you think you would need to follow in order to effectively prepare to function in this capacity.

NAME

WORK SHEET

DATE

HEALTH AND NURSING LEGISLATION

1. The current movement toward changing abortion laws in many states has caught the attention of the communications media so that papers are being presented, articles written, and programs presented. What is the law in your state? When was it passed? In your opinion does it meet the needs of your society?

2. Mental health is a national problem. How has your state and your community utilized the Community Mental Health Acts?

NAME

WORK SHEET

DATE

THE GRADUATE NURSE'S FIRST JOB

1. Assume you plan to go to work in another city following your graduation and receiving your license to practice nursing. Write a letter to a hospital or other health agency to apply for a position as a staff nurse.

2. In addition to salary, what are some aspects of a job that should be given major consideration by a person seeking a position? Do you believe a nurse is justified in refusing to work anything but a straight forty-hour week, with no weekend, evening, or night duty?

3. In the event you marry soon after graduation and do not continue in active nursing, what obligations do you have to yourself and to the profession?

WORK SHEET

NAME ______________________________

DATE ______________________________

OPPORTUNITIES FOR PURSUING A CAREER IN NURSING

It can be said that education, like time, in itself has no worth. The true value of both depends on the use made of them. As you prepare to leave the school, make a few final surveys that will help in opening the doors to the future. Here are some suggested projects:

1. Make a list of the *major* problems faced by student nurses that you have observed and would like to see corrected in the future. Place an asterisk before those which you would be especially willing to help overcome. (Avoid including personalities or situations within your immediate environment which are beyond your control. Consider the preparation and welfare of student nurses in general.)

2. Whether you choose a career in one of the six federal government services or not, you will still be functioning as a professional nurse in a democracy. What does the request of our late president, John F. Kennedy, mean to you?

   "Ask not what your country can do for you—
   but what you can do for your country."

3. To be a member of a profession such as nursing requires that each nurse grow and change and develop her highest potential in the service of people in need. Nursing is a *continuing* profession with *continuing* opportunities for professional improvement and advancement. You owe it to yourself to spend enough time and effort to choose the type of nursing and the specific job best suited to your needs and interests. Ideally, a plan encompassing both immediate and long-term goals should be plotted before the student's graduation from the nursing program.

Making a wise decision about the choice of a career involves two major tasks: first, a careful analysis of job opportunities in your area of interest and second, analyzing your personality traits and relating them to the job opportunities available. In terms of *your* interests and the type of nursing *you* would like to do, explore the possibilities in your chosen field and present the results of your explorations in the form of a project.

The following suggestions may help you to choose your career area in nursing and in the development of your project. Investigating areas of nursing practice and job opportunities (this is accomplished largely through research)

a. What are the fastest growing specialties in nursing?

Studies have shown that among BSN grads specialty areas are rated as
(1) Med Surg
(2) Pediatrics
(3) Ob Gyn
(4) Psych

b. In which areas is the need for nurses likely to be the greatest in the coming years?

c. What educational preparation and work experience requirements are needed to function in your area of special interest?

d. Is it likely you will be able to meet these requirements? How long will it take, as you view your present situation and commitments? Can these requirements be accomplished in stages?

e. What financial help will you need to plan for? Are scholarships available?

4. Analyzing your personal assets, interests and needs (this necessitates some soul-searching and an honest examination of one's feelings, motives and attitudes)
   a. Do you feel more comfortable in routine situations?

   b. Do you enjoy being "in charge"?

   c. Are you at a loss when you must cope with emergencies?

   d. Do you become impatient when things do not run smoothly?

   e. Do you have a facility for writing?

   f. Does speaking before a group come easily to you?

   g. Will the job accord you the professional and personal contacts that will be satisfying to you?

   h. Will the job you aspire to consume more time and energy than you are willing to give to it?

NAME ________________________

WORK SHEET

DATE ________________________

THE OFFICIAL NURSING ORGANIZATIONS

Obtain the following information about your specific nursing associations:

1. American Nurses' Association OR National Federation of Licensed Practical Nurses
   a. Who is the present president?

   b. Where are the headquarters?

2. State
   a. Who is the present president of your state association?

   b. Where are the headquarters?

   c. What sections are functioning at this time?

   d. When and where will the next convention be held?

3. District

a. What district association do you have the privilege of joining after you become a RN? or LPN/LVN?

b. Where are the headquarters of this association?

c. Who is the present president?

d. What are the dues at this time? Determine how fees are divided among local, state, and national organizations.

e. How often and where are meetings held?

4. National League for Nursing OR National Association for Practical Nurse Education and Services

   a. Who is the present president?

   b. Where are the headquarters?

   c. When and where will the next convention be held?

5. Constituent League

a. Who is the present president?

b. Where is the executive office located?

6. Give a reliable source for obtaining information about your state association and the American Nurses' Association or your state association and the National Federation of Licensed Practical Nurses.

WORK SHEET

NAME ____________________

DATE ____________________

AMERICAN NURSES' ASSOCIATION POSITION PAPER

1. Survey a health facility in your community for nurse utilization. Is there a shortage of nurses? Are the nurses employed at that facility placed in the position for which they are qualified?

2. Read the American Nurses' Association Position Paper on Education as it appears in the December 1965 issue of the *American Journal of Nursing.* Interpret the "implications" on page 111 of the article as they are reflected in a health facility used by your school for clinical laboratory.